*"We first make our habits,
and then our habits make us."*

JOHN DRYDEN

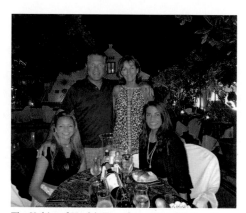

The Habits of Health Transformational System is dedicated to the memory of Lori Lynn Andersen. She changed the lives of thousands of people by spending almost two decades coaching and leading the mission to create optimal health and wellbeing.

The impact of her loss for our family is indescribable. She was an unbelievable mom, always put us first, and provided a loving environment for our girls to grow into adulthood. As my business partner, best friend, first mate, and soul mate, she has left an indelible imprint. Not a day goes by that I do not see her smiling face and long to hold her just one more time.

Lori, the world is a better place because of you. Our dream to create health and wellbeing for all that desire it is alive and well. I know you can see how you have changed us all forever.

All our love,
Wayne, Savannah, and Erica

Dr. A's
HABITS
OF
HEALTH

DR. WAYNE SCOTT ANDERSEN

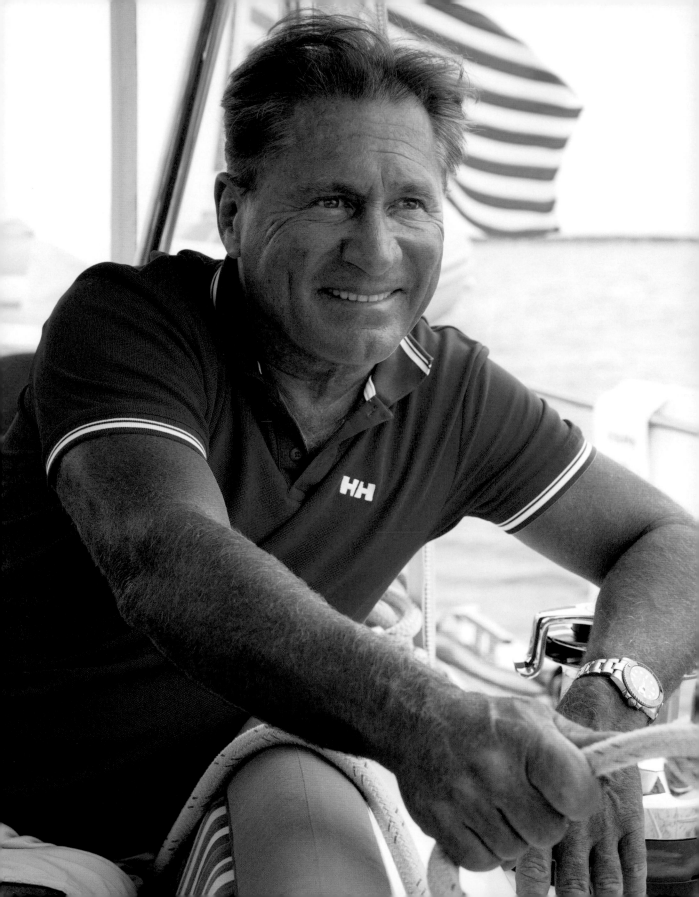

Dr. A's
HABITS
OF
HEALTH

*The path to
permanent weight control,
optimal health, and wellbeing*

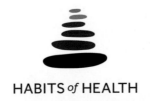

HABITS *of* **HEALTH**

CONTENTS

At the very essence of this book and the evolution of the Habits of Health Transformational System is the union of two powerful forces: medical science and the personal drive to become a higher version of ourselves. For this reason, I have asked two important thinkers in their respective fields—Robert Fritz, international bestselling author and leading authority on the creative process and Dr. Lawrence Cheskin, founder and director of the Johns Hopkins Weight Management Center—to share their unique perspectives and insights by contributing forwards to this text.

FOREWORD BY ROBERT FRITZ

Dr. A's Habits of Health may be one of the most important books you will ever read. By following Dr. Wayne Andersen's advice, you'll be able to redirect lifelong patterns that are leading you down the wrong path and replace them with new, helpful practices that will enable you to build better and better health over time.

This isn't yet another book trying to motivate change through fear, warnings, shame, and images of disaster. Dr. A knows the difference between a process that allows you to *create* the state of health you truly want versus a process that merely addresses health problems. Dr. A is a true leader and original thinker who considers the complete question of health: what it means and how to create it. He has advanced a new vision in his belief that a person can reach his or her optimal level of health. Creating health is an entirely different approach than trying to heal once you get sick. And Dr. A continues to refine his approach as the evolution of the Habits of Health has become a transformational system that provides multiple touch points to help assist the individual in their journey.

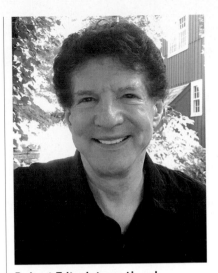

Robert Fritz, international best-selling author, international award-winning film and screen writer / director, creator of Structural Dynamics.

This book continues to be the compendium of health and wellbeing and advances the idea of taking charge of your health so you can become the dominant force in your life. It is now joined by *Your LifeBook* and Habits of Health App designed to provide support and give you more tools to help you create your new life.

Why is Dr. Andersen's vision and system so important to the future of healthcare?

Unfortunately most of the medical establishment today is problem-driven. You need to get sick before they become involved. Doctors are against illness, but ironically they don't think in terms of creating health in the first place. Yes, there are a slew of pharmaceutical and medical advances that help slow the progression of heart disease, high blood pressure, high cholesterol, and other life-threatening conditions. But while we're all grateful that this technology exists, this is an orientation that has profound limitations when it comes to actually creating optimal health. As people in the pharmaceutical industry tell us in every one of their TV ads, there are side effects to their products.

While treating illness surely has an important place in our lives, doesn't it make sense for each of us to create the highest level of health possible before we face life-threatening problems? While the logic of this is indisputable, many in the medical community think that it's virtually impossible for people to change their ways and that people simply aren't able to develop new habits. And while, as this book will show, these opinions are false, they're clearly steeped in physicians' own experiences. Throughout the years, their warnings have gone unheeded by patients.

What are they left with but an ongoing search for therapies that address the consequences of destructive habits? Too often, the medical establishment has concluded that people will not change their lifestyles, even if their lives depend on it.

Dr. A understands how to help people accomplish real and lasting change in their lives. He understands that it's not a matter of willpower, or reactions to dire warnings. He knows that if it's hard to change a habit, people won't do it. So he's developed processes that are easy to adopt. And he knows that even if the process is easy but the logistics surrounding that habit are challenging, change won't happen either. So he's developed straightforward, manageable, and clear logistics that anyone can handle.

Dr. A isn't going to give you a pep talk or a gloom-and-doom tirade. Instead, he'll show you how to design an overall strategy to accomplish one of the most important goals you will ever have: optimal health. And his approach isn't an ivory tower theory. He's already helped tens of thousands of people create and sustain optimal health in their lives over the last number of decades.

You'll find that one of the nicest things about this book is Dr. A's down-to-earth voice, which is fun, friendly, warm, and personable. The material he presents is full of science, wisdom, valuable insights, and practical advice, all brought to light in a highly readable and thoroughly enjoyable style.

I've known Dr. A for a number of years, and I'm privileged to call him a friend and colleague. We have written a book together: *Identity*. So I know firsthand that he is highly creative, open, quick-witted, and upbeat.

Dr. A is dedicated to other people's success. As you read Dr. A's Habits of Health, you'll find yourself developing a personal relationship with him. He'll become your health coach, your guide, your teacher, and your friend.

Dr. Wayne Scott Andersen has had a remarkably distinguished career that ideally positions him to forge new territory in the realm of creating optimal health. A board-certified anesthesiologist and critical care specialist, he has served as chairman of the Department of Anesthesiology and director of critical care at Grandview Medical Center, which is one of the top 100 hospitals in the country. He graduated first in his class from medical school and completed postdoctoral work which includes residency training in cardiovascular anesthesiology at the Cleveland Clinic and fellowship training in surgical critical care medicine at the University of Miami.

As the tenth board-certified physician in critical care in the nation, he helped pioneer the emerging subspecialty of intensive care medicine. It was in the course of this work, upon observing the pivotal role that nutrition plays in recovery from illness, that Dr. A determined to redirect his focus into the preventative arena of nutritional intervention and lifestyle management.

He is highly sought after for his innovative thinking in creating sustainable health and wellbeing and is currently scholar in residence at Mount St. Mary's University in Los Angeles. He is also helping to develop the University's wellness advocates, as well as the design of their massive new wellness pavilion with the goal of equipping college students to embrace optimal health and wellbeing as prerequisites of thriving in our constantly changing world.

Dr. A's life is about helping you create the highest state of health available to you. He can help you, just as he's helped a multitude of people reach a healthy weight, which is one of the first building blocks for creating optimal health. But his goal isn't merely to help you reach your desired weight. It's to install habits in you that support a lifetime process, which will allow you to achieve the highest state of health possible and make it last.

This book can be a major contributor to the goal of creating optimal health if you allow yourself to study it, follow its design and insights, and let it be your manual for reaching your optimal health goals. So get ready to transform your life, learn profound lifebuilding lessons, and reach a higher state of health than you ever thought possible!

ROBERT FRITZ

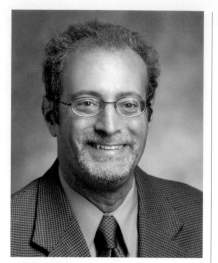

Lawrence J. Cheskin,
MD, FACP, FTOS
Director, Johns Hopkins Weight
Management Center; Associate
Professor, Health, Behavior
& Society, Johns Hopkins
Bloomberg School of Public
Health. Joint appts: Medicine
(GI), Nutrition, Public Health
Studies, Nursing; Director of
Clinical Research, Global Obesity
Prevention Center at Johns
Hopkins.

FOREWORD BY LAWRENCE J. CHESKIN, MD, FACP, FTOS

Let's start with why the new, revised Dr. A's Habits of Health is so critical to readers, and indeed to the world:

- In the U.S. alone, obesity and inactivity are responsible for at least 300,000 deaths every year.
- This is because obesity adversely affects virtually every organ in the body, and increases the risk of heart disease, type-2 diabetes, stroke, osteoarthritis, and even many cancers. Obesity now accounts for over 10% of all healthcare costs.
- Seven out of 10 American adults are now overweight or obese, and obesity is increasing at an even faster pace among children. As a result, the coming generation may actually have a shorter life span than their parents for the first time in American history.

Undeniably, we have a collective problem in the U.S. today. While the underlying causes of this epidemic of obesity are complex and still much debated, genetics, socioeconomics, environmental factors and learned behaviors all play a role. But of these, only learned behaviors can be altered by us as individuals in a meaningful way—in particular, what we eat and how we respond to stress and other triggers that lead to inappropriate eating. In this sense, behavioral factors appear to be the most important contributor. What causes someone to make poor decisions about food in today's obesity-generating environment?

According to research, on average, we make at least 200 food choices every day. Learning to make better choices in terms of specific foods, portion size, as well as in terms of physical activity, could maximize our ability to counter the pervasive environmental influences that make attaining and maintaining a healthy, stable weight so difficult.

In the end, though, hard facts and theoretical concepts like these aren't really all that useful or motivating for those of us who struggle daily with the battle against weight gain.

What is useful, then? The goal of Dr. Andersen's groundbreaking new book is to shift the emphasis away from passive reaction to disease and toward individual responsibility for health. He encourages people to create health in the first place, rather than stand by while the negative forces of our society erode their health.

As the founder and director of the Johns Hopkins Weight Management Center in Baltimore, a clinical and research program devoted to helping people who are obese, I've treated thousands of individuals with weight problems. I was also chairman of the Scientific Advisory Board of Medifast for the past 10 years. In the course of my work, I've become convinced that we must move toward a new era of medicine—one that focuses on fostering optimal health and preventing health problems before they appear. Dr. Andersen shares this vision.

Unfortunately, we are still in the minority in our current healthcare system. Ironically, even today, patients rarely receive insurance coverage for weight-control services, despite ample coverage for all the medical consequences of obesity that could be avoided by losing weight to begin with!

Dr. Andersen's book offers a refreshing new paradigm—a simple, practical way for people to change their habits and lifestyle by building on small, easy, and almost imperceptible steps. While this may go against our tendency to view change as a dramatic break from the past, change is in fact often easiest, and easier to make permanent, when it's gradual.

In the journey that you're about to take, reaching a healthy weight is a starting point, not an end point, and this realization helps create the momentum that moves you forward toward change, rather than backward into old behaviors. The ultimate goal is to continue this forward movement toward optimal health. As Dr. Andersen explains, that goal will look different for each of us, but the decision to take our health into our own hands is the critical first step.

You'll find this new, totally revised book, interactive journal, and accompanying App replete with all the tools that will help you on this journey to a new, better approach to health and a more fulfilled life. These include a variety of revealing self-assessment techniques and questionnaires, and exercises to help you change those ingrained, lifelong habits that make it so hard to break free. You'll learn to make daily choices that support your goals through creating your own "microenvironment of health", a healthy eating system, a movement plan, and strategies for invigorating rest and sleep. Dr. Andersen reveals tried-and-tested dietary tools that can serve as an important shortcut to healthy weight, and explains how the support of a like-minded community of people can help you reach and maintain your goals. The new *Dr. A's Habits of Health* also takes advantage of the latest discoveries in the science of human motivation and behavioral neuroscience to assist you to make positive and lasting changes in your life. There is even the potential to achieve both a longer and happier life with the tools provided by Dr. Andersen.

The book also contains a series of innovative ways to reflect on your goals and monitor how you respond to life's changes and stresses. After all, it's often not so much what we face that stymies us, but rather our reactions to these challenges. Dr. Andersen is a master at helping you look at situations in the most positive way possible— a valuable tool indeed in your journey toward optimal weight and health.

I urge you to look at this journey you're about to embark upon under Dr. Andersen's guidance with eager anticipation. Facing and overcoming something that has challenged you, perhaps for your whole life, with an open mind and heart, with determination and conviction, is a wonderful gift that only you can give yourself. I invite you to now take the first step of your journey, and enjoy the results!

LAWRENCE J. CHESKIN, MD, FACP, FTOS

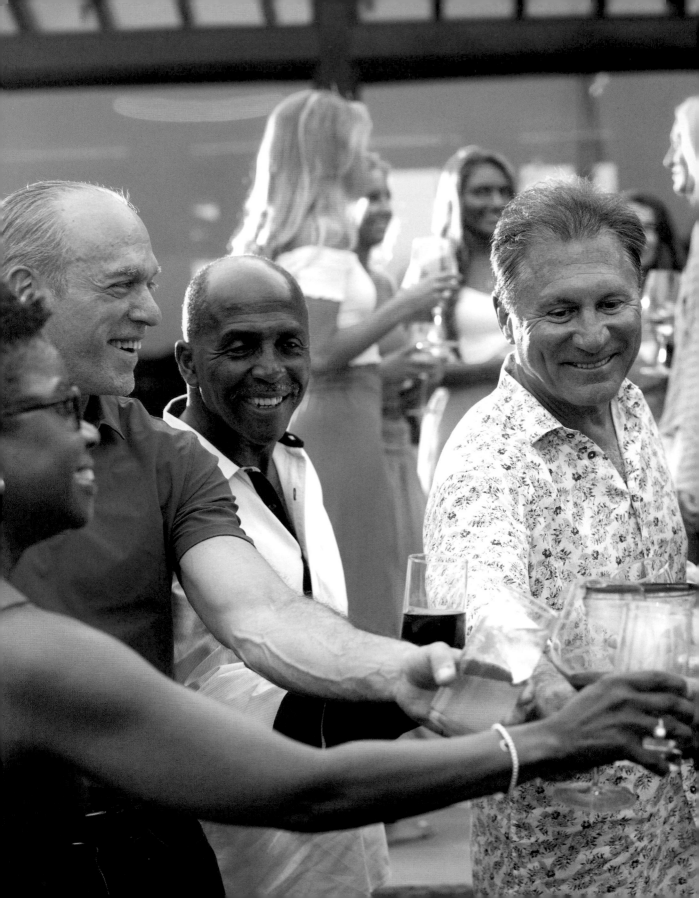

WELCOME TO THE HABITS OF HEALTH 2.0

Almost a decade has passed since the first edition of Dr. A's Habits of Health. The following year I followed it up with the companion guide, Living a Longer Healthier Life. If you were to judge the system by its popularity and acceptance as a resource for those that want to improve their health and wellbeing, you might say it was an overwhelming success.

In the last 10 years or more since it was published, we have reached over half a million people, thereby positively affecting the lives of countless individuals.*

*Based on book sales to date.

This past decade has changed me forever. It has brought tears of gratitude that a physician who has spent most of his career focused on treating and reacting to disease and its accompanying suffering is now part of a new movement and way of thinking that creates joy, vibrant health, and thriving lives for so many. Hearing the countless stories about lives that have been changed and reading the daily emails and letters sent to me by people describing their transformational stories is humbling and incredibly gratifying.

It's also fueling a burning desire to improve and to provide an even more practical and effective way to help people change their lives. So why has the first edition been so powerful and life changing for so many? It was a refreshing and comprehensive approach to reaching and maintaining a healthy weight. Making the move to optimal health was innovative, simple, and explained in a way that made sense to people.

It made bold steps too. It exposed the futility of dieting, the ineffectiveness of the food pyramid, and the need for more movement than an hour in the gym a few times a week. It introduced the vital role of sleep in weight loss and health and the key role that support plays in any long-term success. From its basis in sound clinical science, along with questionnaires and exercises, to its innovative new ways of eating, moving, sleeping, and creating a more relaxed, healthy mind, the system worked together to help individuals take control of their weight and their health.

But that was then and this is now. Many things have changed over the last 10 years, and I am very excited about sharing what I have learned with you.

The science of human motivation and behavior, as well as the area of neuroscience, have seen rapid and remarkable expansion. Our understanding of how the brain and mind influences our behavior continues to increase at a breathtaking pace.

Unfortunately, this rate of change is making it harder for us to adapt. Many people feel their sanity, health, and overall wellbeing slipping away.

That reality—the challenge we all face—has been the impetus and central focus of my work over the last decade. In fact, there is one question I have been seeking to answer: how can I help those that desire better health, happiness, and wellbeing make sense of it all? How can we transform to a more optimal way of living that supports radiant health and vibrant energy when everyday it seems like we are falling further behind in our weight, our health, our relationships, and our zest for life?

Well, the good news is that it is actually all there, hidden in our habits—the "software" that determines almost everything.

Beyond scientific advances, I've had an extraordinary opportunity to help tens of thousands of people face their reality. I've watched people tackle these challenges in their own lives and I've been able to fully comprehend the subject I've written so much about.

The Habits of Health are the answer. They can change everything.

Obesigenic:

Likely to cause someone to become excessively overweight or obese.

> *If you don't own a copy of Your LifeBook, visit the Habits of Health website, contact your coach, or you can start your own journal in the notebook of your choice.*

Real, tangible, lasting change. I have passed the 10,000 hours of practice and experience that Malcolm Gladwell suggests it takes to become a master of something, and I believe I have the authority to make the following statement: if you are willing to take responsibility and stay the course, we can help you predictably change your health and wellbeing.

The book you are reading will be your guide. If you are new to my work, then let me offer you a warm welcome. If this work and thinking has helped you in the past, I promise you are in for a treat. This sequel is simpler yet more powerful than its predecessor. I've worked hard to make it better, more effective, and more in line with today's challenges. It will guide your mind and your body in equal parts. Its comprehensive approach will help you make the changes in both your health and wellbeing that may have eluded you in the past.

Alongside the writing of this second edition, I have evolved the Habits of Health companion workbook into an even more important and useful companion and tool. Used in parallel, it will allow you to build a new story, create a healthier you, and give you space to document your achievements and progress in a style that will help the transformation stick.

That is why it's called *Your LifeBook*. It's the record of your journey, your goals, your ups and downs but mostly it's your path to your desired health and wellbeing.

Together they are a highly effective system to create predictable transformation in those that decide their health is important to them.

Let's take a few moments to reflect on the wider challenges we face as a world. In the first edition, I started the preface by stating, very clearly, that we live in an obesigenic world (a world full of factors that are causing weight gain).

Sadly, over the last 10 or so years, nothing has changed in terms of our access to seductively tasty, cheap, convenient, but unhealthy food. It's still here. In fact, it's more available and more affordable than ever.

Energy saving devices have become even more absurd. Activities such as shopping, learning, working, and entertainment that previously required physical energy can now be accessed from the comfort of our own homes, on a train, or sitting in a café. Our way of life is killing us.

Yet when it comes to our own lives, certainly in the developed world, everything has changed. The fabric of society has changed. Our lives have become more chaotic.

Just coping with the ever-increasing pressures of everyday life is pushing people to irresponsible actions. Irrational behavior—from violence, crime, and public defiance to acts of personal and social irresponsibility—is eroding a long-range common sense approach to modern living. The result is a growing cost to every aspect of our society and a direct effect on both our physical and mental health.

At the time of writing, the U.S. leads a worldwide trend in weight gain: almost 70% of the population are overweight or obese.[1] The resulting acceleration of sickness and disease is having a catastrophic effect on the nation. For the principal cause, look no further than the advancement of technology. We will build a case in Part 1.1, *It's Not Your Fault That You're Struggling,* that adapting both physically and mentally to the continuous impact of technology has caused significant collateral damage. The role that processed food plays (in terms of quantity and quality) and the havoc it wreaks on our energy management system is no secret.

You can also factor in that the average American spends 95% of their time indoors.[2] Combine this with the progressive trends toward urbanization and mechanization of almost all labor and it's no surprise that we see more and more marshmallow bodies. The reduction of physical activity and lack of exposure to the natural world is resulting in a worldwide human migration. We are truly becoming a species that lives in the Great Indoors.

Today, kids spend less time outside than prison inmates: the average child plays freely outside for just four to seven minutes a day.[3]

The aggregate effects on our health and wellbeing are not good. Estimates suggest that by the year 2020, depression will be the second leading cause of disability throughout the world—the first is heart disease.[4]

Despite all the apparent benefits of modern life, a recent survey said that we are the first generation that has a significantly lower quality of life than every generation before us.[5] Clearly our inability to handle the pressure and stress in our lives can have a devastating effect on our attempts to create optimal health and wellbeing.

It affects our children, our teachers, our schools, our jobs, our relationships, our neighborhoods, our communities, our countries, and our planet. So you might reasonably ask why I'm bringing this up in the Introduction to a book about health and wellbeing?

The answer is simple. We will need to spend time addressing your own current relationship with the world and how you respond not just to the good days, the vacations, and the great job you did at the office, but to those days when you feel that the air has been let out of your balloon.

It's on those days that we all need some help in order to get our minds to operate in a way that can effectively support optimal health and wellbeing. A strong infrastructure of support for our thinking and doing and interacting with others is crucial to create sustainable success.

So, in the evolution to *Habits of Health Transformational System 2.0,* we will include significant amounts of new information and equip you with new ways to interact with the world in a more effective way.

Put simply, the world cannot change quickly enough to better serve the health and wellbeing of man. The Habits of a Healthy Mind and Healthy Relationships will help you respond differently.

Our goal is to give you a blueprint for taking personal responsibility and adapting to change. I have always thought that

Charles Darwin's most significant contribution to mankind was not the premise of the survival of the fittest but instead the proliferation of those that are most adaptive. And for the human race, I fear that unless we make an immediate adjustment to the escalating pace of change, our future existence is in question. This book is an important step in that direction.

In the following pages, we will outline—step by step—how you can reach and sustain a healthy weight. I will start by helping you learn and install a new set of habits that will create sustainable transformation. I will equip you with the strategies, tools, and support necessary to take the challenges this rapidly changing world presents to you on a daily basis and have you gobble them up like energy bars.

Our goal is to provide you with an owner's manual that will help you thrive as you continue this crazy journey called life.

So if you're ready, let's start the process of taking control of your future health and wellbeing.

IN HEALTH,
DR WAYNE SCOTT ANDERSEN

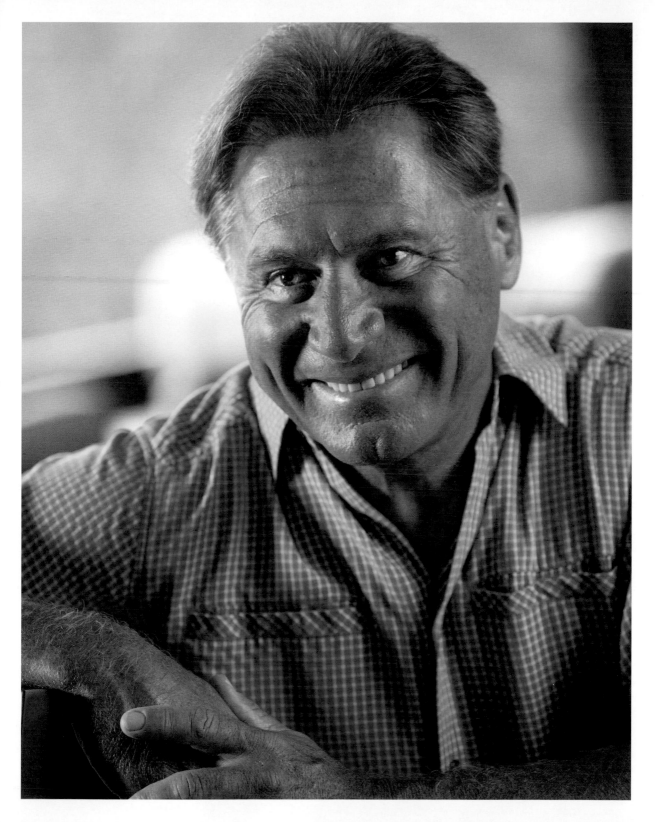

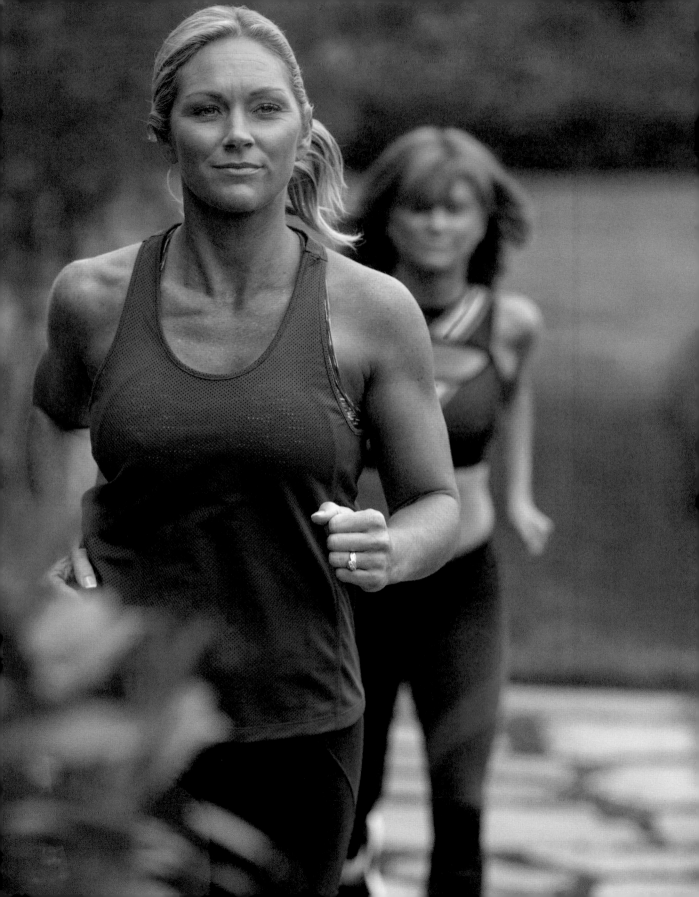

INTRODUCTION

BEATING THE ODDS

When I wrote about how abysmal diets were at creating successful long-term weight control a decade ago, it was news! Most people had no idea that many people who dieted would regain the weight they'd lost and become heavier than their pre-diet weight. More disturbing was the fact that many studies indicated that dieters suffer from worse long-term health compared to non-dieters.

Today, more and more people realize that dieting is an ineffective solution, yet a recent survey revealed that almost 50% of woman are currently on a diet.[1] People are desperately trying to lose weight but are relying on an outdated and ineffective approach.

The desire to lose weight is more pressing than ever. In the U.S. alone, almost two-thirds of the population is either overweight or obese, and levels of obesity are spreading at a frightening pace.[2] The worldwide prevalence of obesity nearly tripled between 1975 and 2016: Globesity is truly becoming a pandemic, with no resolution in sight. The planet's population of overweight people (over a billion) outnumbers the hungry (roughly 700 million).

The health implications of weight gain are alarming. Its ability to generate chronic disease is unprecedented. Weight is a factor in the fact that almost half of all adults are suffering some form of cardiovascular disease, including heart attacks and strokes, as well as high blood pressure, type 2 diabetes, some cancers, gastrointestinal problems (including gallbladder disease), osteoarthritis, poor bone health, and breathing problems (including sleep apnea and asthma).[3]

The unacceptably high rates of chronic disease that are caused by being overweight or obese have persisted for more than two decades and continue to create havoc with our health, our minds, our pocketbooks, and our overall wellbeing with no definitive answer on the horizon.[4]

But I have a feeling that you may already know this. What you really want to know is how to do something about it. Obesity (too much body fat) is a symptom of a much more complex system of mismatches between the way our body was designed to function and the world which we now find ourselves in. One of the goals of this book is to help you remove the excess weight caused by body fat, which robs you of your energy, stamina, and health.

Yet, the main purpose of this book is much bolder and will have a broader impact. Our purpose is to help you reach optimal health and wellbeing, so you can thrive in all the key areas of your life: achieving vibrancy in your physical health, fully enjoying your work, your play, your time with your family and within your community.

This book will help guide you in making optimal health a reality. This may seem like a stretch if you are currently overweight, or obese, permanently tired, sleeping terribly, always stressed out, or feeling utterly alone. But let me share a little-known secret.

The goal of optimal health and wellbeing is possible for all of us. It is the difference between allowing yourself to be guided by your current story versus our ability to work together through this book to create your new story. We are going to show you a different perspective on what is possible, exploring what you really want in your life, and help you to make the necessary corrections and daily choices that will, over time, produce the results you really want.

NEW GUIDING PRINCIPLES FOR YOUR LIFE

The goal of optimal health and wellbeing will determine your actions. The means of reaching that goal will be different for each and

*85% of people who go on a diet without behavioral support gain the weight back within two years.**

*Dr. A's Habits of Health, published November 2008

> *Do you have a history of yo-yo dieting? According to studies, you are likely to gain more weight than your non-dieting friend and have poorer health.*

every one of us. Being optimal for a 20-year-old marathon runner is different from being optimal for a 75-year-old with a history of heart trouble. The point is that when you focus on creating a future that is as good as you can be, it changes everything. It will inform your day-to-day in new ways and create the impetus to shift your behavior.

And since reaching a healthy weight, becoming fit, sleeping better, and having a robust support structure are all vital pieces of reaching and maintaining health, we will help you continue these new behaviors for the rest of your life.

Each day, gradually, you will become healthier by building self-efficacy with slow, steady progress until one day you will be as optimal as you can be. The key to this becoming a reality is not a focus on the goal of optimal health or wellbeing (which may seem unattainable) but instead having laser focus on building your day and influencing thousands of almost imperceptible choices you make every day.

We'll start by meeting you where you are now and discovering what you are capable of right now. We'll then take baby steps and make the necessary adjustments in a way that doesn't dominate your already overwhelming days. That's because an optimal life starts with more optimal mornings and more optimal evenings which add up to more optimal days.

Okay. You may still be skeptical that we can make all of this a reality. You've heard big promises and claims from health gurus in the past, and those didn't meaningfully change your life. So what's different about now?

Let me state with 100% certainty that it does not rely on a high-tech solution that has emerged from a research laboratory, an innovative surgical procedure, or a fancy new exercise device.

It isn't a tool you can buy and yet it is extremely effective at combating the temptations in our modern world. It doesn't matter if you are exposed to highly addictive packaged food or devices that pretend you can achieve what you want without expending energy and effort. Once you understand and can harness the power of this tool, you will be impervious to this nonsense.

What is this powerful force? They're called habits. Habits are responsible for almost 50% of every action you make every day. If you look at your current health and wellbeing, it is the result of your past and present habits. And because they are operating at a subconscious level, you might not even be aware of them.

When we analyze our choices across the whole spectrum of our day, it becomes apparent that we spend most of our time sleepwalking through the decisions we make. Whether it is what we are putting in our mouth, how we move (or don't), the quality of our sleep, or the way we handle difficult conversations with our boss—most of it is happening without conscious input.

In isolation these choices have little effect on our health and wellbeing. But when we add them up they make all the difference in the world. They start developing when we are children and eventually become the operating system that guides us every day.

In this guidebook, we'll explore this complex tapestry of beliefs, thoughts, and habits. These habits are hardwired into your brain, and they've had the time to convince you that this is who you are and what you do. Authors and authorities will tell you most people are not capable of making the changes necessary to transform their lifestyles. Others will give advice and sell you a quick fix or potion that will miraculously repair you.

They won't. Only one path can transform your health and wellbeing and make sustainable changes in your life—you have to change your habits.

Looking to buy something that will make things better is human nature. The reality is that making things better is an inside job, but without a strategy or the skills, tools, and support to make real change, it is very difficult to go it alone.

The good news is that there is a system that has used design thinking to provide real life answers to help make change a reality. It's called the Habits of Health.

THE HABITS OF HEALTH TRANSFORMATIONAL SYSTEM

The Habits of Health is an owner's manual and it's a pity that none of us received a copy when we were born. The Habits make the necessary adaptations to optimize our operating system and counter the negative effects rapid change is having on our health and life.

The Habits of Health Transformational System is comprehensive. It provides key components that can create predictable transformation in individual health and wellbeing and, if you are willing to learn and adopt the habits and make them part of your daily life, you will change. I believe that as long as you continue to apply the principles outlined here, these changes will be permanent.

There is one central caveat to success. You.

The X-Factor is your willingness to make a decision and take individual responsibility for your success. If you're prepared to do this, then I know it can work.

Hundreds of studies show that our health improves if we adopt a healthy lifestyle, and better health improves all the areas of our life within our overall wellbeing. You are more likely to enjoy your job, be successful financially, have healthier relationships with your family and friends, and be spiritually and mentally sound.

As a physician, I rely on evidence based science and the literature and the research is clear—change your lifestyle and you will change your health and wellbeing. The challenge has been the lack of a predictable way to make the necessary changes. It just seems too hard and the low success rate of people trying to make that change validates this conclusion. What has been missing is a successful system.

When I designed the original lifestyle program, Habits of Health 1.0, I focused on how to make lifestyle adaptation simpler and easier

This plan is about much more than weight loss. It's about reaching and maintaining optimal health and wellbeing.

to apply. I packaged it into one system with consistent, verifiable components and I dispensed with gimmicks or logistically impossible tasks. These principles still remain at the heart of the system today.

Let's go back to the caveat. I have been helping thousands of people achieve optimal health, and the most important variable on whether the *Habits of Health Transformational System* works or not is you. This new version, the Habits of Health 2.0, is a vast improvement on the original and addresses many of the areas where people fell short of complete transformation. But success or failure is still dependent on you. I'll provide cool strategies, tools, skill sets, and easily adopted techniques to make the journey easier, but you still need to do the work.

So, if you are ready to make a change but are not totally convinced that this system is right for you, let's take a look under the hood and explore what Dr. A's Habits of Health is all about.

IT STARTS WITH YOU AND I WORKING TOGETHER

We're going to be spending a lot of time together and, because of this, I think it's important you understand what makes me qualified to help you. I was born to a low-income family. I was the first member of my family to go to college. I spent my whole childhood traveling as a military dependent. The constant travel, adjusting to new locations, and making new friends helped me recognize what is needed to adapt to a life of constant change.

I was in one of those many new locations when I read a book about surgery. Straightaway, I knew I wanted to be a doctor. I convinced my nanny to take me to a medical supply house in downtown Seville, Spain where I acquired surgical instruments and ether. At 10 years old, I was putting frogs to sleep, then opening them up and observing their hearts beating; this gave me a head start on the practical aspects of anatomy and physiology.

When I was old enough, I went to college, then medical school, and I took internships and residencies to finally become a cardiac anesthesiologist with a specialty in surgical intensive care.

I demonstrated enough skill as an intern to study and become a specialist in one particular organ, but I had already realized something fundamental to human health. I could see—very clearly—that a critically ill patient, with organs close to failing, needed to be taken care of by a physician who was watching the organ systems in an integrated way, not as separate pieces.

That realization set me on a path to help pioneer the emerging specialty of critical care. Three years later, I was awarded certification in critical care. I was the tenth physician in the country to be board certified in this new holistic approach. For the next 18 years, I ran a teaching hospital in the Midwest, learning as I taught about the pivotal role of nutrition in healing and how the body's organ systems needed to be integrated into a specific plan to help a sick patient recover. They were some of the most amazing years of my life up to that point.

In those two decades, I saved many patients' lives but never helped even one patient create health. Before I left traditional medicine, I had a growing concern that our approach was really only treating symptoms that were a result of poor lifestyle choices. And I was personally aware of the problem as I was gaining weight that could be conveniently hidden by the drawstrings of my scrubs. I could see that lifestyle was more important than medicine in terms of our health.

One of the most important things I learned was about integrated, holistic care and how our system works as one in good health and ill health. When I realized the full magnitude of what determined the health of a patient it was clearly so much more than biomedical measurements. It involved the full interplay of chemical, neurological, psychological, environmental, and social systems.

What I grasped was this: if I really wanted to make the biggest difference in the lives of my patients, I needed to move upstream and use the talents and medical acumen I had gained to help people manage the way they interacted with their world. I truly believe people don't want more medicine or surgeries. They want to live, long, healthy lives and to have the time and resources to be able to organize their lives around what matters most to them.

This realization has taken me a long way from the intensive care unit. Today, as a physician, I am fully engaged in helping patients, clients, and anyone who raises their hand to create optimal health and wellbeing in their life.

Back in 2002, when I first spoke about these ideas, I was among the very few that thought this way. Many of my peers thought the idea was far-fetched but now more physicians are starting to realize that the current medical system—in the context of developing general health—is broken.

Over time, more and more healthcare providers have joined our mission to move medicine into a new era—one where we do what is best for our patients and partner with them to help them create optimal health and wellbeing.

We've started the new American College of Lifestyle Medicine which has a focus on addressing the key areas that can help people change their health and lives. Our aim is to continue to push the envelope to improve the social responsibility of the food and pharmaceutical industries, and to help develop the understanding of holistic health in big businesses and those that design and run our cities.

It is only a matter of time before our medical community takes back business control of our domain and traditional medicine becomes focused on acute injury and to help with those rare diseases that are not a result of lifestyle. But let's not get ahead of ourselves. If today, you have made a decision that you are sick and tired of being sick and tired then I am afraid that you are still mostly on your own in an obesigenic, unhealthy world. Or, rather, you were. From today, I can help you get a head start on your health and wellbeing, starting by describing how this book and its integration with the *Habits of Health Transformational System* can make that a reality.

THE JOURNEY TO OPTIMAL HEALTH AND WELLBEING

We're embarking on an exciting and incredibly satisfying journey. It's also challenging and a bit scary. What I do know for sure is that you are going to love how much better you are going to feel and look and how your physical and overall wellbeing is going to improve.

I need to reassure you on a couple of things. If you've tried to make changes before, you might, like many, have started off with fanfare and great intentions only to see yourself going back to your old ways and, as a result, you felt like a failure. If that has happened to you, then rest assured you're not alone.

Whatever has happened on your previous attempts to get healthy, one thing you might not have had at your side was a plan. Like making a journey to an unfamiliar place, you need guidance from someone that has been there before. Without it your chances of reaching your destination are reduced and you will become more anxious.

You can think of the journey to optimal health and wellbeing in a an expert way, I'll guide you to create a strategy by empowering you with the skills, tools, and support to help you successfully transform your health and your wellbeing.

Over time, we'll build a different kind of relationship to the one you have probably had in the past with a physician. I am not going to use prescriptions, warnings, or fear tactics. Instead, I will be your coach, your guide, and your partner. Together, we will build a path to taking permanent charge of your health.

Let me be clear about one thing: this won't be easy. Changing lifelong habits takes effort. It might even be stressful. If that happens, you should remember that this book isn't solely the product of medical research or the knowledge and experience I have gathered in 38 years as a physician. It is also about a journey that I have taken myself and through which I have guided thousands of people. I have learned as much from all of these amazing patients and clients as they have from me. These real-life experiences have forged an understanding of what it really takes to reach and maintain a healthy weight and live a healthy life. Believe me, I know what is involved in dealing with the naysayers, the pressure of family dynamics, the remembering of past failures, and the voice in your head that just screams self-doubt.

I have helped people fight through those struggles and been there to celebrate when the hard work has finally paid off. Some of these amazing individuals started this journey as many as 17 years ago.

What I have seen over the last two decades leaves me in no doubt. We have validated the sustainability of a system that has been designed to meet you where you are and take you where you want to go. The journey you're about to embark on has three parts.

Part One: Preparing for Your Journey

The first part is preparing you for the journey and equipping you with what you will need. We'll explore why it is so hard to reach and sustain a healthy weight. We'll examine how our modern life is negatively affecting our health and our wellbeing, and we'll consider why your 10,000 year-old design and today's environment need to be realigned.

We will explore the power of habits and how they work and then jump right into the microHabits of the *Habits of Health Transformational System,* which will help you realize you are no longer focusing on problem solving but organizing your life around what matters most with the tools to help you accomplish it.

Part Two: Your Journey to Optimal Health and Wellbeing

The second part is all about doing. All the ideas and understanding you will have gained can do nothing to improve your health unless they are accompanied with a series of new habit installations. We'll start with the simplest and most important areas: the keystone habits. Reaching a healthy weight and learning how to eat, move, and sleep better are the foundational categories of the Habits of Health that set the stage for long-term health and wellbeing. When we have these in place, we will move on to optimizing your overall health and wellbeing. Our goal? For you to become the best you can be with what you've got.

Part Three: The Keys to Longevity

The third and final part will put you in the best possible position to live longer in a healthier state. We'll explore the ongoing science, research, and ideas related to longevity, and with the help of rapidly expanding technology, we will keep you on the leading edge of health and wellbeing.

THE HABITS OF HEALTH TRANSFORMATIONAL SYSTEM

I have asked one question almost every day in the evolution to the Habits of Health 2.0: What does it take to help people change their health and lives and make those changes permanent? Asking and answering that question has led me to many discoveries and insights that I know will help your journey be more successful.

Beyond this book, there are support pieces that are vital to your chances of success, updated with my latest thinking and the latest health research.

The original Habits of Health System (or 1.0) developed as a book, and I added the companion workbook the following year to help document what people were learning through a means of a series of exercises.

These new versions are much more synergistic. Using the same design-thinking process that companies like Apple use to develop their products, the Habits of Health is now a complete Transformational System and, in my opinion, more effective at helping you optimize your transformation because it's founded on the stories of thousands of people that have made the change.

Each piece can be used independently, but each piece also functions at a different level of learning with a unique role in the overall system. When used together, they create a synergistic approach to help guide you to success.

Dr. A's Habits of Health is the compendium on health—the definitive guide to optimizing your health and wellbeing. It's the book you have in your hands at this very moment.

Your LifeBook is a personal journal and modular learning system to make sure that you are hitting the milestones on your health and wellbeing journey and provides documentation of your new and developing story. You may not have used a journal before, but there's evidence to suggest that those who write down their goals and use a journal to monitor their own progress are more successful.

The Habits of Health App is a companion piece of the system, designed to act as a habit installer. It is a way to set day-to-day reminders that help make sure you are consistently building the microHabits that will transform your health.

This book can help you take control of your health and be a catalyst in improving your wellbeing. It is full of stories about people from every walk of life who set out on their own journey to health from the same point you are at now. As you will see, they are thriving thanks to the *Habits of Health Transformational System*. They did not reach their goals overnight but, because of this, they have remained healthy for many years and continue to become healthier and enjoy a higher state of wellbeing.

Many have had the help of a coach and some have actually taken that next step and decided to help others. We will talk a lot about the extra benefit of support.

Your story begins today, and there is every possibility that yours will be as powerful, transformational, and as long lasting as theirs.

Starting with baby-steps, we will teach you how to create lifelong Habits of Health. If we do this one small habit at a time, everything is possible. So, now it's time to join me as we walk the path to optimal health and wellbeing.

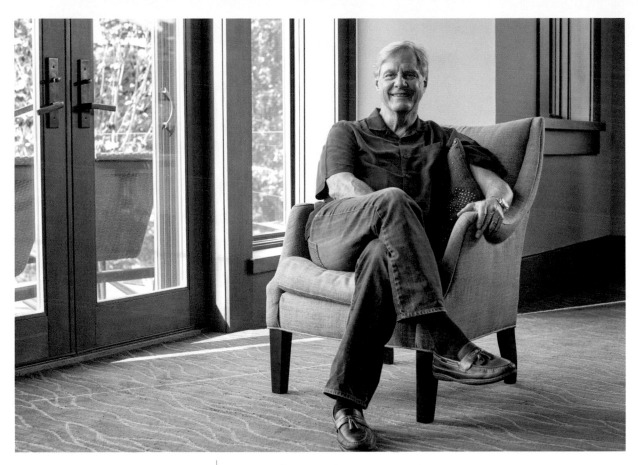

TRANSFORMATION: DAN BELL

I've always had an interest in health. I was an athlete growing up and I tried to have healthy habits as I've gone along but, like so many people, I didn't have the whole picture. I tried many things and, of course, as I got older, I started to gain weight. I tried a lot of different things to lose weight and again, but Dr. A put it in a package that made sense to me.

I have a background in science, so I understood the Habits of Health from a scientific vantage point, and it just made a lot of sense. And then when you implement it and look at how these MacroHabits cumulatively affect your overall health, it's about deciding what health do you want to create in your life.

I haven't been a perfect practitioner of the Habits of Health, but I have adopted these habits, and they've helped me in my life by keeping me healthier and off medications. I just went in for my annual checkup at the Mayo Clinic, and my physician went, "Man, your cholesterol is lower than it was the last time you were here. Whatever you're doing, keep doing it." That's how the Habits of Health have impacted my life in a very, very positive way.

> "
> I tried a lot of different things to lose weight, but Dr. A put it in a package that made sense to me.
> "

PREPARING FOR YOUR JOURNEY

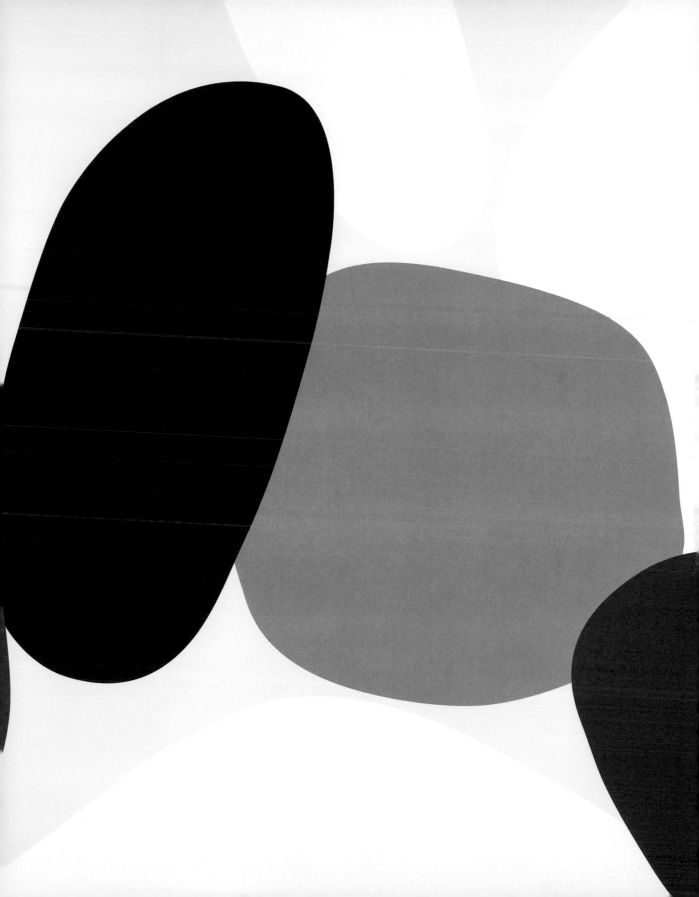

The world is changing at a blistering pace, and there is a real danger that we will not be able to keep up. There are signs everywhere that we are failing to adapt.

There is no area more profoundly affected by change than our health and wellbeing, so it's no wonder that so many of us feel our health slipping away as our days leaves us disorientated and even scared.

It doesn't have to be this way. But putting balance back into our lives is going to require a shift.

Achieving optimal health in today's world requires us to take charge of our own health but the places we normally turn to for help are actually making it harder for us to get healthy.

The food industry offers us tasty, cheap products that are addictive and unhealthy. The medical and pharmaceutical industries are more intent on curing sickness than promoting health. Even the preventative healthcare movement takes a passive approach by focusing on avoiding and reducing the risk of disease rather than helping people achieve the best health they can. Our approach, by contrast, is about actively creating health.

In Part One, we are going to start by pausing and reflecting on what is happening to us and why it is happening. This will start the process of reconnecting to what is most important to us and help us imagine a better path and a satisfying journey to optimal health and wellbeing.

So, let's start by going back in time...

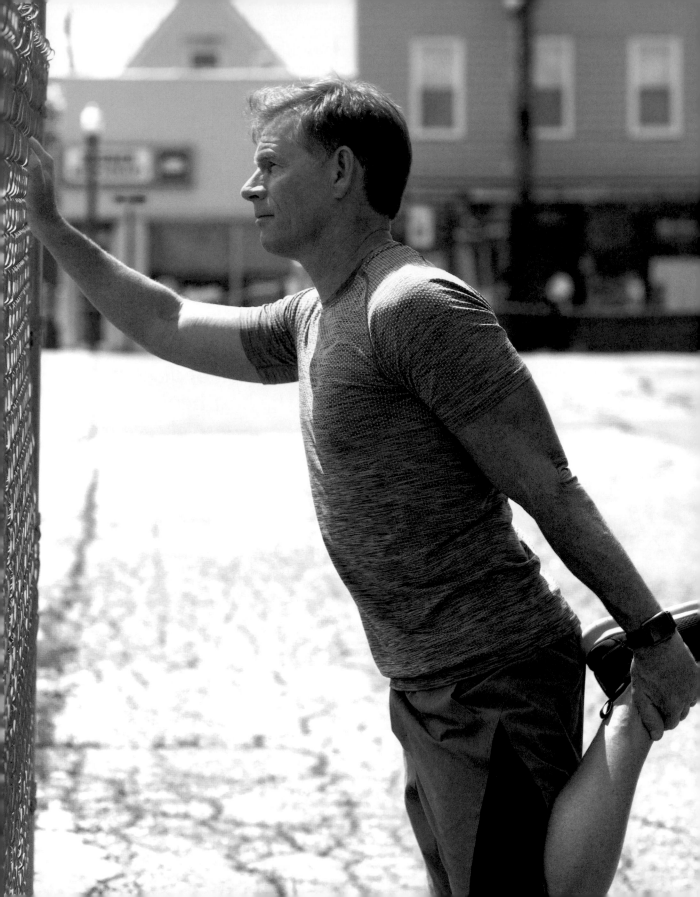

IT'S NOT YOUR FAULT THAT YOU'RE STRUGGLING

10,000 years ago there was no obesity, heart disease, or type 2 diabetes. Just getting enough to eat was a struggle. We foraged for food most of the day. If you found a bush full of ripe berries, you ate them right away because who knew when or if there would be more. If you caught an animal, you and your clan ate the whole thing then and there.

10,000 years ago, being overweight would have meant you were an extremely successful member of the tribe. Your ancestors may have made you leader. It would have taken a lot of ambition to have a body mass index (BMI) above 25.

When I hear someone say, "I went to a party and before I knew it I'd eaten a whole bag of potato chips" I think "well, of course you did" because your body was designed that way.

With so much nutritional energy right in front of you, your 10,000-year-old programming insists you eat it all, especially if you're distracted by a conversation at a party or what's on TV. Your cravings are being fueled by some of the most addictive substances on earth, and I can say with certainty that your next hunting trip to the refrigerator will be 100% successful. You'll bag something full of fat, salt, or sugar.

Ancient humans used their energy to stay alive. If they wanted to get somewhere, they had to walk, climb, run fast, or paddle. If they wanted to eat, they had to gouge roots from the ground, find vegetables and fruits, or grind up grasses and grains. Cooking meant carrying water, gathering wood, and building a fire. So our bodies evolved to be extremely efficient at using energy. If they hadn't, none of us would have survived. To this day, our bodies fight to hold onto every calorie of energy we take in. We're programmed as if our survival is still in question.

The same is true of sleep. 10,000 years ago, when the sun went down, we gathered around a fire winding down from a day of surviving. The amount of physical activity by day and the lack of nighttime distractions would lull us into a long restorative sleep. We'd wake up in perfect balance with our circadian rhythms. Today, for most, the digital sunset doesn't occur until late in the night. Until then, we are bombarded with light and energy. The blue light of TVs, computers, and phones flood our brain with light and stimulation and disrupt our ability to initiate and sustain healthy sleep.

Campfires served another purpose. They helped us build a strong communal bond—nurturing a sense of belonging, compassion, empathy, and shared safety crucial to wellbeing. Today, the communal fire has been extinguished by a digital world that creates constant contact and instant sharing of information but fails to create the deeper connections that are so important to our souls.

Last but not least, the world of 10,000 years ago was full of imminent danger. As a result, we were designed to respond without thought. We would flee the scene and reflect on what happened later. Faced with a genuine threat, our bodies triggered a stress response that released chemicals and hormones that allowed us to run away from danger. Today we are surrounded by perceived dangers. Most are without merit, but they still trigger our ancient programming. The result is that the same threat-induced chemicals swirl around in our bodies and bloodstream but, without the need to flee, they are simply left to keep us in a highly stressed state. The fight without the flight.

Today, we live in a state that evolutionary biologists would describe as being of mismatched conditions where an organism that is not well suited for the conditions in which it exists. We are, as the saying goes, like "fish out of water". Dr. David Katz, a Yale obesity epidemiologist, uses the example of a polar bear in the Sahara as a metaphor to describe the conflict between our 10,000-year-old design and the current world in which we are expected to live. The polar bear was designed to endure the brutal cold conditions of the Arctic

> *To reach and maintain your ideal weight, you need to get on top of the inherent battle between your 10,000-year-old biological predisposition and your desire to be healthy.*

IT'S NOT YOUR FAULT THAT YOU'RE STRUGGLING

Our bodies are programmed to hold onto calories for the sake of survival, so when you try to "diet", you are really fighting your own nature.

(at least until recently). When transported to the desert those same adaptations would accelerate their demise.

The same is true of the modern world which is why we need to talk about the disconnect between the world we were designed to live in and the land of chaos we find ourselves in. You will see that it is not your fault you are struggling with your weight, health, and wellbeing.

THE STORAGE FACTOR

Our bodies are designed to store and conserve fat and calories for those times when we can't find food. It's a storage system made up of over 40 billion adipose (fat) cells, which provide a virtually unlimited storehouse to help keep us alive. We can also store small amounts of carbohydrates in our liver and muscles. But the ability to stockpile precious energy as fat is our most critical survival mechanism. We're here today because 10,000 years ago our ancestors' bodies got very good at storing fat because they never knew when the next meal was coming.

But what happens when this perfect, biologically balanced creation is dropped into the twenty-first century? Getting food today takes almost no effort at all. You drive to the supermarket, throw your packages into a cart, roll the cart to your car, and drive home. The only real effort will be carrying your shopping from the car to the house. That's hardly tending and harvesting your own crops from dawn till dusk.

Perhaps you get food at a local fast food restaurant? You pull in to the drive-thru and use a button to lower your window. You've used two calories so far. You shout into a speaker and place your order. Another two calories. You drive to the pick-up window, grab your supersized burger, fries, and drink and place them on the seat next to you. You might use eight calories lifting a big order. Three minutes later, it's all eaten. How far we've come from our days as hunters and gatherers.

So let's do the dietary math on that hunting trip. Calories consumed: 1,500. Calories expended as energy: 12. Can you see what's wrong with this picture?

THE SUPERSIZED GENERATION

You might have noticed that serving sizes have grown. Restaurant portions are now as many as eight times the standard serving size listed in the FDA's dietary guidelines. Let me say that just once more, just so it sinks in.

Restaurant portions are eight times bigger than they used to be.

Restaurants can be irresponsible too. One steakhouse chain takes a 70-calorie, root vegetable (an onion), full of vitamin C, antioxidants and healthy phenols, and transforms it into a 2,400-calorie, 134-gram fat-fest called a Bloomin' Onion®. And that's before the entrees.

The fact is that you don't have to look hard to see that the calories we consume versus the calories we use are dangerously imbalanced. We're surrounded by food that's larger portioned and more calorie dense than anything we could have imagined even 50 years ago. We're also surrounded by labor-saving devices that help us conserve the energy we once had to exert. It's no wonder that more than two-thirds of Americans take in more calories than they can ever use.

Let me stress once more: this is not your fault. It's not your fault that you were born in a time of unparalleled plenty and physical ease, or born with a body that stores and conserves energy. It's not your fault that you're confronted by food that's more plentiful and addictive than at any other time in history, with a day-to-day lifestyle that finds us at a desk or on the couch in front of the TV.

A 10,000-YEAR-OLD BODY IN THE TWENTY-FIRST CENTURY

Hopefully I've demonstrated that there's a lot more that determines the current state of your health than any lack of willpower or resolve. Our bodies inherited instincts that are no longer useful but are still a force to be reckoned with. How do you manage competing tendencies: the ancient instinct to eat whenever you can, and the modern aspiration to live a long and healthy life?

This is the simple truth that's so critical to understanding why being overweight is not your fault.

One thing's for sure. All the pep talks in the world won't help you. "Lose weight, go on a diet, exercise" are words you might hear from your healthcare provider. It's sound advice, but it's not very useful without a road map to guide you, especially for the long term. Your family may have felt compelled to give you the latest diet books (some or all of which you've probably tried). If you take the advice from those books but then fall into a yo-yo pattern, what then? Even if you agreed with what you'd read, you just aren't sure you can pull it off in the real world. There's old-time positive thinking too. "If you think you can, you can!" sounds powerful if shouted loud enough. But what happens when your boss has been screaming at you, and you find yourself face to face with a pint of Ben and Jerry's® ice cream? Your 10,000-year-old biological instinct says "Eat it all right now!" as your brain repeats its timid mantra "I am a positive and healthy person" Then the tub is empty and you feel powerless to change your life.

You're not powerless.

To reach and maintain your ideal weight, you need to get on top of the inherent battle between your 10,000-year-old biological predisposition and your desire to be healthy.

You don't have a willpower problem or a negative thinking problem. You have a simple conflict between two real desires: the desire to achieve your health goals, and the desire to satisfy your instincts. Dr. A's Habits of Health takes this conflict into consideration and empowers you to take charge successfully, safely, and permanently.

HOW THE FOOD INDUSTRY SABOTAGES YOUR HEALTH

The food industry isn't your friend. Between sodas, snacks, and slices of bread, the average American consumes 26 spoonfuls of refined sugar every single day, while your body only needs the equivalent of one teaspoon of sugar in order to operate your entire bloodstream.[1]

Americans consume an average of 156 lbs of sugar each year. That's an increase of 47 lbs per person in just 20 years.

A century ago, our average consumption was only five pounds per year. So why does twenty-first-century food have so much sugar in it? Simple. Sugar makes food taste good, and food companies need to sell food.[2] The problem is it being consumed in such excess.

Once upon a time, food businesses made profits by offering high-quality food that earned the long-term loyalty of customers. If the butcher sold you a bad piece of meat, you would stop shopping there and let everyone in town know about it. If the greengrocer sold you rotten vegetables, you wouldn't go back. The food industry used to be run by people that took pride in their products. The butcher knew his beef, lamb, and pork; the greengrocer knew his fruits and vegetables and the farmers that supplied them. The food industry was personal. But as food became bigger and bigger business, the focus moved from quality to profit.

Today's food industry is run by accountants. The numbers they love most—costs—are the ones they can control: lower costs mean higher profits. One way to cut costs is to get a better deal from suppliers by buying in larger quantities. That's how Amazon can offer the same book at lower prices than a corner bookstore.

Businesses can also cut costs by using cheaper ingredients. To an accountant, buying cheap and selling high is a recipe for success. In the early 1980s, high-fructose corn syrup replaced sugar in Pepsi and Coke because it was cheaper. Soft drink companies could super-size their eight-ounce bottles and offer 64 oz for the same price. That's great value. Or is it?

Not really. High-fructose corn syrup, like table sugar, is highly addictive (as addictive as cocaine in fact[3]). Your body gets used to it and starts to crave it. If I were an accountant thinking of ways to sell more soda or cakes it would be simple. I would add something that creates a demand for more of my product and keeps Wall Street happy.

A sweet tooth may be good for business, but it's not good for health and wellbeing. Our 10,000-year-old body can't handle wave after wave of sugar and other high-glycemic carbohydrates indefinitely. Refined sugar and carbohydrates flip all kinds of metabolic switches that turn on fat storage and open unhealthy inflammatory pathways and people suddenly discover that they're pre-diabetic (a position that 86 million people in the U.S. alone find themselves in).[4]

So our 10,000-year-old body must deal with a modern world that profits by selling us the most addictive and unhealthy food there is. It's easier to go to a fast food chain than to a healthier, more expensive restaurant or to prepare a healthy meal at home. If we do go to the supermarket, we're confronted by products that are so overly processed they offer very limited nutritional value. They might taste great, they're certainly convenient, and they're definitely cheap and easy to prepare. What a shame they're also unbelievably bad for you!

Moss wrote an amazing expose on the efforts the food industry was making to optimize the taste, smell, feel, and addictive qualities of junk food. Howard Moskovitz, a Harvard Ph.D. dramatically advanced individual consumption by engineering food that had a very specific sensory-specific satiety. In layperson's terms, this is the tendency for big, distinct flavors to overwhelm the brain, which then responds by depressing your desire to have more. Intentionally mundane foods—like white bread—will never get you too excited, but you can eat lots and lots of it without feeling you've had enough. In essence, Moskovitz manipulated our brain's response to food so that its salt and fat content create a constant craving. It gives us a particular crunch and taste that makes us want to keep eating. However, no matter how much we consume, we never feel satisfied.

Put very simply, the food industry is not your friend.

THE KITCHEN HAS BECOME THE LIVING ROOM OF THE PAST

As a baby boomer growing up in suburbia, kids were not allowed to hang out in the living room for fear we would ruin the upholstery. You could describe it as an early form of staging. Slipcovers kept the dust off, and a velvet rope kept us out. The living room was a show piece, reserved for adults, and only used when there was company. Some things never change.

Kitchens seem to have gone the same way; Sub-Zero™ refrigerators, exotic granite surfaces, copper pots and pans, and Viking Ranges™ that look like showroom models create exhibition rooms to be admired but not used. We eat out almost as much as we cook our own food. In 1900, two percent of meals were eaten outside the home.[5] In 2010, 50% were eaten away from home. And one in five breakfasts is bought at McDonald's.[6] Even when we do eat at home it doesn't look like the gathering place of my youth, where we would congregate around nourishing home-cooked meals.[7]

Today family meals last less than 20 minutes and take place (on average) three nights a week.[8] On top of that, time together as a family, which has been proven to increase the success of our

Sugar is Not Evil

We were born with a preference for sweets, and our taste buds prefer sugar because we can safely digest it and it supports our body functions. Breast milk is sweet because we need a concentrated fuel to develop our bodies and grow our brains. Our brains connect sugar with pleasure because that relationship has allowed us to survive.

A Habit of Disease: The Fast Food Habit

Did you know that eating too much unhealthy fast food—even for a single week—can cause noticeable damage to your body?

In a study published online in *Gut*, the international journal of gastroenterology and hepatology, 18 healthy adults ate at least two fast food meals a day. It doubled their daily intake of calories. The study also limited their exercise. In just one week, half of the group had elevated levels of ALT enzymes—a common indicator of liver damage. By the end of the study, the entire group had gained an average of 14 lbs per participant. The conclusion? Our bodies just aren't made to handle more than occasional fast food.[10]

children, is degraded by watching television or texting.[9] More meals are eaten in the minivan than the kitchen.

According to data from the Bureau of Labor Statistics, Millennials alone spend 44% of their food dollars eating out. That's an increase of seven percent from the tail end of the Baby Boomers.[11] What we know is that a habit of eating out on fast food is perilous.[12]

- Eating fast food and processed food may increase your risk of depression.[13]
- Eating foods filled with sodium, like many fast foods, can increase your risk for headaches.
- The carbs and sugar in fast food produce acids that can destroy tooth enamel leading to dental cavities.
- Carbs, not grease, can trigger acne.[14] Carb-heavy fast food like French fries, hamburger buns, and potato chips may lead to acne breakouts.
- Elevated cholesterol and increased blood pressure are two of the top risk factors for heart disease and stroke.
- Extra calories can turn into excess pounds. Without exercise to counteract the increase in calories, obesity will follow.
- Obesity can cause shortness of breath even when you do very little physical activity.
- Fried foods are filled with trans fats. These fats are known to raise LDL (bad) cholesterol levels.
- Fast food is typically sodium heavy, which can elevate blood pressure or aggravate existing heart disorders, including congestive heart failure.
- Fast food can lead to frequent insulin spikes. This can lead to insulin resistance and type 2 diabetes.
- Your body may retain water if you eat too much sodium, leaving you feeling puffy, bloated, and swollen.
- People who eat at fast-food restaurants tend to take in an extra 187 to 190 calories per day.

Along with a more sedentary lifestyle, there's been an alarming increase in our daily ingestion of calories since the early 1980s. The result is a rise in fat accumulation that leads to pre-obesity and obesity. The following chart shows this trend is expected to accelerate into the next decade. If that's not scary enough, a new computer model in the *New England Journal of Medicine* suggests that the majority (60%) of children growing up in America today will be obese by age 35.[15]

How did this happen? Well, you could argue it was economics. The overworked, time-starved workforce of the early 1980s spurred the food industry to produce convenient, pre-prepared products and easy-to-access, affordable restaurants. It created more variety but also added more calories to our diets. The Reagan Administration hastily deregulated the agriculture industry, which made food cheap, abundant, and more energy dense. Finally, continued demand for

The Science of Food Addiction:
Padding the Pockets
of the Food Industry,
Paving the Path to Disease

Try this simple experiment. Read the labels on the products you eat. See if you can find how many contain high-fructose corn syrup or table sugar. According to the U.S. Department of Health and Human Services, added sugars show up on food and drink labels under various names and so it may be described as one of the following:

Anhydrous dextrose, brown sugar, cane crystals, cane sugar, corn sweetener, corn syrup, corn syrup solids, crystal dextrose, evaporated cane juice, fructose sweetener, fruit juice concentrates, high-fructose corn syrup, honey, liquid fructose, malt syrup, maple syrup, molasses, pancake syrup, raw sugar, sugar syrup, and white sugar.

Other types of sugar you might commonly see on ingredient lists are fructose, lactose, and maltose. Fructose is sugar derived from fruit and vegetables; lactose is milk sugar; and maltose is sugar that comes from grain.

If you look at original recipes for these same foods (perhaps the recipe used by your parents or in cookbooks from a generation ago), you'll see very few of them contain sugar, much less high-fructose corn syrup.

Why is our food full of this stuff? Well, because when you add high-fructose corn syrup to salty foods like ketchup or lunch meats, we eat more of it and that means more money for the food industry. Your internal appetite control center is designed to tell you that you're full when it senses specific quantities of certain nutrients in your blood. But food scientists, working for food companies, manipulate the ingredients in processed foods to prevent you from reaching the "I'm full" feeling. And it's working. When food science began as a discipline in the 1970s, Americans were spending six billion dollars a year on fast food. Today, we're spending 200 billion.[16] The math is simple. Unfortunately, the truth may be even more diabolical than we thought.

An article in the *Chicago Tribune* by Patricia Callahan describes a collaborative effort by Phillip Morris and Kraft Foods to use the brain research on cigarette addiction to explore how brain scans could show the way the brain processes tastes and smells. Kraft's interest in how the brain is rewarded by sweet and fatty foods led to a tantalizing glimpse of the interplay between food and tobacco scientists.

The Side Effects of Eating Fast Food[17]

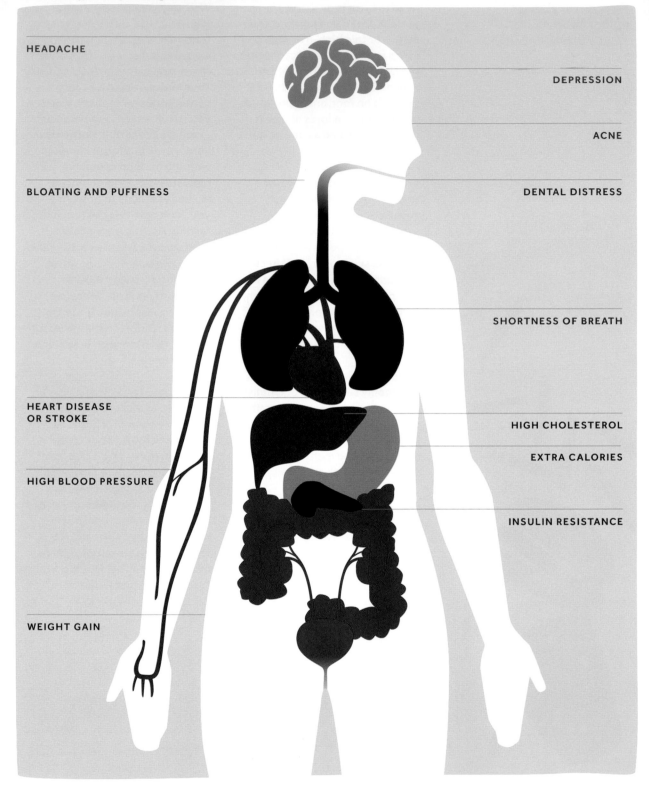

HEADACHE

DEPRESSION

ACNE

BLOATING AND PUFFINESS

DENTAL DISTRESS

SHORTNESS OF BREATH

HEART DISEASE
OR STROKE

HIGH CHOLESTEROL

EXTRA CALORIES

HIGH BLOOD PRESSURE

INSULIN RESISTANCE

WEIGHT GAIN

higher short-term returns on investments by Wall Street stockholders forced food companies to expand their reach into schools, bookstores, and just about any other location humans could be found. I'd wager there has been at least one marketing director that has said "If we can introduce a delivery system to feed our customers while they sleep, then we can tap into a seven-hour-a-day niche that no one owns!"

The food industry continues to lobby hard in Washington. They sponsor journals and special interest groups to market favorable viewpoints of their goods. In the supermarket—today's great common marketplace—consumers seek out sound nutritional advice but are instead faced with the communications of for-profit enterprises, which are guided in turn by their need to return profit to stockholders.

THE NUMBERS TELL THE STORY

The math couldn't be simpler or the impact of what it tells us more deadly: consume more caloric energy than you use and the excess must be stored as fat. Keep that up and those extra pounds quickly lead to pre-obesity and obesity—an insidious disease that leads directly to premature death.

THE ANSWERS ARE RIGHT IN FRONT OF US

There is no need to spend any more time researching the causes or thinking about the solution to this overwhelming problem. In 1993 McGinnis[2] published the most significant causes of death in the U.S. in the *Journal of the American Medical Association*.[18] The top three causes of death were smoking, overeating, and a lack of exercise. They are all causes that are within our control. Today not much has changed. All recent studies reach the same conclusion. The only new news is that the modifiable behaviors of eating too much and not being active enough are catching up with smoking in causing disease and death.

Although we're learning more about metabolism and the inequality of different sources of calories with regard to how they switch on our natural fat storage capacity, the facts and the fats remain the same. If our daily choices create unhealthy dietary patterns and if we subscribe to a sedentary lifestyle we can predict the following: we will gain weight, become overweight and obese, and shorten the quality and the quantity of our lives.

So where is medical technology in all of this? Sadly, it's focused on sick care, not healthcare. Its focus today is where I was a long time ago—delivering new technologies and life-saving breakthroughs in operating rooms and intensive care units. The problem is, no matter how remarkable these developments in critical care are, they are too

Research shows that children who have regular meals with their parents do better in every way: from better grades, to healthier relationships, to staying out of trouble. They are 42% less likely to drink, 50% less likely to smoke, and 66% less likely to smoke marijuana. Regular family dinners protect girls from bulimia, anorexia, and diet pills.[19]

Family dinners also reduce the incidence of childhood obesity. In a study on household routines and obesity in U.S. preschool children, it was shown that kids as young as four have a lower risk of obesity if they have regular family dinners, have enough sleep, and don't watch TV on weekdays.

IT'S NOT YOUR FAULT THAT YOU'RE STRUGGLING

High-glycemic carbohydrates are starchy foods and sugars that quickly raise your blood sugar to a high level and put the body in a fat storage mode.

What is a Calorie?

Calories are used to measure the amount of energy we get from our food. While different types of calories appear in scientific contexts, in the fields of nutrition and food labeling, a calorie refers to the amount of energy needed to increase the temperature of one kilogram of water by one degree centigrade—hence the abbreviation kcal. For our purposes, we'll use the terms calorie and kcal interchangeably. Different sources of calories affect the body in different ways but for now a good rule of thumb is to eat what your grandmother ate whenever you can!

far downstream from the source and the start of the problem.

Part of the blame lies in the medical model itself. Sick care today is overseen by so many people with so many diverse interests and agendas that the healthcare provider/patient relationship is no longer the most important component of the model.

The main strategy is the same as it was 18 years ago. Medicine cures illness rather than create health and wellbeing. Most of us have little exposure to the current model until we exhibit symptoms—a sign that we're already a long way down the path to disease. Don't misunderstand me, as healing the sick is a noble cause but it comes too late. We should be asking why disease is present in the first place. We should be working out health creation strategies so that diseases don't get a head start. Medical science, with its emphasis on fighting disease rather than preventing it, just isn't prepared to answer these questions.

It's totally understandable. It's in our nature to be problem solvers. In fact, society encourages it. 10,000 years ago, our hostile world presented one life-threatening problem after another. In order to survive, we had to think in terms of the threats, hazards, dangers, and risks we might face every single day.

So, although we might all be against the idea of disease it doesn't mean we're necessarily doing what's needed to create health and wellbeing. It's a critical distinction that most of the medical profession hasn't made. Today's medications and surgical advances are helping to control the symptoms of people who are already sick, but modern medicine is doing very little to stop the progression from health to non-sickness and disease. The vast majority of us—90% of us in fact—are currently in a less than optimal state and headed in the wrong direction.

The reality—that the current health plan isn't working—is nowhere more apparent than in today's disturbing increase in obesity, diabetes, and hypertension in young people. Even the term adult-onset diabetes has become obsolete. Renamed type 2 diabetes, this debilitating disease is reaching epidemic proportion among people of all ages. It's attacking children as young as six years of age.[20]

The Health Path chart on the next page illustrates the effect that the current medical model is having on our health. As you can see, the forecasted path indicates that in the future more people are expected to become sick at a younger age. Life expectancy is also expected to shorten.

And it's not just our health that's suffering—it's our pocketbooks as well. Despite the fact that the U.S. spends more than any nation in the world on healthcare, we're not even in the top 25 in terms of the health of our citizens. We have made great strides. Our directive on curing heart disease brought about many new advancements, including noninvasive diagnostics and clot-busting medications. The death rate from heart disease has decreased dramatically as a result.

But the cost of these super-advanced devices and advances is bankrupting our healthcare system. In the U.S., we spend 50% of our $3.2 trillion healthcare budget taking care of people who are sick.*

Less than five percent is spent on helping people stay healthy in the first place. And the medications we're using to treat symptoms caused by excess weight and lack of exercise are making us sicker.[21]

So, I think that it is clear that the institutions we depend on to keep us safe are either letting us down or adapting too slowly to the epidemic of obesity.

By contrast, the health plan that is laid out in this book and its original companion guide has already helped tens of thousands of people take control of their health and forge a new health path—one of optimal health, wellbeing, and the potential to live longer.

Current and Projected Health Path

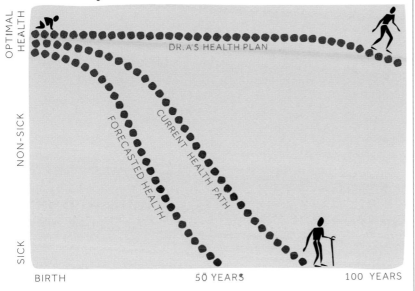

According to the forecasted path (in red), more of us will be getting sicker younger and dying sooner, unless we adopt a new health path

We have discussed the current inadequacies of the food and medical industries in supporting our health and wellbeing. Unfortunately, this tidal wave of unhealthy calorie rich food, labor saving devices, and overwhelming stress is negatively affecting every area of our health and wellbeing. And, as you will see in the following diagram, it is more urgent than ever that we get out ahead of it or we'll go the same way as the dinosaurs.

Thomas Friedman, best known for his work *The World is Flat*, recently published *Thank You for Being Late* in which he talks about acceleration. "Today," he says, "is the slowest change will ever be." He states that our ability to adapt to change is lagging behind the speed that technology is changing.

*In 2016 U.S. healthcare spending increased by 4.3% to reach $3.3 trillion, or $10,348 per person.

Medication: A Double-Edged Sword

Did you know that medications are now among the leading causes of death in the nation? According to a study in the *Archives of Internal Medicine*, the number of serious adverse drug events (those resulting in disability, hospitalization, birth defects, etc.) more than doubled between 1998 and 2005, and the number of adverse drug events resulting in death nearly tripled.[22]

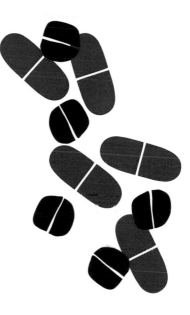

IT'S NOT YOUR FAULT THAT YOU'RE STRUGGLING

There is a group of healthcare professionals who are starting to devote more time to looking at what is necessary to educate their patients on how to improve their lifestyles. I am very proud of the growing group who are joining our team to help coach patients and clients on how to transform their health and wellbeing.

There is a general movement in the Centers for Disease Control and Prevention (CDC) to start focusing on lifestyle and I am also a member of the recently chartered American College of Lifestyle Medicine. Our goal is to move medicine into the third era where our focus is on a holistic approach to health and wellbeing. In time, we may even eliminate the need for traditional sick-care except in trauma and acute illness but, in the meantime, the Habits of Health is our best answer.

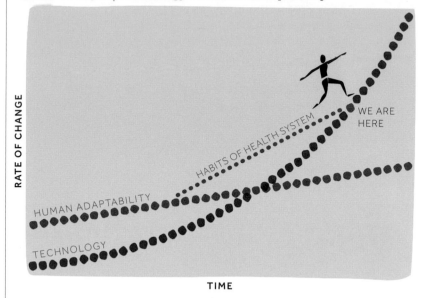

He also says that if humans are going to survive they are going to have to learn how to adapt at a quicker pace. We'll have to learn to deal with change very differently.

This is particularly true when we focus on responding to the factors that determine our health and wellbeing. Each of us needs to take full responsibility for our own health and wellbeing while, at the same time, working collectively to build a new, healthier world. If we demand healthier food from the food industry and real healthcare from the medical industry, we will help move those industries forward.

There are other key areas that we will need to address so that we can control and modify our behavior:

- We know we should not smoke.
- Smoking equals disease and death.
- We know we should eat healthier and move more.
- We know that sleep is not a luxury but a prerequisite to health.
- And we know that wellbeing is disrupted by our technologically advancing world.
- There are so many ways that the modern world is affecting our health and wellbeing.
- That's why this book looks at all the things you can do to start building radiant health and vibrant energy, thereby creating the optimal health we all desire in our lives.

Studies show that most people that start out to lose weight, or get healthy, will fail. In fact, 93% of people that make a New Year's resolution never reach the goals they've set.

They fail because they lack one or more of the following: a sound strategy, a clear process, the skills required, understanding, support, and a proper environment.

I want to reinforce an important point. If you have decided to change do not go it alone! The role and purpose of this book is to put those things together in a simple, achievable system that will help you create optimal health and wellbeing in a predictable way.

We'll be addressing all the key areas that determine your health. Reaching a healthy weight is a natural endpoint that will come from learning the Habits of Health and using the creative process to help you focus on organizing your life around what is most important.

We are going to build you a new house of health and wellbeing, brick by brick this new structure will be built on enough bedrock to endure whatever this constantly changing world throws at you.

So, before we go on, let's look at why so many people fail.

" Diets that put your nutritional balance out of whack nearly always fail and can actually make it harder to lose weight in the future. "

THE FAILURE PATTERN: DIET VS. EXERCISE

Your healthcare provider tells you to lose weight and sends you off to the hinterlands to look for answers. It's like sending a lamb to wolves. There are a million "miracle" weight-loss products out there and just as many opinions on how to lose weight. Every miracle cure we read about has its proponents. But, for now, forget the cabbage diet, lemon juice diet, water diet, colonics, purging, and other unhealthy methods, and let's just take a look at the two major routes to better health: diet and exercise.

In moving you toward your goal, diet pundits tell you to focus on diet and exercise pundits tell you to focus on exercise. Of course, both sides pay lip service to the other but, ultimately, they're invested in supporting their own interests.

The fad diet folks tell you to lower your calorie intake and manipulate macronutrients (protein, fat, carbohydrate). That's where we get the "low-fat diet", "low-carb diet", and "high-protein diet"—all of which create an abnormal ratio of nutritional intake. But the food fight among these diet gurus as to who's right and who's wrong is an exercise in futility (no pun intended). At the end of the day, your body doesn't work the way they think it does.

If you lower your carbohydrates, fat, or protein by the wrong percentage, your body will develop cravings, and your chance of maintaining weight loss is like a dog trying to stay away from a porterhouse steak.

If you make it through this first phase of weight loss—and many people don't—the irony is that you will have lowered your total energy expenditure per day and therefore lowered your metabolic rate.

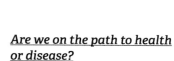

DR. A SAYS...

To lose weight through exercise alone, you'd need to work out strenuously for 90 minutes every day.[23]

Are we on the path to health or disease?

It is beyond argument that excess weight is associated with earlier risk of obesity-related disease and death in adulthood. Perhaps one of the most sobering statements regarding the severity of the childhood obesity epidemic was published by the American Heart Association last year when former Surgeon General, Richard Carmona, characterized the threat as follows:

"Because of the increasing rates of obesity, unhealthy eating habits and physical inactivity, we may see the first generation that will be less healthy and have a shorter life expectancy than their parents."

By not picking precisely the right fuels and foods, you'll lose muscle— the bane of periodic cycling (yo-yo-ing). Your body's furnace has been reset at a lower level than it was when you began your diet and this can actually lead to obesity. Without going through a recalibration process, you're likely to slip into your old eating habits and gain the weight back but with a less effective metabolic furnace.

The result? A heavier weight, a higher percentage of body fat versus muscle, a lower metabolic rate, and less inclination to be active, all of which making it even harder to lose weight next time.

The exercise enthusiasts try to exercise themselves to a healthy weight. But people who focus on exercise tactics will find themselves as disappointed as the dieters. There are health benefits associated with exercise but it's hard to lose much weight through exercise alone.

To really lose weight, you would need to do 90 minutes of strenuous exercise a day, according to the U.S. Institute of Medicine. A daunting task that would be impossible for most to fit into their schedules! So, while exercise is critical for long-term success, it has to be one part of a comprehensive process. Once you begin to lose weight, you'll naturally become more active. At that point, we'll increase your activity incrementally through fun choices that increase muscle mass with effects that can last a lifetime.

Hopefully, this explains why you gain back weight after dieting alone. As tough as it sounds, there's just no simple solution to reaching and maintaining a healthy weight. That's not to say it's difficult to do, but there's a lot more to it than just diet or exercise. It's not your fault that, like the polar bear, you and your body and brain were designed for a world that is long gone, and you need to survive in a world that is changing every day.

If we choose to wait and watch, our health and our lives, and those that we love and cherish, will all be negatively affected one way or another.

Or, you can make a different set of choices, following a path that will teach you how to create permanent health and wellbeing. The path to optimal health is paved with the Habits of Health. In the next part we will start to explore this new path to optimal health and wellbeing.

HABITS OF HEALTH

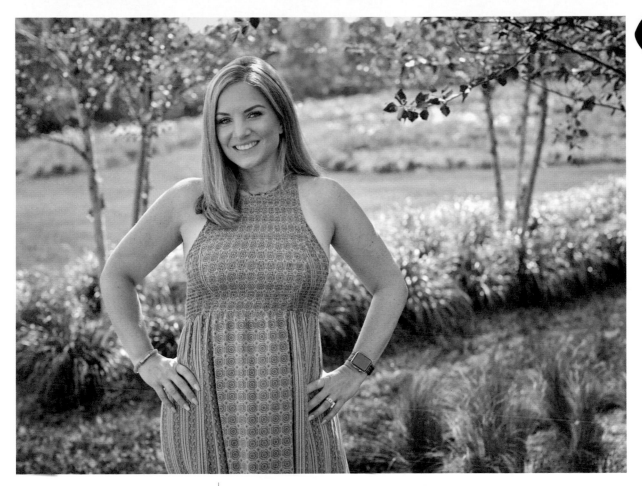

TRANSFORMATION: SUZY HEYMAN

> "
> *My energy level is very different, and our lives are just completely changed.*
> "

I decided to do Dr. A's program with my husband. It was one of just many that we've been on, and little did we know our lives would change. In the past three years, we've been able to change our health completely. My energy level is very different, and our lives are just completely changed.

In the past, what we've done is diet after diet after diet. What we now know is that diets mostly fail. This means that we have undergone a lifestyle change, and we've ingrained these healthy habits that we didn't even really know about. Because of that, we're able to embrace our health and we don't feel like it's a diet at all.

Learning the Habits of Health has affected me so much. Dr. A has been able to enforce those habits and show us why we want to have them in our lives—everything from the amount of water that we drink, to how to fuel ourselves properly, and the habits of sleep. By becoming part of this community and being exposed to Dr. A, we've seen what's possible and learned how to become the highest version of ourselves.

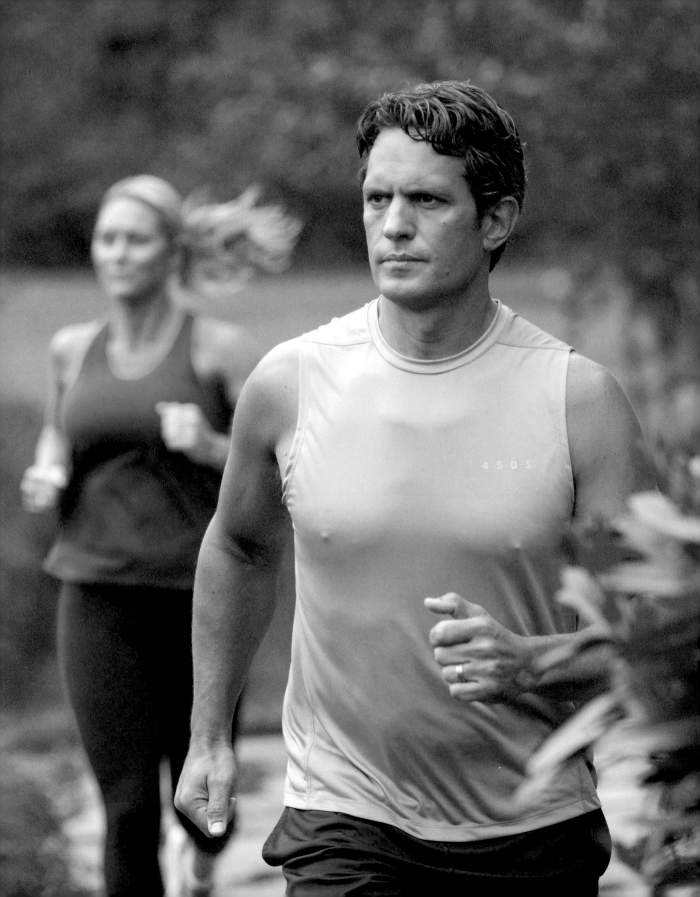

PART 1.2

THE PATH:
THE CREATION OF
OPTIMAL HEALTH
AND WELLBEING

If you had the choice to thrive in your health and life, would you take it?

I'm not asking you if you think you can do it. I'm only asking if it's important to you. I know the thought of being healthy might seem a long way from where you are right now. If your motivation for buying this book was to lose some weight, the goal of optimal health and wellbeing might seem like a fantasy. Let me assure you, it really isn't.

You can definitely create optimal health in your life. You just need to learn how. The insights you will gain in this part will lay out the path.

Understanding that your body is no stranger to optimal health is important. Most of us are born in pristine condition. But once we leave the womb, everyone's life takes a slightly different path.

We are thrown into a world that is intrinsically unstable. That's why entropy—the natural tendency of things to lose order—is important. Weeds take over gardens, rooms get messy, cars rust, our carpet gets old and so do we. Our health and our wellbeing determine the trajectory and the speed at which we age and get sick.

The good news is that we can fight entropy. We can weed our garden, organize our room, wax our cars, clean our carpets, and so on. And when it comes to human entropy, we can make different choices, change the environment we live in, and the people we associate with.

So, how about we kick entropy in the rear?

YOU'RE GOING TO MOVE FROM HEALTHCARE TO SELF-CARE

First, I don't (and can't possibly) know how well you have done to this point. You have been subjected to so many influences that shape your health and your life. Enablers have either helped or hurt your health. The journey from infancy to childhood, those difficult teenage years, and the development into adulthood exposes us to many variables. Along the way, we adopt values and beliefs that become the primary drivers of our thoughts and actions. They help us negotiate everything life throws at us. This programing is influenced by our parents, family, friends, teachers, and mentors (or the lack of them).

Environmental influences are also powerful determinants of our current health and wellbeing. They include where we live, our socioeconomic status, our education, and institutions like the food, transportation, technology, and medical industries—all of which are designed (at least in theory) to serve us.

All those influences have brought us to this point in our life's story. Your story determines how you respond to your world. And your story is driving your current behaviors and your choices, most of which are made without conscious effort.

Are those choices currently driving your health and wellbeing in the right direction? For most, the answer is no.

IS "NON-SICK" YOUR WAY OF LIFE?

We used to think "If you're not sick, you must be healthy." That's how much of the medical world saw it too. But that's changing. In the last few years, medical research is starting to validate what the *Habits of Health Transformational System* has been preaching for a decade: non-sick and healthy are vastly different states of being.

The year after the first edition of *Dr. A's Habits of Health* came out, a key study was published in the *Arch of Internal Medicine*.[1] They evaluated over 25,000 people and concluded that by adhering to four simple lifestyle factors, you can reduce your risk of developing major chronic disease by 80%!

Those lifestyle factors are:
- **Not smoking**
- **BMI less than 30**
- **Perform 3.5 hours a week or more of physical activity**
- **Adhere to dietary principles such as a high intake of fruit, vegetables, whole-grain bread, and lower your meat consumption**

Non-sickness is like purgatory—surviving, not thriving. It is caused by eating an excess quantity of nutritionally barren, calorie-rich unhealthy food which overworks the pancreas and facilitates your body's storage of fat. Non-sickness is a state in which your muscles become weak and flabby, you don't get enough sleep and you're always stressed.

Non-sickness invades your thoughts and feelings and takes the joy out of your days. It's a state that leads you to progressive dependence on medications to relieve symptoms that are merely your body's way of telling you you're not healthy. If you drive your car off the showroom floor and on your way home the oil warning light came on, would you cut the wire and keep driving? No, you would take it straight back to the dealership.

So, that begs the question: why are we suppressing our body's warning signals with industrial size bottles of Tylenol? A blue-light special on 1,000 capsules of painkillers is not a good thing. By concealing symptoms, you are ignoring physical and mental signals that something is wrong.

The same stores that sell you over-the-counter medicines are also selling chips, sodas, candies, alcohol, cigarettes, and many other disease-causing products! To say it's hypocritical is a generous assessment.

These choices—part of the Habits of Disease—lead first to non-sickness and eventually cause life-threatening illness. The road to obesity starts with a state I call pre-obesity—a more apt description than the innocuous sounding overweight. Excess weight and a sedentary lifestyle take their toll and can lead to metabolic syndrome,[2] which affects one in three Americans. In a state of non-sickness, time is not your friend because one day you will be so fatigued that you finally go to your healthcare provider and find out you have diabetes.

If any of this sounds familiar, please don't worry. You're not alone. Close to 90% of our population falls somewhere in this non-sick category. The good news—or dare I say, the great news—is that if you make the decision to change, this non-sick state can be overcome, and you can usually reach optimal health in a relatively short period of time.

CHOOSING YOUR HEALTH PATH

Let's look at the health path most people find themselves on. Too often, non-sickness progresses over time to sickness and disease—a descent accelerated by our modern lifestyle (take a look at Part 1.1, *It's Not Your Fault That You're Struggling,* if you need a reminder!). But this decline isn't inevitable, you just have to realize life isn't a reality show—it's real, and it's the only life you've got. Waiting for healthcare providers, weight-loss gurus, or drug companies to come up with a solution won't work. Your health is not a spectator sport.

You need to create focus and expend energy to create stability, structure, and simplicity. In essence, we're fighting entropy and creating health. Let's start by asking a few questions to determine your current direction:

- Is your health improving every day?
- Are your daily habits creating greater health and vibrancy or draining your battery and putting you on an accelerating path toward disease?
- Are you already in a non-sick or sick state?

The answers will tell you whether you're on the path toward illness or health.

What if you're already descending to a state of disease? Is it too late? Not at all. Even if you've tried time and time again to lose weight and create health but only to fail, your future is still far from determined. You can change your path. You just need to take the right actions, begin to adopt new healthy habits, and build momentum.

You're not predestined to get sick, despite what pharmaceutical commercials tell you. In fact, as you can see in the next illustration, the further you are from optimal health, the more dramatic your change in health is likely to be.

Changing Your Health Plan

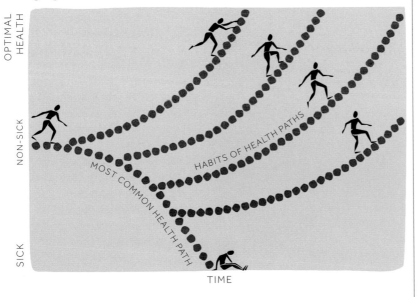

Remember, the goal is to be much more than "non-sick": It's to be healthy and to thrive in all the areas of your life. And your daily habits—your Habits of Disease or Habits of Health—will determine that direction.

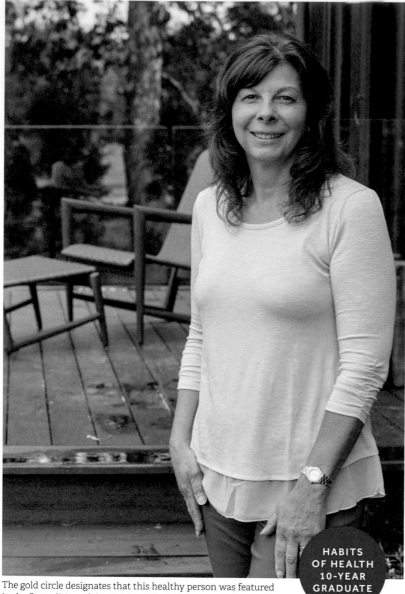

The gold circle designates that this healthy person was featured in the first edition of the Habits of Health 10 years ago!

HABITS OF HEALTH 10-YEAR GRADUATE

TRANSFORMATION: RITA TARINELLI

At 41 years old, I was not feeling very well. I was overweight and had gone to my physician and was looking at taking some medications for various things that were going on in my body. I was very unhealthy even though I was young and I looked good; I just didn't feel very good at that point.

I was introduced to the Habits of Health and changed my habits. Over the years, they've become second-nature. I have just been exercising more, eating well, and sleeping better—all those things that we're taught that we don't put into action. I finally put them into action to work for me, and they have been great over the years.

For me, the Habits of Health was a lifestyle change. It was more about eating better and eating every few hours instead of just really big meals and feeling tired all the time. It was about exercising, but exercise in moderation and not overdoing it. I wasn't sleeping very well, so sleeping played an important part of my health, as well as being more active, and doing a lot of things with the children.

> "
> *I was very unhealthy even though I was young and I looked good.*
> "

THE PATH TO OPTIMAL HEALTH AND WELLBEING

A lot has happened in the world of research since I wrote the first edition of this book. The Healthy Living Study, as well as a series of new studies, validate the importance of a healthy lifestyle in staying healthy and improving our quality of life.[3-9]

What needs to happen is the wholesale adoption of a healthy lifestyle across America and the rest of the world.

Over the last 10 years—as researchers have been validating that healthy habits make the difference for sustainable transformation in health—we have been figuring out the *what* and *how*, constantly improving our methods to provide practical solutions and, in the process, transforming thousands of lives.

In Part 1.1, *It's Not Your Fault That You're Struggling,* we discussed the conflict between our own biological design and the modern world. We also realized that if you are going to change your health and life, then you are going to have to be the master of all your habits. You won't be alone: I will be here with you, and I will suggest other things we can do to build your support. But it has to start with you.

Let's now look at the key areas of focus and how we will approach them every day.

THE HABITS OF HEALTH: AN OVERVIEW

Every aspect of my system—*Dr. A's Habits of Health Transformational System*—is designed to form a long-term partnership that helps you to optimize your health and wellbeing and, in doing so, develop and sustain a healthy lifestyle. I want to build a level of trust and a positive rapport with you so that you can enhance your self-motivation and self-regulation to navigate a journey of change. We will explore your current position and where you want to go. The habits themselves are health promoting behaviors that focus on your physical, mental, and overall satisfaction.

The Habits of Health cover the areas necessary to allow you to improve and eventually thrive in your life. They will address the key aspects of healthy weight control including healthy eating, movement and fitness, healthy sleeping, stress management, and your overall relational coherence: how you deal with both your inner and outer world. We will help you build the new life skills to develop this personal blueprint for optimal health and wellbeing and give you the ability to implement it.

Since we take a whole person approach to health and wellbeing, you will have the opportunity to pick and choose where you want to start and what you'll focus on.

" *A microHabit of Health (mHoH for short) is a habit that's small, easy to do, and almost impossible to fail at.* "

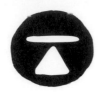

HABITS OF HEALTHY WEIGHT MANAGEMENT

Over two-thirds of us will want to start our journey here. We'll make the beginning simple so we can quickly build efficacy to create early success for you. As you feel better, have more energy, and are losing weight safely, you will be motivated to discover more ways you can improve your health. As you continue to reach a healthy weight, we will add more new habits that will help you maintain your ideal weight. It's an eating plan that is specifically designed to move you through a fat-burning stage to a recalibration stage to an optimizing stage in which your metabolism is working at its most efficient.

It's easy to do, and you won't have hunger pangs or food cravings.

HABITS OF HEALTHY EATING AND HYDRATION

The Habits of Health will continue developing the behaviors that you started installing as you reach a healthy weight and will encompass a number of healthy eating and hydration behaviors. We will talk about portion control, meal frequency, and eating a balanced diet. We will continue to improve your fuel sources so your body is receiving the right vitanutrients in simple steps as you enjoy the benefits of one of the most helpful habits you can adopt. We will help you discover the foods that add flavor and texture (and that you actually like), which support optimal health for the rest of your healthy life.

We will also address the importance of water and proper hydration, as well as help you optimize the efficiency of your body, even if you are struggling to drink enough water at the moment.

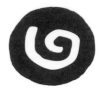

HABITS OF HEALTHY MOTION

We'll ease you into the right amount of physical activity at the right time. While your movement plan may include formal exercise, the Habits of Health are more often made up of activities and clever strategies that make moving your body easy and fun—including some you may not have considered. We pioneered the importance and ability to create activity throughout the day with our NEAT (more on this system later). Studies are starting to support the need for this daylong movement to counter the disease producing effects of a progressively sedentary society. Even among those that exercise greater than seven hours a week, those that spent the most time sitting had a 50% greater risk of death from any cause!

Put simply, all day motion is a necessity.

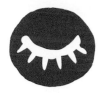

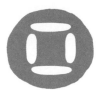

HABITS OF HEALTHY SLEEP

The effect of regular sleep patterns on health is often underestimated, but sleep is one of the most critical factors in creating overall health and wellbeing. It also has a direct impact on losing weight and keeping it off. Skipping that necessary extra hour of sleep decreases your wellbeing, productivity, health, and your ability to think. When you master the Habits of Healthy Sleep, the benefits ripple throughout all areas of your health: from weight management to your relationships with friends and loved ones.

We will also address energy management and how you can optimize your attention, focus, and productivity throughout the day. We will create your own Habits of Health clock to help you have more optimal days.

HABITS OF A HEALTHY MIND

Your long-term success depends on choosing the best strategic actions to support your health. These include examining how you make choices, understanding your patterns and triggers, and helping you maintain a sense of calm and resilience. With greater self-awareness, we will increase your capacity to thrive in a changing world. We will help you adopt new behaviors by enabling you to master the art of habit installation, so you will no longer have to rely on willpower to avoid unhealthy behaviors. We will help you focus and through mindfulness help you put your mind where you want, anytime you want, in any situation. We will build self-efficacy by creating generative motivation, thereby supporting what is most important to you and working within your current ability to change and improve your key life skills.

HABITS OF HEALTHY SURROUNDINGS

The people, places, and things you surround yourself with can enhance or diminish the success of your other Habits of Health. I'll show you how to build a "health bubble" which will help you take control of your personal environment and create conditions that support long-term health. This will be particularly important in helping you establish support systems. As with any good strategy, the first steps make the next steps easier to do. I'll help you build the support system that works best for you, whether that's me, your coach, a friend, a group of friends, or a whole network of people. This will help build great lasting relationships and a stronger sense of connection.

And once we have you well on your way to optimal health and wellbeing, we will continue to grow new Habits of Health that will support your potential to live longer in a healthy state.

THE PATH: THE CREATION OF OPTIMAL HEALTH AND WELLBEING

> *Time and daily choice are our most powerful agents of change. Our choices can be powerful allies or an erosive force that takes our health from us.*

Most people come to us with an immediate need to become the boss of their own weight management, so I will start our journey with healthy weight management and continue with the other key categories as we outline the Habits of Health at a macro level. You need to be in charge and be given the new patterns of thinking, doing, and relating that allow you to determine your future health and wellbeing. Through the system of the Habits of Health and a variety of easy daily activities, we will use these powerful habits to put you on track for sustainable lifelong transformation and help you attain optimal health and wellbeing.

ALL TOGETHER NOW

You may have tried to improve some of these habits in the past with limited success. You may be doing some of them really well. Maybe you've reduced your daily intake of calories, but you aren't in the habit of putting your body in motion every day. Or, you're exercising and taking vitamins, but you're not getting enough sleep. Well, we're ambitious. We want to harness all of the recuperative power of your body. For that to happen, it's essential that the habits work together.

Now, by this point, if you're like most of my clients or patients, you probably have some questions.

"Can I adopt these Habits of Health?" Yes, you can.
"Will they work for me?" Yes, and better than you might imagine.
"Is it hard?" No. The structure and the science means you'll find it easier than you might expect.
"Do I need willpower?" Not in the usual sense. You won't be manipulating yourself through willpower or pressure. Instead, you'll learn how to make strategic choices that support your aspirations.
"If I lose weight, will I yo-yo and gain it back?" No. Most programs can help you to lose weight. But what they're missing is the crucial way the Habits of Health work together to reinforce long-term success and sustainability.

YOUR DAILY CHOICES AND YOUR CURRENT HEALTH

You probably haven't escaped the effect of too much food and too little activity. You're not alone. Two-thirds of Americans are either pre-obese or obese.[10] By reading this book and deciding to make a change, you're already on the path to a powerful transformation.

At each phase of your journey, you'll be making choices that fit your lifestyle. Whether you're 20 years-old and not eating right, 40 years-old and seriously overweight, or 60 years-old with diabetes, high blood pressure and a previous heart attack, the habits I'm about to teach you will create a blueprint for your daily life and will advance you from your current state of health toward optimal health. As you lose weight and increase your energy, you'll find that it gets easier and easier to make the healthy choice.

THE MODERN WAY OF LIFE—OR DEATH?

Let's say that today at lunch you ate a greasy cheeseburger, onion rings, and supersized soda, and then had a near-fatal heart attack. Would you wake up tomorrow and order the same thing? Of course not.

Yet every day, millions of us are eating foods again and again that are destroying our health. It may not happen right away, but after days, weeks, months, and years of poor choices, heavy loads of saturated animal fats, trans-fats, and excess high-fructose corn syrup— along with a lack of healthy vegetables—leads to an insidious rise in insulin, cholesterol, triglycerides, and a sinister state of inflammation.

These substances, aided by our own immune system, lead to the formation of an atherosclerotic plaque, causing the artery wall to weaken. And one Monday morning, a stressed-out executive grips his chest in excruciating pain, and all those poor daily choices that didn't seem to matter much at the time begin to matter a lot. The coronary artery ruptures its endothelial lining and platelets quickly gather around the tear, forming a clot and cutting off the heart's blood supply. He collapses as a result of a massive heart attack. He's only 50. Yet everyone's surprised. He seemed so healthy.

Here's the thing: eating one cheeseburger didn't kill him. The body has an amazing ability to handle a few bad choices. What killed him was making similar bad choices day in and day out over the course of all those business lunches, year after year. Our health is our most precious asset, yet the daily choices most of us make directly conflict with our ability to preserve it.

Why? Because the negative results aren't obvious right away. Eating a cheeseburger today or bypassing the treadmill on your way to the couch won't cause a noticeable downturn in your health in that moment. By the same token, choosing a healthy vegetable for lunch today or going to the gym once or twice in January won't create a noticeable improvement either. In a flood, every drop of water matters, but you probably don't think much of a single raindrop.

Today's instant society wants immediate gratification. We're always looking for the next breakthrough, the next cure, the next pill that will help us lose weight fast. That's why people rush out and have gastric bypass surgery or buy the latest prescription—often with no regard to long-term health risks or side effects. Take my word for it, there are always side effects.

Drugs may lower your weight for a short time, but without changing your Habits of Disease—the cheeseburger, the salt, the lack

On average, a habit takes 66 days to become an unconscious part of your routine.[11]

Drink one extra glass of water today, working your way up to a total of eight glasses of water a day (eight ounces each).

Changing Our Focus

In an instant-gratification society, we think of weight loss as a destination. In fact, weight loss is really just a first step. Optimal health is a journey. This requires a reorientation from merely hoping to lose weight to creating health by allowing our minds and bodies to work together. This is different than focusing on weight loss alone.

of exercise, the six-pack (of beer)—medications are nothing but a symptom reliever. Let me be clear—there is no breakthrough drug on its way that will cure obesity.

However, there is a powerful solution available to you right now and it starts with the compounding effect of choice. Just as your small Habits of Disease add up to create a big heart attack, small daily Habits of Health can create big rewards. When you make those choices today, and tomorrow, and the next day, day in and day out, the benefits compound. And, in the end, you will gain a treasure far more valuable than weight loss alone in the form of optimal health and wellbeing.

Over time, those choices make all the difference in the world—the difference between death and radiant health.

Your Health Path

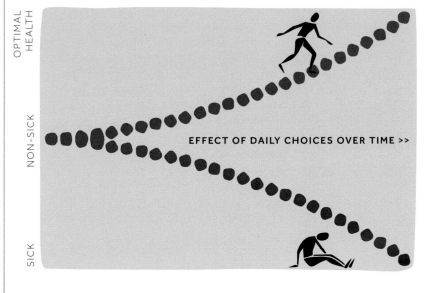

EFFECT OF DAILY CHOICES OVER TIME >>

THE PATH TO OPTIMAL HEALTH AND BEYOND

As I take you through the phases of your journey to optimal health, a number of improvements will begin to occur throughout your body. If your health is like most people's, your body is probably in fat-storage mode right now, with progressive weight gain and an associated high insulin level. These unhealthy physical conditions create an inflammatory state that's a major contributor to heart disease, cancer, and premature ageing.

As you start up your new path, we'll focus on your energy intake and the foods you're eating—things we can change immediately. Beginning in Phase I, we'll transform you from a fat factory to a fat-burning machine, stabilize your insulin, douse the inflammatory fires, and start building habits that support health. Here's a snapshot of some of those improvements as you journey through the phases toward optimal health:

The Path to Optimal Health and Beyond

	FAT VS MUSCLE	BODY MASS INDEX (BMI)	HABITS OF HEALTH
YOUR CURRENT STATE OF HEALTH	FAT STORAGE	BMI HIGH	HABITS OF DISEASE
PHASE I BEGINNING THE WEIGHT-LOSS PHASE	FAT BURNING	BMI DECREASING	HEALTHY EATING AND ACTIVITY HABITS
PHASE II INCORPORATING THE HABITS OF HEALTH	MUSCLE BUILDING	BMI <25	HABITS OF HEALTH
PHASE III OPTIMIZING YOUR HEALTH	MUSCLE OPTIMIZATION	BMI <25	HABITS OF HEALTH AUTOMATED
PHASE IV LONGEVITY	EXTREME LEAN MUSCLE	BMI 20 – 24	SPECIFIC LONGEVITY STRATEGY

But before we begin, let's look at the choice you're making to create optimal health. In order to reach and maintain your goals—weight loss, better health, a more fulfilled life—it is essential to understand where you are right now, where you need to be, and just what's standing in your way.

12 years ago, I was a burned out, stressed out, overweight cardiologist. I didn't have time with my wife or my family, I was very out of shape and, most of all, I felt very out of balance because I went into medicine to help people, and what I discovered was that I really wasn't able to help them that much.

I was living very unhealthy habits of life in the middle of a healthcare system that's supposed to model health and wellbeing. It took me a while to accept the fact that I was in a very unhealthy environment, and I was unhealthy myself. A large part of that was the only time I had restful sleep was when I was on vacation, and that didn't last long because I was worried about when I'd have to go back to work.

As a healthcare professional, I had a lot of facts and knowledge, including information about weight and obesity. I was trained and paid well to treat and manage disease. At the same time, I had a very unhealthy mind and I was unhealthy myself. Dr. Andersen created a science-based methodology to take all that theory and knowledge and actually get results.

I've learned new habits, I eat healthy, I hydrate well, and I sleep really well. I work out all the time, and I love it. I have peace and balance in my mind and in my life. And when people understand that the power is in the choices that they make, then they can become the architect of their lives. We have a science-based methodology; this is evidence based. I'm part of the evidence. People can do this.

I'm now 70 years old and I'm stronger than I've ever been in my life. I have more balance, joy, freedom, and fulfillment in my life than I have ever had. What Dr. Andersen shared with me and many others was really the understanding that the power is in the choices we make each and every day, whether they're the small choices or the bigger choices that over time lead to healthier habits.

My life is completely different. I'm the best doctor I've ever been. I think of myself now as a true health professional and a true physician because I'm not waiting for people to get sick and simply reacting to disease. I've learned how to teach people and guide people using the Habits of Health to empower them to create healthier lives.

> *I went into medicine to help people, and what I discovered was that I really wasn't able to help them that much.*

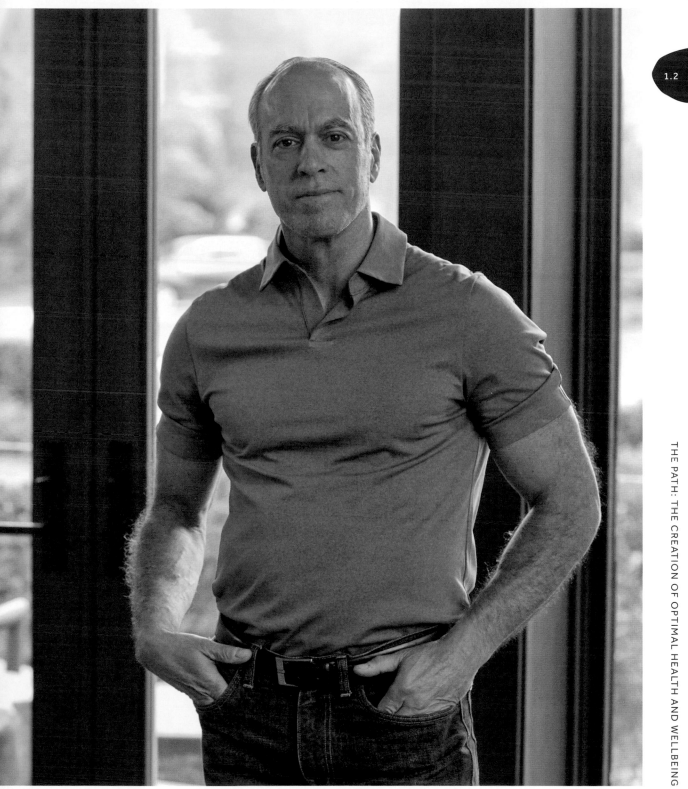

THE PATH: THE CREATION OF OPTIMAL HEALTH AND WELLBEING

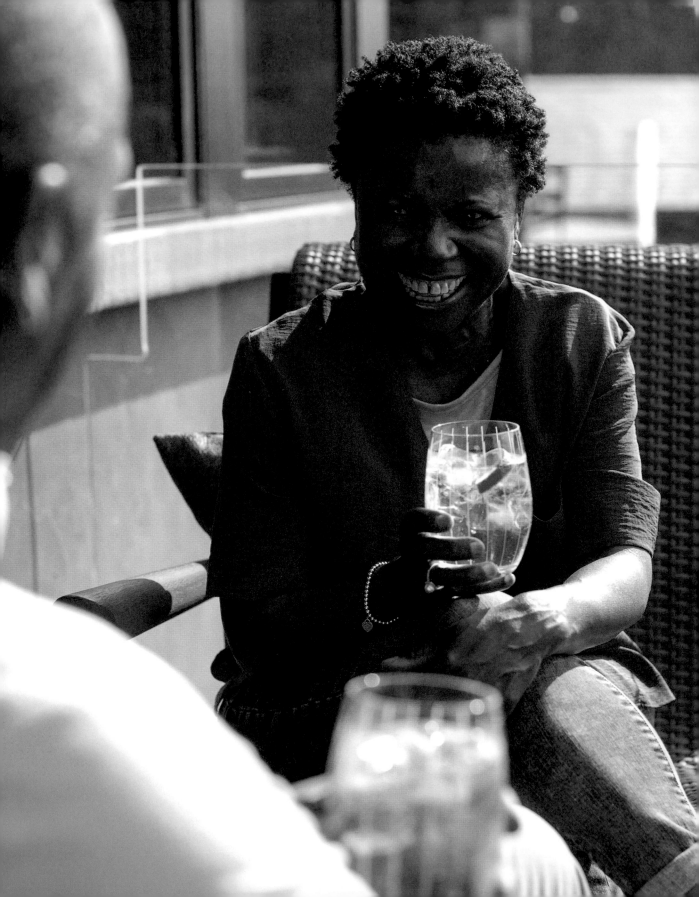

PART 1.3

ARE YOU
REALLY READY
TO CHANGE?

I ask this because one of the most important factors in successful change is determined before we even start: do we want to change in the first place? If we want a higher level of health and wellbeing, we have to be ready to change.

If we are not prepared to shift our mindset and focus on the necessary behavioral changes, then we're set up to struggle, fail, or quit.

THE READINESS FACTOR

In almost two decades of helping people transform their health and their lives, I've seen a pattern to people who truly decide to make a change. They move from a stage of not thinking about changing a habit or behavior to thinking about changing and, over time, they plan for change before they start acting on it.

It's important to understand this for two essential reasons. First, if you are not prepared to begin the journey, we need to examine your current level of motivation and help you decide if this is the right time to start. Second, you may be ready to change one aspect of your health or life but unwilling to work on others. If so, I'll help you understand each key Habit of Health and why it is vital to improve that habit and awaken your desire to make a change.

Once you have decided to change, we will help you through the process and explore what areas you are willing to address to create a plan to install those new behaviors. You might be willing to start a walking program but unwilling to give up late night TV. You may be willing to work on your emotional resilience but not quite ready to start meditating.

The Habits of Health will allow you to progress through a series of habit installations that will create predictable transformation, but self-awareness of your level of desire for change is important. You need to be sure your motivation is aligned with your desire to improve your health and wellbeing and that you have the ability to consistently make the new, daily healthy choice.

Are you ready to change your behavior?*
1. *"I am not ready to change."*
2. *"I am thinking about changing."*
3. *"I am preparing to make a change."*
4. *"I am in action."*
5. *"I am sustaining this new positive behavior."*

I'll assume you're reading this book because you're thinking about changing or preparing to make a change. You may already have started making changes and taking action. We'll use the five stages of readiness as a general guide and checklist as you start your journey and as a review to see if you are ready to add a new behavior. This allows us to address your state of readiness for any new habit installation. The good news is the momentum you generate as you adopt a new habit creates momentum in other areas of health and wellbeing. This is called the Halo Effect and it is a powerful lever that will awaken your desire to change in other areas.

Let's review the stages of readiness.* They will give you the opportunity to discover what stage you may currently be stuck in or whether it's a green light to start your new habit installation.

*Note: this is a practical progression of an individual's thought and action based on the predictable and stages of change as outlined by Prochaska et al.

> " *When you try to change in order to get rid of negative feelings or situations, you will slip up once things get a little better. It just does not work long-term.* "

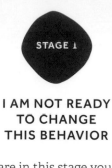

STAGE 1

I AM NOT READY TO CHANGE THIS BEHAVIOR

If you are in this stage you are probably saying "I won't" or "I can't" because you do not think there is a problem or you have tried before and do not believe that you can try again. Either way, I am not going to try to convince you if you're not ready. However, I will be forthright and remind you if you are reading this book your need or desire to change is already awakened. Read on, and we will support you.

STAGE 2

I AM THINKING ABOUT CHANGING THIS BEHAVIOR

This stage means you are probably thinking about improving your health or life and changing unhealthy behaviors. In this state of mind, you are weighing the benefits of change versus the effort it will take. When the pros outweigh the cons, you will be ready.

Once we understand the immediate as well as long-term benefits of making changes, we can move onto making a plan for action. We have been building a case of why you desire to change. My goal in this book is to create a mind-shift so that you decide that you are ready.

STAGE 3

I AM PREPARING TO MAKE A CHANGE IN THIS BEHAVIOR

Most readers are at this stage. This first section of the book is preparing you to start the change process—helping you move from thinking to doing. During this stage, we'll investigate your motivations for change, explore what the change process looks like, and how we will use the power of habits to help you make the changes permanent. We will identify where you are in your health journey and envision what the desired outcomes are for your health and wellbeing.

STAGE 4

I AM IN ACTION, CHANGING AND CREATING HEALTH AND WELLBEING

At Stage Four, you are working on building new health behaviors and installing the Habits of Health in a series of small habits. You are refining your lifestyle to reach and support long-term health and wellbeing, as well as finding the balance between your daily motivation and your ability to consistently install the new habit. It's when you're re-molding your environment, your relationships, and building your mental and physical strength to stay on track. The more modes of support we can surround you with, the easier and more consistently you can move along the path to transformation.

STAGE 5

I AM SUSTAINING THIS NEW POSITIVE BEHAVIOR

At this stage, the new behavior has become a habit—you're doing it automatically. This is the holistic integrated approach of the *Habits of Health Transformational System*. We know that lifelong transformation only occurs if you create a new set of habits. These transformational habits are all available to you and I know that you can master them. These sustainable behaviors continue to be improved as you continue on your health journey because your new orientation allows you to get better in order to become the best version of yourself.

I will show you how to install the Habits and make it easier than you imagine.

STAGE 6

FORWARD AND BACKWARD, LAPSE AND RELAPSE

In these stages of change there are lapses and relapses. Lapses can occur in both the action and the sustaining stage of change. Life will dish out challenges. You may be traveling, or your environment or job may change. The key is to quickly recognize that there has been a slip and refocus on your goals. In a moment, we will discuss why it is unusual for this to happen once you are fully using the *Habits of Health Transformational System*. Relapses in traditional programs can be more challenging because an individual may fully abandon the new behavior and lose the health and wellbeing benefits. In essence, if you experience a lapse or relapse it simply means that you need to make a course correction and get back on the path and refocus on your desired outcome of optimal health.

Course corrections are just part of the journey. Remember: you're only human, and it is going to require focus and work to dial in this transformational process. We are going to spend a lot of time helping you build a growth mindset. In this state of mind there are no failures. Instead, there is just a natural curiosity to figure out why you had a slip and what we need to do to get better. No judgement, no blame, just a focus on learning the new habit. Isn't that refreshing? It starts by really understanding why you want to change.

Changing our emphasis from what we're against to what we're for can have a dramatic impact.

Each time you think about what you don't want, reframe the thought by focusing on what you want to gain with a choice instead of what you want to lose.

THE MOTIVATION FACTOR

Why do you Want to Change?

Motivation: the desire to do things. In order for me to help you create sustainable optimal health and wellbeing, you must realize that I am helping you take charge to fully determine your future health and wellbeing. Only by equipping you to take full responsibility will you be able to reach the highest level of motivation, engagement, ability, capacity, and resilience to thrive and be successful.

At the very core of that success is the source and substance of your motivation. There are generally two sources of motivation: external and autonomous.

External Motivation

This is often when someone other than ourselves—our spouse, our boss, or our parent—tells us what to do. Our spouse demands that we lose weight. To avoid conflict, you say "I am on a diet because my wife will get upset if I eat that fast food." You are being compliant to avoid conflict. You are trying to solve a problem. We internalize the external pressure without really wanting to make the change or aligning it with our personal values and desires. It sounds like "I ought to" or "I should start to watch my weight." This external pressure may work in the short-term, but it won't last.

Autonomous Motivation

This source of motivation is sustainable. It's good for our future. We decide because we want the energy to make a difference in our lives. We want to live longer in a healthy state because we want to play with our grandchildren. We voluntarily decide to make this change. We want to become good at it, and we want to share this change with, and be supported by, others.

This self-motivation is a powerful source of energy that is aligned with both our biology and our deep desire to survive, belong, connect, and make a difference. Recent studies show that those without a deep sense of meaning and purpose are more likely to get sick. When we look deep inside ourselves and align our desires with our values, we are much more likely to create sustainable results.

Throughout your journey we will come back to why you are doing what you are doing. It is a key determinant of your ability to make the changes and whether those changes will be transient or lead to the transformational power of the Habits of Health.

So, let's return to the question: why do you want to change? The answer might seem so obvious that we don't often think to ask the question or to properly consider the answer. If you're overweight, have poor health, feel tired, and lack energy, the obvious answer is that you want to change in order to solve those problems.

That's true of most changes we try to adopt—they're based on solving a problem or trying to get rid of an unwanted situation. This type of motivation almost never leads to lasting change.

Typically, you make some changes at first, but later you fall back into your old ways of behaving. Why? Because whenever you experience emotional conflict and feelings of negativity you want it to stop. Who wants to feel uncomfortable? You think about your health problems, and about how much you hate the way you look, and your natural response is to feel terrible. In order to end that discomfort, you take actions that make you feel better about yourself—maybe you go on a diet, get off the couch more and start exercising. But those actions aren't motivated by what you want and so they lead you into a predictable cycle:

1. *Emotional conflict leads you to act.*
2. *Because you've acted, you feel better—even if the situation hasn't changed much.*
3. *Feeling better takes the pressure off, thereby lessening the emotional conflict.*
4. *Less emotional conflict means there's less reason to continue doing the things that reduced the conflict in the first place.*
5. *Since you feel better, you no longer feel a pressing need to follow through on your actions.*
6. *And the original behavior returns.*

Here's another way of looking at this cycle. Your bad feelings (intense emotional conflict) motivate you to take action, which reduces your emotional conflict:

Emotional Conflict

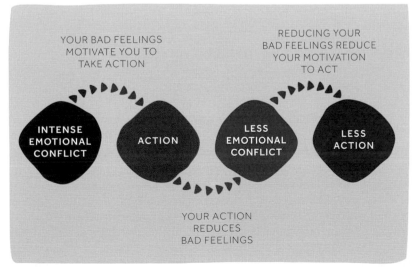

The right eating approach is vitally important, but it's just the first step. For long-term success you need the right motivation.

But once you experience the relief of less emotional conflict, your motivation to change weakens and you have less need to act. It's a typical yo-yo pattern. And the most natural thing in the world is to fall back into your previous habits: eating, smoking, or whatever it is you're trying to change. In fact, it's more than natural—it's inevitable. Here's a truth that's worth committing to memory:

Conflict-driven motivation is one of the major reasons people yo-yo. And what's reinforcing this pattern? Look at healthcare providers, warning patients about the ill-effects of eating the wrong foods, of not exercising, of smoking, or of not taking care of themselves in lots of ways. You leave their office ready to do anything to avoid the terrible things that could happen to you if you don't change your ways. Doctors mean well. But, unbeknownst to them, they're setting a yo-yo pattern in motion by using threat to force a change in their patients. Their intentions are good but their approach floats like a lead balloon.

Despite the fact that relying on self-control is nearly impossible and unlikely to lead to long-term success, most of us regularly use this sort of conflict manipulation to try to lose weight. It just doesn't work long term, especially if you're an "emotional eater" that's why we're going to change the way you motivate yourself and, in the process, create a fundamental new Habit of Health.

The more effective mindset is to think about what you gain by choosing health. Yes, you might want to lose weight, but really your desire runs much deeper than the numbers on a scale. What you really want is to be able to keep up with your children, enjoy a long hike, or gain a level of confidence that you might never have had. This is the more powerful way to think about your health. This is tapping into autonomous motivation in a deep and profound way.

Lasting motivation comes from focusing on what you want to gain and not what you want to lose.

PROBLEM SOLVING VS. DESIRED OUTCOME

Let's say you have two choices. You can:

1. *Think in terms of trying to fix your bad health (a problem orientation), or*
2. *Shift your focus to creating health (an outcome orientation)*

Most diet books fail to understand the difference between a problem-oriented motivation and an outcome-oriented motivation. The first is about solving a problem, like being unhealthily overweight; the second involves creating a desired state, like being optimally healthy. In the first, you're motivated to take action to get rid of a problem; in the second, you're motivated to take action to bring what you truly want into being.

Changing our emphasis from what we're against to what we're for has a dramatic impact. Are we merely against something, or do we want to create an important result? Let me be clear: I'm not talking about "positive thinking" but rather about the fundamental reason we act, with no spin on it, positive or otherwise.

Researchers regularly report the success of certain diets, all the while warning that the subjects on these "successful" diets couldn't sustain weight loss for more than two years on average.[1] And they always blame the diet itself for this long-term failing because they don't know any better. The one factor that's never named—and which is almost universally ignored—is that the dieter's motivation is usually a problem-solving, conflict-driven reaction to emotional anxiety.

You could adopt the healthiest diet that ever existed but if your motivation is to fix a health problem, you'll be back to your old tricks in two years (or less) with your weight back on and in worse shape than ever. No wonder so many people feel helpless after trying time and time again to lose weight. They don't know why they can't pull it off. They're sincere about wanting to lose weight and they know the stakes are high.

As you'll learn in Phase I, choosing the right way to eat is one of the most critical factors in creating health. But how do you go about making this new approach a true transformational lifestyle change? As vital as the right approach to eating may be, that alone isn't going to do it. And that's why reaching your healthy weight is only the beginning of our journey. The motivation factor is what makes all the difference between yo-yoing weight loss and creating optimal health by adopting healthy habits you can live with.

Think back to the last time you unsuccessfully tried to lose weight. Remember how easily you reverted to your old eating habits once the pressure to change diminished? It's not unusual for someone who's spent months losing weight to celebrate their accomplishment by running to the local burger joint.

Welcome to human nature! Soon enough you're back to where you were before, or worse. Study after study shows the negative impact of dieting once the diet's over. As you yo-yo from one diet to the next, you put yourself at higher risk for cardiovascular disease, more weight gain, and a myriad of other problems.

It's not your fault. You simply didn't know that your problem-solving motivation was your downfall all along.

A TEACHABLE MOMENT

So what do you do if you bought this book with problem solving in mind? Don't worry, you're not doomed! Your starting point is where you begin, not where you finish. You can recalibrate your motivation right now.

To figure out how to reach optimal health, we have to look at where we are. The space between these two points creates the tension that motivates us to change.

This is a teachable moment! And here's why it's possible:

1. **You're about to take a step forward.** *You've made the decision to begin losing weight. Even if that first step is a reaction to the emotional conflict you feel, at least you're committed to getting healthier. We just need to keep you going in the right direction on the path to optimal health.*

2. **You're open to allowing the change process to succeed.** *Until this moment, you didn't know how important motivation was, but now you can see the profound difference between avoiding bad stuff and supporting good stuff. With this new insight, you're able to make a major shift in your motivation and, as a result, dramatically improve your chances of success.*

3. **You truly want a positive outcome.** *Sure, there are problems you'd like to solve and future problems you want to avoid. But, even more, there's a life you want to build. Think of it this way: even if those problems disappeared tomorrow, you'd still want to have the life you desire, right?*

Imagine how your life will look once you've created optimal health for yourself. Optimal is the most desirable or favorable state possible. It's the perfect word for us. After all, we're all different. One person's optimal health might mean running a four-minute mile or breaking the record for weightlifting. For someone else, optimal might mean being able to play tennis or run a few miles every day. And for another it might mean they can play with their grandchildren and live a healthy, normal life.

Your optimal health profile—your personal best—is one of our most important goals but it is not the only one. It all begins by shifting your motivation from being against bad things to being in favor of good ones. This will align you with your values and what matters most to you on your journey to optimal health and wellbeing.

Structuring Your Success
Having goals is a good first step, but goals alone aren't enough. We need to position those goals within a structure that supports them. With the right structure, our chance of success goes up. With the wrong structure, our chance of success goes down.

We need to know our starting point. If our goal is optimal health, our starting point is our current state of health. This is because having a realistic picture of where we are now helps us to see the steps we need to take to get to where we want to be.

The Importance of Structural Tension
Over the last 15 years I have studied, lectured on his principles, and been a close personal colleague of Robert Fritz, best-selling author of *The Path of Least Resistance* and many other important works that have changed the way we understand human motivation and the structure of change. Robert is a dear friend and we collaborated for

many years to help people create meaningful change in their lives. We have recently co-authored a book, *Identity*, which we feel debunks the myths of the importance of self-esteem in the lifebuilding process.

Robert describes how the difference between our desired state and our actual state creates what he calls structural tension. It is as if we've stretched a bow and aimed the arrow. The tension in the bow makes reaching the target possible, and even probable. It's the type of tension that helps us take the actions we need in order to get the results we want.

In nature, all tension strives for resolution. So, by establishing structural tension, we've created a powerful dynamic to help us achieve our goal. It's as if nature herself is on our side, and we find ourselves capable of working on behalf of our goals.

Granted, our goals for optimal health aren't easy to accomplish. If they were, we'd have done it years ago. The fact that we've tried to reach these goals in the past and failed makes them even more daunting. However, with the right approach, within the right structure, we can change that pattern.

TRACKING YOUR PROGRESS

Where are you right now in relation to your goal? Remember, your current reality is constantly changing, so it needs to be regularly updated.

The actions you're taking right now have an impact you can measure to see if you are making effective progress. If one of your goals is to weigh 140 lbs, how much do you weigh now? Weigh yourself weekly to track your progress. If your goal is to fit into that tight pair of jeans, how close are you? Try them on every few days to find out.

You may have other health goals, each one with its own current status. Maybe it's blood pressure, cholesterol, or blood sugar, or a goal for increased energy and stamina, which can be measured by how far you can walk, jog, or swim. Each of these is one part of your optimal health picture, and each one should be tracked and updated as you manage the relationship between your actual situation and your desired goal.

We will take a look at your current and desired health and wellbeing in the next few parts and assess where you are in the key areas. Hopefully, you have started using *Your LifeBook* and are documenting and progressing through the Elements we are beginning to unpack.

BEING HONEST WITH YOURSELF

Honesty is crucial to achieving our goals. But what exactly do we mean by honesty?

mHoH

Be honest with yourself. Honesty is crucial to achieving our goals, so be clear on your goals and what you want to gain with your choices.

In the previous edition of this book, I wrote about how learning better ways to cope with emotional eating may be one of the most important factors in overcoming obesity and enjoying successful long-term weight loss. That thinking is supported by a study in the journal, *Obesity*.[2]

Researchers at the Miriam Hospital's Weight Control & Diabetes Research Center compared a group of overweight individuals who reported eating due to internal factors (like loneliness, self-comfort, or as a reward) to those motivated to eat by external factors (such as a party or holiday gathering). The "emotional" eaters lost less weight over time and experienced more weight regain.

New research published in *Neuron*[3] has found that we are all prone to emotional eating. Researchers observed the brains of participants when forced to choose between healthy and unhealthy foods. When the participants were subjected to stress, the part of the brain responsible for self-control began to "shut off", leading participants to value taste and gratification over health. Even though this study was small, the findings are not surprising.

Later in this book, you will learn how to overcome the challenge of emotional eating with mindfulness exercises. These help us to recognize the choices we make and eliminate the stressors that trigger our desire to give in to emotional eating in the first place.

One aspect of honesty is being clear about our goals—we shouldn't lie to ourselves about what we want. Another is separating what we want from what we think is possible—we need to describe our current reality both honestly and objectively.

Most of us aren't trained to be as honest with ourselves as we need to be. But being honest is an important Habit of Health. And like any new habit, it takes practice. The more you do it, the more it becomes part of who you are. This is one area where a coach can help you understand your current reality and develop new habits.

THE POWER OF CHOICE

Choice means it's your call—you can do it or not (whatever "it" is). Choice is the power to make a decision.

Now, if you just want one thing, making a choice is easy. But what happens when two things you want are in conflict with each other? Most of us never learn how to deal with this sort of conflict. In fact, most of the time we're not even aware that a conflict exists, but the reality is that we face situations like this all the time: you want optimal health and you also want to eat a banana split.

Those two desires are mutually exclusive. You can't have both. You need to make a choice. But how? The overall principle is this: make the choice that supports the more important desire. Of course, that means you need to sort out which desire is most important.

THREE TYPES OF CHOICES

There are three distinct types of choice: primary, secondary, and fundamental. I'll discuss primary and secondary choices here, and leave fundamental choice for the next part. Primary choice is something we want more than anything else.

When we think about optimal health and the vital habit category of healthy eating versus a banana split, the question is: what's more important to us? The benefits of a long and healthy life or the short-lived satisfaction of eating something that can harm our health? Of course, the prospect of a long and healthy life is a far better proposition. But when confronted by a banana split, we sometimes forget our larger goal and succumb to temptation. We're only human, but it's also human to become a bit savvier in distinguishing the things that support our health from the things that harm us.

Secondary choice concerns the actions or secondary habits we take to support our primary choice, even if we don't really want to do them. We're motivated to take these actions not because we like doing them but because we like the result they bring. Dorothy Parker said "I like having written." In other words, she didn't like the process of writing, but she was willing to do it in order to produce a piece that she liked.

Once we know what our primary choice is, it's easy to figure out how to make our secondary choices support our primary choice. If optimal health is our primary choice, what secondary choices do we need to make to support it? These choices fall into two categories:

1. *Doing some things we don't like doing*
2. *Not doing some things we like doing*

Many secondary choices aren't things we would normally choose to do. In fact, if it weren't for the primary choice, we wouldn't do them at all. And yes, this may include the habit of exercise. Some lucky people love to exercise. But many more people don't like to exercise but do it anyway. Why? To support their higher, more important goal of creating health. So they adopt an exercise program—a secondary choice that falls into the category of doing things we don't like doing, but do anyway to support a higher goal.

Now, that doesn't mean we can't try to find exercises that are as fun as possible or make healthy eating easy and enjoyable. In fact, making things easy and enjoyable increases our tendency to do them and supports our higher goals—in this case, optimal health. Making things easy and enjoyable is a big part of my plan for you, but we must never lie to ourselves about our motivation. The reason we're doing things we don't want to do is because it supports something we really want. The real power of choice is not in doing things that are easy and enjoyable but in doing things that are strategically critical to our goal.

That's important to keep in mind. We make secondary choices to support our goal, not because we particularly like the actions but because we like the outcome.

To support our goal of optimal health, we may find that we no longer choose to do certain things—smoking, eating the wrong foods, being a couch potato, and other Habits of Disease. If you use conflict to stop, the moment the pressure's off, you return to the unhealthy behavior. However, by understanding our primary choice and making strategic secondary choices, we discover a whole new ability to support ourselves.

So, what goes on in our heads when we're confronted by the need to make a secondary choice, such as eating a banana split. Here's the internal conversation:

"I like the look of that banana split."
"Yes."
"I could have it".
"That's right, you could."
"I want it."
"Yes, you do."
"But I also want to support my long-term goal of optimal health."
"Sure."
"I could eat the banana split or not."

"

Primary choice is about deciding that we want one thing—optimal health, for example—more than something else. Secondary choice is about taking the daily actions that support our primary choice— for example, choosing not to have a banana split.

"

1.3

To support our primary goal (optimal health), we do things we wouldn't otherwise do, like exercising or eating right. We may not always like doing these things, but we like where they take us.

"That's true."
"If I ate it, it would be harder to create my goal."
"That's true too."
"What do I want more: the banana split or optimal health?"
"Optimal Health."
"Therefore, while I could have the banana split, I choose not to have it to support my more important goal."
"That's right!"

And what goes on outside? Here's the external conversation:
"Would you like a banana split?"
"No thanks."

One thing's clear: you are very aware of what you're doing when you make these choices. And that's part of the power of primary and secondary choices. You're not doing things unconsciously. Quite the opposite. You're becoming much more tuned in to what you're thinking and doing. If you don't have that type of conversation with yourself when temptation rears its head, you'll eat the banana split and then regret it later when your senses return. Mindlessness is the enemy. And we will pay lots of attention to helping you make mindfulness a critical habit of health.

THE KEY TO DISCIPLINE

Throughout your life, you face situations that demand a choice. Even by not choosing, you've made a choice. But the choice not to choose usually isn't in your own best interests. Knowing how to determine what's primary—and, therefore, what's secondary—enables you to rise above any situation, however hard, to support your greater good.

It's in the relationship between the primary and secondary choice that the key to discipline is found. Once you know how to manage this relationship, you'll be able to accomplish more than you ever thought possible.

Now that you are both ready to change and know why you want to change, let's start laying out your future and setting in place the process to begin your journey

In the next part, we'll organize your life around Optimal Health and all of the rewards it brings.

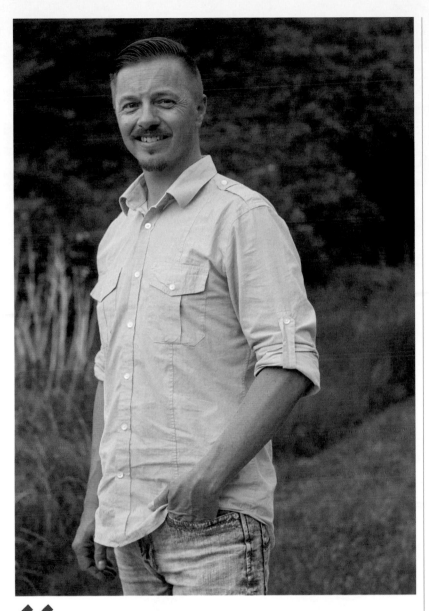

TRANSFORMATION:
ADAM ECHOLS

I watched my mom have a heart attack at 50 and inside I was thinking, well, what's going to happen to me when I'm 50?

Getting myself healthy allowed me the opportunity to actually go out there and be physically fit and be able to be with my kids. I take them on hiking trips. We go backpacking. We go swimming. I'll tell you what: before the program, for many, many years, I would go to the swimming pool and be that guy in the pool with his shirt on. I was embarrassed, seriously embarrassed and ashamed, that I had to wear a shirt into the pool.

Now I'm very comfortable going out and spending time out in the sun. It's an amazing thing to not have to worry about it at this point. The Habits of Health have really given me long-term health, and it's actually helped me to again be the best dad that I can be.

> " I'm creating long-term health and it's actually helped me to again be the best dad that I can be. "

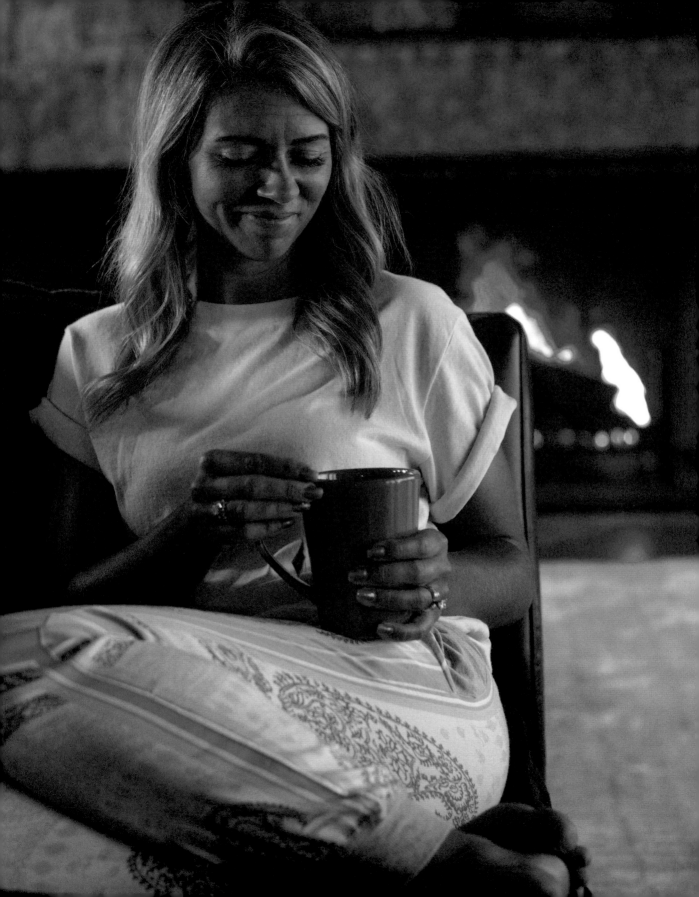

PART 1.4

HEALTH IS
ALL ABOUT
CHOICE

In the previous segment, we discussed the importance of being ready for change. If you've followed the book up until this part, I'm going to assume you're ready for change. Congratulations on making that decision. It will change everything.

If you need more information to help pull the trigger and begin, then this segment will break down the strategy we'll follow. It will also go over some of the tools we will use to help make that change simple, doable, and fun.

HOW TO TAKE CONTROL

We have talked about creating specific goals and making the primary choices, which are the big goals of transformational habit change. In addition, we laid out the actions we have to take to support those goals—our secondary choices. We will use the relationship between our primary and secondary choices to install the key Habits of Health as we move along the path to optimal health.

But there's another type of choice that's equally important: fundamental choice. Robert Fritz calls it "the choice upon which all other choices rest."[1]

FUNDAMENTAL CHOICE

Fundamental choice is what defines our state of being. It's where we stand. It's our choice to be free and healthy. It's what we're willing to fight for.

Let's start with an example. Let's say you try to quit smoking, but you've never really made the fundamental choice to be a non-smoker. Fundamental choice means choosing to make this change, not because your husband or wife or healthcare provider wants you to, but because you want to. Without making that fundamental choice, nothing will work, even if you follow methods that others have found successful. You'll soon be back to your two-pack-a-day habit. However, if you do make the fundamental choice to be a non-smoker, just about any method will work and you'll be attracted to the methods that work particularly well.

It's the same with any fundamental choice. Once you make the choice to be healthy, you've made it your business to act in accordance with your goal. You're taking full responsibility for your actions rather than letting circumstances drive your decisions. You become the author of your own life story. This is the whole idea behind *Your LifeBook,* which is to build the first year of your new story by bringing what is most important into your life in a truly authentic way.

One of the most important aspects of fundamental choice is that you have to accept that no one can do it for you. People can help with their advice, good wishes, medical insight, and understanding of human patterns and motivation. But it will always come down to you. If you're thinking, "I'll do my best, but it's really someone else's job to make it work", then you haven't made a fundamental choice.

Fundamental choice is also important because most of us have been raised to react to circumstances. We haven't been taught to believe that we can adopt a fundamental, self-generated resolve. But this is how we take charge of our lives—by realizing that no matter the circumstances, no matter the temptation, we can do what we know is right.

We know it because we've taken a stand for the choices we hold most important. This is what Deci et al. describe in their self-

"

Is anything in life more important than health? When people realize that they are dangerously ill, the answer to that question becomes clear.

"

determination theory, which is based on helping an individual reach their highest level of motivation, engagement, performance, persistence, and creativity.[2]

THE FUNDAMENTAL CHOICE OF OPTIMAL HEALTH AND WELLBEING

Today, whatever your circumstances may be, you can make a profound, fundamental choice for optimal health. Begin by asking yourself this question: "Do I want to be optimally healthy?" Most likely, the answer is yes. (Notice that I didn't ask you if you thought you could be optimally healthy. I asked whether if you could have it, would you take it!)

Let's think about it for a moment. Is there anything else in your life as important as Optimal Health? As you ponder that question, let me give you a little perspective.

As Director of Surgical Intensive Care at a large teaching hospital, the patients I managed would very likely have died without the interventional care they received. They had the benefit of every piece of next-generation medical technology, constant and invasive monitoring, potent intravenous medications, and sophisticated nutritional intervention.

These vulnerable patients came from all walks of life: some young, some old. But they all knew that at any moment they could die. They shared a universal realization that changed them in profound ways: at that moment, surviving and getting healthy was all that mattered. All of a sudden, optimal health became everything. It was more important to the millionaire than his portfolio. It was more important to the executive than his job promotion. It was more important to the teenager than his new car he'd just wrecked. Reality can be very enlightening.

In fact, health deserves to be right up there alongside freedom and the pursuit of happiness as one of our most prized possessions. It's certainly my most prized possession. I want to be healthy to go skiing with my girls. (Authors note: I started heli-skiing three years ago, age 63, which they have not done yet, in order to stay ahead of them!) I want to watch them graduate from college. I want to see them get married and my grandchildren go to school. I want to sail around the world and I want the world to be a healthy thriving place where everyone has the opportunity to determine their health and wellbeing. I want these things more than anything I own. And they're all possible, as long as I make optimal health my top priority— my fundamental choice.

I hope you have decided that optimal health is your fundamental choice. Once you've made that choice, you simply need to arrange your primary and secondary choices to make it happen. Sound simple? It really is.

Our task now is to:
- Review the foundational categories that support optimal health and wellbeing: our MacroHabits.
- Understand the roles of primary choices as core Habits of Health in each category.
- Understand the role of secondary choices (the steps that will inform and support those primary habit goals).
- Use our knowledge of choices to understand and begin to build skills and self-efficacy through the process of habit formation.

By making these actions and creating new choices as part of your daily life, you'll begin to embody Dr. A's Habits of Health.

Foundational Categories for Optimal Health: MacroHabits of Health
Now that you've made health your fundamental choice, we can work on achieving your goals. I'll be your guide, but it's up to you to actually do the work to create optimal health. We will start by focusing on the primary areas that will support your fundamental choice.

Optimal health and wellbeing are built on a foundation of behaviors that together create a lifestyle that restores your body and mind, as well as optimizes its ability to function. The basic components of a healthy lifestyle—what I describe as the foundations of health—are the MacroHabits outlined below:

MacroHabits of Health: The Foundations of Optimal Health and Wellbeing Categories
- Habits of Healthy Weight Management
- Habits of Healthy Eating and Hydration
- Habits of Healthy Motion
- Habits of Healthy Sleep (Including Energy Management)
- Habit of Healthy Mind (including Habits of Emotional and Personal Mastery)
- Habits of Healthy Surroundings (people, places, and things, including Habits of Healthy Environment, Support, Relationships, and Community)

When integrated, these are the major areas of focus that determine, deliver, and sustain the fundamental choice of optimal health and wellbeing. Their installation requires a series of primary choices, or Habits of Health, which create optimization in a specific major area of behavior that is a determinant of our health and life. You may already recognize and even practice some of these, such as having a healthy weight or living an active lifestyle, but our approach will help you solidify them. In addition, when all of these critical components come together in an integrated way it will help you generate and energize a lifelong transformation.

We will approach each category in detail throughout the book; however they do share common characteristics:

- Deep work in both installation and focus
- Usually approached one at a time
- Require selective discipline for installation
- Assess readiness and motivation in each category
- Create a Halo Effect and have an overall influence on physical and mental health
- Specifically engage brain-mind-relationship health to create lasting transformation

In the previous segment, we looked at health in a new way. Rather than thinking of issues, such as your weight or your blood pressure as problems to solve, I outlined the importance of thinking about what you really want out of life—the things you stand to gain through optimal health. I also showed you how to use this new motivation to adopt behaviors that support your health goals. Those behaviors are the Habits of Health.

This system is all about creating lasting, radiant health. It starts with an assessment of your current state of health and wellbeing, which are the direct result of your past and present habits. In order to transform your health and life, it's essential you understand where you are now in these foundational MacroHabits because it creates a baseline and helps identify which area you are most interested in changing first. You can take the Habits of Health assessment on line at HabitsofHealth.com at anytime to evaluate your current reality in terms of your MacroHabits.

ENVISIONING OPTIMAL HEALTH AND WELLBEING IN A MACROHABIT

In order to prepare you for the process of change, we are going to tap into the creative process. It is a powerful force for moving you from where you are now to where you want to go in your health and your life. We will use the structural dynamics described in the last part to initiate our strategy, tactics, action, and support to reach our desired outcome.

As we address each of the MacroHabits categories in this book we will discover several primary choices or Habits of Health that will transform our health and wellbeing in each category. Many of those will have an impact in multiple areas of your health and wellbeing.

I realize that at this point you may not know which Habits of Health support your journey. That's OK—it's my job to help teach you how to adopt the powerful Habits of Health that will help you do just that. In order to demonstrate how the creative process can structure your journey let's use a real life example. Most of us struggle a bit when it comes to our weight; so let's pick one of the primary Habits of Health in the MacroHabit of Healthy Weight Management category.

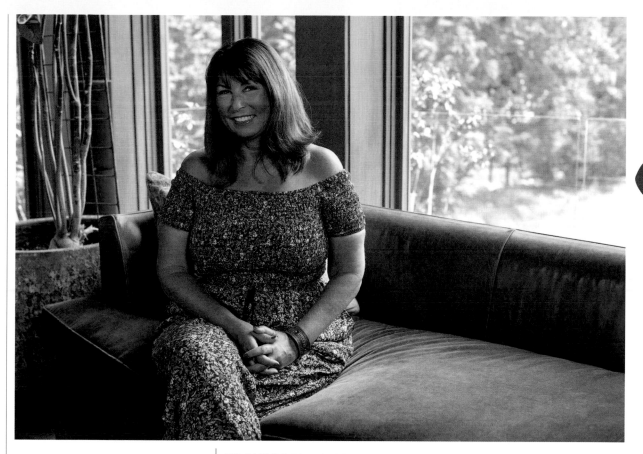

TRANSFORMATION: TERRI MILLER

> "
> *I became more awakened to actually be the person that was making the decisions about my health.*
> "

I was introduced to the Habits of Health just before I turned 40. I had tried a multitude of different types of programs to lose weight. I'm pretty hypoglycemic, so every time I tried something, I didn't feel well. It was pretty devastating when I wasn't successful, and I would beat myself up for failing and then use food to soothe myself.

The reason that utilizing this program with the Habits of Health worked is because I was able to learn reasons why I was choosing food to solve things. Stop. Challenge. Choose.™ was my favorite because it gave me the ability to be in control of my choices and empower myself. Even if I didn't necessarily make a good choice, I knew it was a choice I had made.

I was trying to get off some medications and lose weight. I started to actually envision what I was moving towards, and it was very interesting. It gave me a whole new sense of energy.

I realized I could sleep better. I could go on vacation with my teenage boys and actually be engaged with them, swimming and feeling comfortable publicly with them. I even forgot where I had come from. It was more about what I wanted to create.

Desired Outcome: To Reach a Healthy Weight and Waist Circumference

If this applies to you, take out a blank piece of paper or open *Your Lifebook* to Element 03, *How Do You Create What You Want?*, and write down what it would look like to be at your own optimal weight. Since we're all at different stages of health, it will look different for each of us. That's fine.

Describing Your Current Health Reality

Take a moment to write down where you think you are currently in terms of your actual weight and waist circumference. Be objective. You can use the ruler in Element 02 in *Your LifeBook, Knowing What You Want to Accomplish,* to give you more specific guidance, or you can simply reflect on where you see yourself today. In this case, I am 195 lbs and have a waist circumference of 35 inches.

Creating a Structural Tension Chart

A simple structural tension chart for each of the foundational components can be an important tool to help you progress. These charts aren't difficult to make, and they give you a direct, visual way to compare your current reality to your desired goals. As we learned in Part 1.3, *Are You Really Ready to Change?*, the relationship between where you are now and where you want to be creates a dynamic tension that serves as a powerful motivator.

As you go through the book and we address your health one MacroHabit category at a time, you'll have a better sense of your current health reality and will be able to create a more refined structural tension chart for each goal that emerges on your journey. Right now, using the current example, your first goal may be to reach a healthy weight, and you'll soon have a precise idea of your current healthy weight, body mass index (BMI), and waist circumference.

Find magazine pictures that represent radiant health and put them up on your walls to remind you of your goals.

Structural Tension: Three Months to Reaching a Healthy Weight

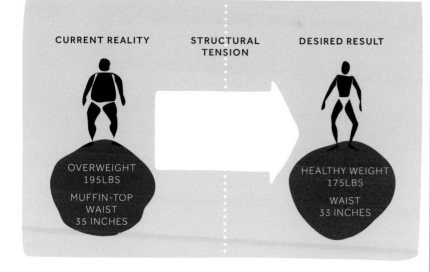

CURRENT REALITY	STRUCTURAL TENSION	DESIRED RESULT

OVERWEIGHT 195LBS
MUFFIN-TOP WAIST 35 INCHES

HEALTHY WEIGHT 175LBS
WAIST 33 INCHES

> *"Make a list of the reasons you started your journey to optimal health and remember to pull it out when you need a little positive reinforcement!"*

Now that you have a list of the foundational MacroHabits for optimal health and a framework for creating goals, it will be much easier to map out your future. We will use structural tension in every habit setting exercise to set your direction towards each new habit. We will focus on what you're creating. Remember, this isn't "positive thinking", but a matter of writing and visualizing where you're going, thereby creating the magical tension that needs resolution.

As you move forward, your current reality will change. You can use these charts as a road map to help you understand where you are in relation to your goal at any point and to give you important feedback on your progress. Along the way, you will discover, learn, invent, and install daily activities to move you to your desired outcome.

SECONDARY HEALTH CHOICES: DAILY CHOICES AND SMALL DISCIPLINES

Secondary choices—the action steps that support your primary choices—are the day-to-day behaviors that build your path to optimal health. They're not always fun, and we wouldn't necessarily choose to do these things if they weren't organized into our hierarchy of choice to support our higher goal.

Let's say you decided to become a world-class violinist. What would you do every day? You'd practice, of course. Even if you came home from work tired and would rather grab a drink and kick off your shoes, you'd make the secondary choice to practice because it supports your primary choice—your goal of becoming a world-class violinist.

Make no mistake, spending long hours practicing the violin isn't easy. But maybe it's a little easier when we know that we're supporting a goal we really want. And maybe that also applies to a 30-minute walk, a healthy low-glycemic dinner, and going to bed at 10:00 p.m. instead of watching The Late, Late Show. Being a great violinist is a lofty primary choice, but it pales in comparison to your choice of optimal health.

Get started by pinpointing those secondary choices: your Habits of Health. You'll be learning step-by-step in the next few parts and then practicing for life.

Identifying Your Secondary Choices

How do we determine whether our actions are likely to move us toward our goal? Here's a checklist of questions to ask yourself. Let's examine them in the context of the sample structural tension chart below with our goal of a healthy weight and waist circumference in three months.

1. If you take these steps, will you achieve primary goal? For example, "If I eat healthy once a week, will I reach my three-month goal of a healthy weight and waist circumference?"
2. Are your action steps accurate, brief, and concise? Picture the action step and then write it down in a couple of sentences— for example, "I will learn and use portion control by either prepackaged fuelings or Dr. A's Plate system."
3. Does every action step have a due date? For example, "I will eat one lean and green meal everyday."

Structural Tension Chart Choices

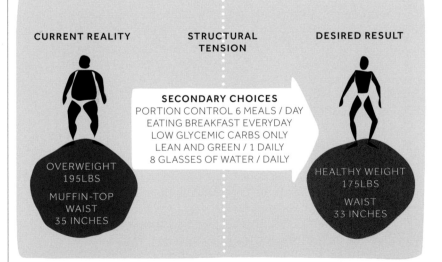

CURRENT REALITY · STRUCTURAL TENSION · DESIRED RESULT

SECONDARY CHOICES
PORTION CONTROL 6 MEALS / DAY
EATING BREAKFAST EVERYDAY
LOW GLYCEMIC CARBS ONLY
LEAN AND GREEN / 1 DAILY
8 GLASSES OF WATER / DAILY

OVERWEIGHT
195LBS

MUFFIN-TOP
WAIST
35 INCHES

HEALTHY WEIGHT
175LBS

WAIST
33 INCHES

These secondary choices—daily, mundane activities—might seem insignificant in and of themselves. They might seem easy or not. It does seem that most people are living in a world of impulse, with no regard to the effect their choices have over time. Well, time is the great equalizer. It's either on your side, helping you build and maintain a thriving, vibrant life, or it's slowly but insidiously draining your overall health, stamina, and resilience against disease.

People fail to understand that today's cheeseburger won't make a difference. Neither will substituting a salad. And that's part of the problem.

We live in a society that's focused on instant results. Flip a switch and we're online, talking to people on the other side of the world. That same mentality is what makes us believe that medicines will make us healthy or reduce our fat. The truth is that the process of creating health takes time in the real world.

After taking your action steps day in and day out, you'll begin to enjoy optimal health, and through feedback you'll know that your real work is already done. You'll have taken control of your daily choices and beaten the negative consequences of our modern lifestyle. It's the same lifestyle that causes the "widowmaker" (a lesion named for its ability to cause instant death by blocking the blood flow to the heart). When a conference I attended showed an angiogram of just this kind of lesion, the hall gasped when it was revealed the lesion was in the body of a 17 year-old boy.

It doesn't have to be this way. And it's never too late to start, but it's all up to you. Our small almost insignificant daily choices are the underlying power of the *Habits of Health Transformational System*.

We are going to change the trajectory of your health and those around you by your actions, and over time your actions will become your ally.

Daily Choices Chart to Optimal Health or to Disease

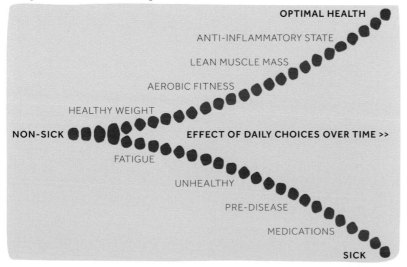

Life of Optimal Health Arrow Chart

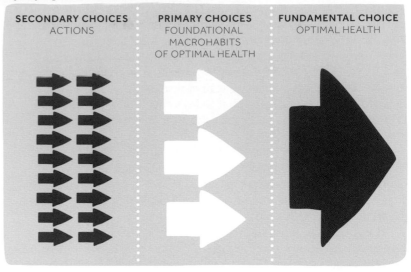

In order to have a more precise idea of your starting point in your current health assessment, log in to HabitsofHealth.com to take a health evaluation that will define your exact location on your health path in much the same way that a GPS device helps you plot the most efficient path to your destination. Exploring current behaviors in your MacroHabits that affect your health—how you react to stress, how you spend your leisure time, and even behaviors you may have ignored or considered unimportant—is an important step in putting you in charge of your own life's journey.

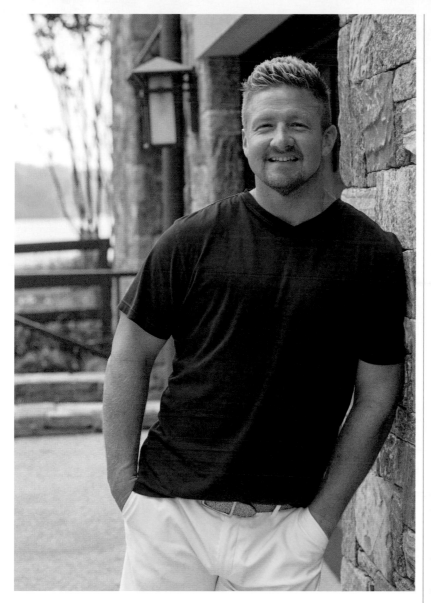

TRANSFORMATION: DOUG WOOD

I was not born in a healthy household. I thought the only way to lose the weight was through exercise. The problem was that it wasn't working. Even though I was gaining muscle, my waistline seemed to be growing, and the frustration began to build.

After trying countless diets, I reached a point to where I thought I was cursed: I was always going to have fat genes, and nothing was ever going to change.

One of the microHabits that has been so important to me was healthy motion and exercise. I thought that health meant I needed to be skinny, but it's actually building health and fitness, and that has been the biggest difference that the Habits of Health have made to my life.

One of the key things that has helped me thrive in my health over the last eight years is being a part of a healthy community and really changing my surroundings. Something the Habits of Health taught me was really to reintroduce a whole new set of habits, which can sometimes include our peer group and the places that we go. I knew that if I wanted to stay healthy, I needed to be around people who value their health as well.

"
After trying countless diets, I reached a point where I thought I was cursed.
"

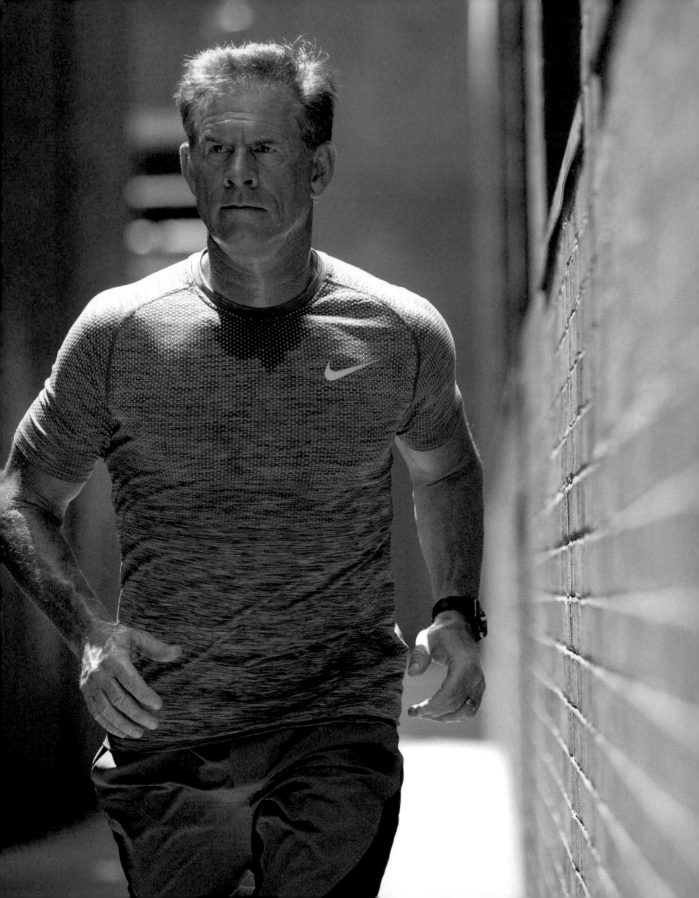

THE BEDROCK OF TRANSFORMATION: SUCCESSFUL HABIT INSTALLATION

Have you ever made the decision to start doing something differently or to put a new habit in your life? And when you did it, did you make a commitment to yourself that this time you're going to stick to it? Yet, a week later you realize that you are no longer doing it at all? You're not alone. I've done it myself many times in the past.

It begs the question, why is it so hard to stick to our goals and form good habits? Simpler still, why is change so hard to achieve? In reading this book, you may have thought that you really want to be healthier and improve your overall life, yet it seems so hard to make any progress.

All I can do is say it again: It depends on you.

I'm putting it all back on you because the most important piece in actually creating the sustainable transformation of your weight, health, and wellbeing is the development of your own ability to take ownership of your choices.

This capability comes from your mastering the ability to create a series of small sustainable changes in your daily choices that will, over time, create long-term change. These are the small daily habits that we'll talk about in this part.

17th century poet, John Dryden describes how powerful habits are in determining our life:

"We first make our habits, then our habits make us."

Modern-day neuroscience supports Dryden's 300-year-old observation. Our brain processes over 10 million bits of information each second and yet, of these, only 50 bits are developed at a conscious level.[1] We are, for good or ill, biological machines, and our interaction with the world works best when we keep things simple. It leaves less room for chance, mistakes, or a breakdown. We are operating on automatic almost all the time.

10,000 years ago, automatic behaviour was imperative to our survival. Without it our voluntary behaviors could have resulted in injury or death.

Today automatic behavior leads us down pathways that are not in our best interest. These behaviors are really out of place in this far more complex world. Without the conscious programming, which I will help you begin, you will find yourself out of sync with modern conditions and you'll be on a trajectory toward the Habits of Disease. Unfortunately, if you are not taking responsibility and reprogramming your choices and habits, your brain will do it for you, under the influence of a range of forces from technology to the company we keep. And you won't even know it.

If this seems far-fetched, let me share some disturbing facts. Almost 79% of all smartphone users check their devices within 15 minutes of waking up.[2] A 2011 study suggested that people check their phones 34 times a day on average.[3] However, industry insiders believe that this number is actually much closer to a whopping 150 checks from morning to night.[4]

Technology's unimpeded advancement might well drive us to extinction, much like climate change finished the dinosaurs. This is happening alongside the catastrophic epidemic of obesity and the increase in diabetes: two significant human events that have been propagated by energy dense food, a progressively more sedentary lifestyle, and a psychological impact that results in isolation and stress.

Initially, I hadn't even considered technology's role as part of the broader problem, but it is short-circuiting even our most fundamental behaviors (I read in a recent survey that a full third of Americans say they would rather give up sex than lose their cell phones).[5]

Now that I have your attention, let's unpack how we are going to eliminate the hidden forces that negatively affect your health and life and start the process of putting you in charge. I need to help you use the power of habits to create the life you want versus accepting that your life is what everybody else wants for you.

We will start with understanding how habits are formed, how they operate, and how you can be a professional-level habit installer. I'll also show you how to adjust the ones that need tweaking and eliminate the effects of those that are not in your best interest.

Vince Lombardi, one of the greatest American football coaches, believed in starting from the beginning. At the start of a new season, he gathered his team, held a pigskin in his right hand and said: "Gentlemen, this is a football." He started from scratch. And so will we.

We need to leave nothing to chance as you develop one of the most important tools and determinants of your life.

WHAT IS A HABIT?

Merriam-Webster's online dictionary defines habit as:

1. *an acquired mode of behavior that has become nearly or completely involuntary*
2. *a behavior pattern acquired by frequent repetition or physiologic exposure that shows itself in regularity or increased facility of performance*

In psychology, the definition goes a little deeper. A habit can be thought of as a link between a stimulus and a response. It serves as a mental connection between a trigger thought or event (stimulus) and our response to that trigger (the response). Repeating this connection time and again forms a habit and affects all subsequent decisions and actions. If repeated often enough, this connection becomes near permanent unless we take conscious action to change it.

Work in neurophysiology coming out of MIT in the late 90s revealed the underlying structure of habits and broadened our understanding of how they are formed. The work also offered clues as to how they run our lives. "We all live mostly by habit," said Ann M. Graybiel, Rosenblith Professor of Neuroscience at MIT. Habits and automatic learned responses such as those used in driving and bike riding, may serve to free up the "thinking" parts of the brain for more creative purposes.

Graybiel began exploring and expanding the idea of habit loops, as these seemed to be the key to habit formation. A region deep in the brain called the basal ganglia was identified as the region responsible for building the automated behaviors that became known as habit loops.

Charles Duhigg popularized the idea of habit loops with a visual diagram to show how habits are formed. The basic habit loop has three parts.

Cue Routine Reward Loop

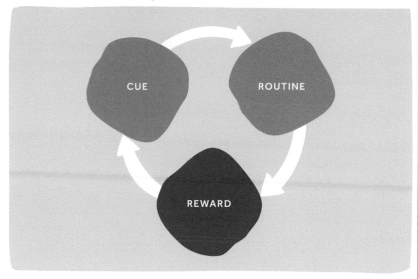

First, there is a stimulus called the *cue*. This tells your brain to select a certain previously developed behavior and then activate an automatic sequence of actions. It's like scrolling through your playlist and clicking the song you want to play from a selection you downloaded to your smartphone.

Second, there is an action or *routine* that can be physical, mental, or emotional. This is activated by the cue and is the behavior or *routine*. This is the behavior or habit that can, over time, become automated.

And finally, there is a *reward*—a benefit that reinforces why the behavior or routine should be repeated in the future. Since most of us own a smartphone, let's use texting as an example of how a simple habit loop is created and then perpetuated. You receive a push notification through a visual, auditory, or vibratory cue or trigger. Your action or routine is to open the text and read its contents.

Your reward is to have your curiosity satisfied, to benefit from information, or feel social acceptance. You are now cued to respond to the same event next time and so you repeat the loop. The first text you received required your attention to open and respond to it, but I imagine that now you do it without even thinking about it. It has become a habituated behavior.

This man-made habit loop is already deeply embedded across millions of people. It has become so highly addictive that we have lost a proper sense of what is important. Families no longer talk at dinner, friends no longer have focused uninterrupted conversations, and the need to respond is creating almost total disregard for the very real risks that come from distraction at the wheel of a car.

The good news is we're going to use this loop for your benefit in installing the Habits of Health. We will use a system that makes installing your new Habits of Health predictable, easy, and so empowering. Much of what we will discuss over the pages ahead has only become fully understood and validated in the last decade with the help of neuroscience, interpersonal neurobiology, group and individual coaching, and lots of observational experience.

The *Habits of Health Transformational System* takes the fundamentals of that knowledge and blends it with the experience I have had in directly transforming thousands of lives over the last decade.

The key to your success is dependent on learning and using the Habits of Health installation system and systematically staying on the path to optimal health and wellbeing. At the core of our system is the very basic behavior of selecting your desired habit and consistently using that new healthy behavior until it is fully automated.

NUDGING THE EQUILIBRIUM OF YOUR LIFE

Your body, mind, and surroundings are in a state of equilibrium based on the life you have created for yourself. It may have happened by chance, but you have also been involved by making choices that have set the current behaviors that guide your life. What you are currently eating, when and how you are moving, the time and quality of your sleep, how you are acting and perform at work and play, your patterns of socializing, and even the way you think are all set in a pattern and driven by routine.

When you go to change a routine, you are disrupting one or more of these forces, and when that occurs the forces of habit will always want to pull you back into equilibrium. In order to create transformation, rather than just temporary change, we will use the only sustainable mechanism for change to build a series of Habits of Health. We are going to make it really easy.

HOW LONG WILL IT TAKE TO INSTALL A HABIT OF HEALTH?

You may have read that it takes an average of 21 days to install a new habit.[6] That number came from a book written by a surgeon who observed that after a limb amputation it would take approximately 21 days to adjust to the change.

That's certainly interesting, but it hardly applies to what we are about to do. The science of change has advanced significantly in the past couple of decades and work coming out of University College London shed light on the variability of habit installation. It was suggested that the time necessary for installation depends on the complexity of the desired behavior. Something as simple as drinking an additional glass of water may take as little as 18 days to install while something as complex as interval training for a marathon may take several months. The research concluded that most habits can be installed on average in 66 days.[7]

Additional research on time to habit installation has shown that ability, motivation, and environment are all variables that can affect how long it takes to learn a new habit.

Each individual Habit of Health will take effort to start and become a routine, but the investment will pay off because you will only need to do it once for each habit installation.

Using an illustration, we can visualize the relationship between the time and effort required for habit installation. In the beginning, it takes some self-discipline and time before the habit goes from being hard and requiring focus and attention to the point where it becomes easier and eventually automatic. Once you reach this point, it becomes much easier to perform the habit. Once the brain has been rewired, your new synaptic connections will endure with almost no attention. They will continue to fire up on a daily basis. This is where your equilibrium starts to shift you toward a healthier state.

In addition, each new Habit of Health installation makes it easier to install the next. Known as the Halo Effect, each new learned behavior builds momentum as your brain and mind start growing and expanding, moving out of mindless thinking and instead awakening the desire, capacity, and ability to create what it is focusing on: the creation of better health which, in the process, creates a healthier, more responsive brain, mind, and body.

Time to Habit Installation: Steep and Hard then Flat and Easy

HABIT INSTALLED:
AVG. 66 DAYS

HARDER AND AWARE   TIME   EASIER AND AUTO (HOH)

Others have described three psychological phases of the ritual of habit installation for more difficult habits that are counter to our natural tendency. This thinking addresses the mental and emotional challenge of disrupting an established routine but I think it has some merit in summing up the amount of discipline you will need to move through the installation.

Phase I: *First third, you want to quit.*
Phase II: *Second third, you are adjusting and it is becoming easier.*
Phase III: *Last part, you are really getting it and it is becoming progressively easier.*

The takeaway message is that you will sense the transition when the habit moves from requiring all of your attention and feels uncomfortable to the moment when you sense you are on the downhill leg and the behavior comes automatically with little effort and no conscious thought. As my grandfather always said, "When you face a challenge, this too will pass."

Having walked through some of the more fundamental thinking on habits and changing routines, let's explore a few ways to make the task easier and reduce the effort it takes to perform it.

THE ROLE OF MOTIVATION AND ABILITY IN HABIT INSTALLATION

We have a tendency to be overly ambitious when we decide to make a change in our behavior. Watching endless TV from the couch on New Year's Day, feeling full, unhealthy, and desperate to do something to overcome the malaise, you rise unsteadily to your feet and declare that you're going to start running every day.

The next day, motivated to make it all better, you dust off your running shoes and leave your couch for the first time in years. You are so fired up that you start down the street and run almost a mile before your body screams out in revolt to stop this nonsense.

You head home satisfied that this is going to be harder than you thought but you congratulate yourself and feel certain that you are on your way.

The next morning you can barely get out of bed, much less walk to put on your running gear because you've now got shin splints. You call in sick for work and your running days are put on hold. Indefinitely.

This may be an exaggerated scenario, but it serves to dramatize that our ambition to change is almost universally foiled by our tendency to bite off more than we can chew. Since the key to habit formation is doing the action or routine consistently over time until it is automatic, our key to installing the Habits of Health will take a very different approach. Our strategy is to make the action simple enough that you have the ability to do it every day.

It really comes down to the dance between how much do you want to do it today and whether you are able to do it today!

Let's unpack that in more detail. In Part 1.3, *Are You Really Ready To Change?*, we emphasized the importance of intrinsic motivation. It defines your level of desire to take action. In order to create long-term success, you will want to be very clear on your most important values and aspirations and your voluntary desire to start and act. We discussed the importance of being ready to change and then picking the correct primary habits you want to change. This informs you of the necessary secondary choices and action steps you will need to begin installation.

These secondary choices or habits are our focus for installation.

We will need to set each of these new Habits of Health into our habit loop and stay the course until they become fully automated.

We also need to narrow our focus from an overall desire to improve your health and wellbeing to a more immediate need: how you will manage each day. We need to make sure you are building in the daily consistency and methodically installing small choices that are building the categories and strengthening your mastery of the *Habits of Health Transformational System*.

When we start installing your new Habit of Health you will need to answer three questions as you begin the step by step journey of transformation.

1. *Is it appealing? Do I want to do it?*
2. *Is it achievable? Can I actually do it?*
3. *Is it easily activated? Is there a prompt that reminds me to do it?*

Let's address each one of these questions.

Appealing: *This is your level of motivation or your desire to take action in the moment. In essence, this asks the question "Do I have a desire to do it?" We know from Part 1.3, Are You Really Ready To Change?, that you have to want the outcome in order to be successful at achieving it. Although we make our secondary choices or habits whether we want to do them or not (because they support what is most important), it is always better to pick actions that are more appealing to us. We will also need to develop habits which we would rather not do which is why we need to look elsewhere to ensure that the daily action and consistency for installation occurs without fail.*

Achievable: *This is your ability to do the action every day, which is the basic building block of the Habits of Health Transformational System. I introduced microHabits of Health (mHoH) a few years ago as a key tool to lower the threshold for daily installation in order to increase the consistency of daily action. My idea was to lower the threshold so that even on days when motivation or desire to do the action was low you would still have done it and*

When it come to the daily installation of these new Habits of Health, we can learn from the marketers and internet gurus who work in the industry of persuasion and manipulation for product adaptation and usage. They have gathered a tremendous amount of data on how to lower the threshold and facilitate people repeating certain behaviors. We will use some of this data in our designs for your habit installation.

The Role of Self-Efficacy

There are plenty of people who talk about self-efficacy as if it is about your attitude, believing in yourself, building self-esteem and believing you can do it. I regard that as a form of harmful self-manipulation.

You will likely have heard it so many times: "If I think I can do it then I can do it and if I think I can't do it I can't." The truth is you don't know if you can do it until you actually do it.

This is why we are focusing on what you want to create and then help you to do it. There is no need to manipulate yourself—you just need to to be based in the truth and do all of this from your current reality.

And since we will make the microHabit so small you will do it everyday. And as you get better over time as you progress and do a little more most days which over time becomes a lot more and build your self-efficacy and eventually install a solid new habit.

avoided breaking your chain of daily habit installation.

A microHabit of Health is by definition easy to do and always within your ability in terms of ease and with an understanding of other limiting factors such as time constraints. It ensures that you will always be able to carry out the habit. Imagine if, by definition, the secondary Habits of Health you pick are such small actions that even on the days when it seems your willpower, discipline, and motivation are almost zero, you will be unstoppable. On the days when your motivation is higher, you'll do more. We set a base level of effort that is so easy and simple, the daily repetition necessary for installation is never in question. You can always do it. It is this consistency and predictability that creates the new behavior.

Activation: Do you have a reminder to prompt and activate your new routine? Until the habit is engrained and becomes a habitual part of your daily schedule you will need reminders. This is the cue in the habit loop structure of habit installation. The nice thing is there are several cues both in your daily surroundings and in your mind that we can latch onto or create to start installing your new habit loop. Eventually, as your new Habit of Health is automatized it will fit into the family of other Habits of Health. In time, these cues will fill in the spaces of existing routines and lead you to more optimal days as your reprogramming takes hold.

We designed the *Habits of Health Transformational System* based on the essential ingredients for predictable habit installation, namely the ability to consistently repeat the habit until it becomes automated. In new habit formation we really need to lower the resistance to activating the behavior, which is why our system relies on microHabits and gradual, sustainable change.

We lower the threshold to initiate and complete the daily habit loop (secondary choice) so that we can effectively install your new Habit of Health. And you won't miss days because we have made it so easy there is no longer a reason not to do it.

This will make you impervious to whatever life throws at you, thereby creating a new level of self-efficacy that will help facilitate success.

And we know that success breeds success.

MOTIVATION VS. ABILITY

Our intrinsic motivation is important in guiding our current choices to support our future desired outcomes. We have to want to get healthier and have a better life in order to set our goals and direction. It is the day-to-day system of habit installation that makes that transformation become a reality.

If we're honest with each other, you know your motivation level is not at a high level every moment of every day. Your willpower is affected by stress, emotional state, internal dialogue, bad day (life happens), lack of sleep, and even hypoglycemia. These all affect the reliable drivers needed for consistent repetition to install a new healthy habit.

The following illustration shows the variability of our daily motivation and how it can easily fall below the level needed to activate the desired behavior.

The bars show that for every behavior there needs to be a relationship between ability and level of motivation for the behavior to be activated. The only thing that needs to be added is a prompt, cue, or trigger that activates the behavior. That activation prompt is your reminder to start the new routine that you have designed to be able to do on a daily basis without fail given your current level of motivation.

Varying Daily Motivation

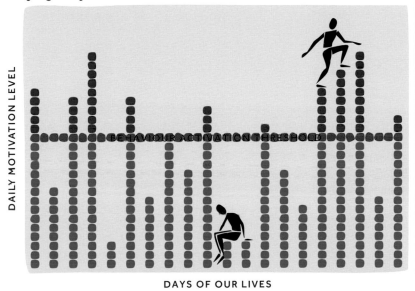

The yellow line is the activation line or the level of motivation that it takes to make sure you do a certain new habit that day. The green dots represent the days you had adequate level of motivation to do the new healthy behavior.

The next illustration shows the situation around an unsuccessful habit installation where the level of motivation, which started out as adequate in the excitement of starting something new fell back as the day to day experience of being human knocked us off our path. Falling below the activation level on progressive days inevitably impacts the consistent repetition required to rewire and engrain the new behavior.

"Think about how easy it is to bite your nails and you can understand that once such a habit is formed, how hard it is to break—you pretty much always have the access and the ability to bite your nails!"

1.5

Daily Habit Installation: Difficult Habit

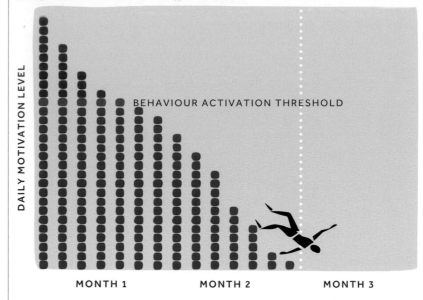

When your motivation is lower than the ability to perform the habit, you won't do it!

The microHabit approach of our system does not rely on your level of motivation but rather on the ease of daily action so that you can be above the activation line every day. Although the motivation level still fluctuates, it is always enough to perform the microHabit action because it is so easy. This is how predictable transformation becomes a reality.

Remember, in order for a new behavior or habit to be installed daily it requires three things. First, there must be enough motivation to have the energy to do the action everyday so it can be consistently installed. Second, it must be easy enough to do on the days when motivation levels are low. And third, there must be a cue or reminder to initiate the new action or behavior.

Habit Installation: microHabit—Making the Behavior Easy to Do Even When Your Motivation is Very Low!

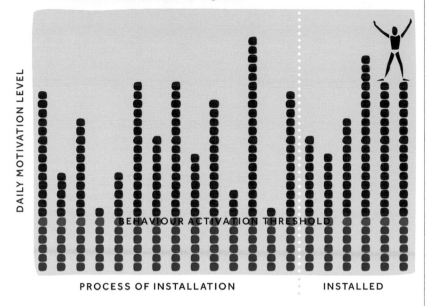

DAILY MOTIVATION LEVEL

BEHAVIOUR ACTIVATION THRESHOLD)

PROCESS OF INSTALLATION   INSTALLED

GENERATIVE INSTALLATION

The Habits of Health installation and your progressive success will help raise your motivational energy and focus, but we are not going to take any chances. Your health is too important for that. We will rely on the key influencer of consistent installation.

This is where the microHabits take each desired habit and decrease its complexity into a small but totally doable daily action which fits into a repeated loop. In the following illustration, you can see we've taken the habit outlined in red and moved it over by making it so consistently easy to do that it is now above the activation line and can be done every day, despite a relatively low motivation level.

The habit loop is activated when there is enough motivation, the ability to do the microHabit, and the cue all present at the same time.

You can see as you repeat and engrain the new habit it increases both your ability and your motivation. And your self–efficacy improves, not based on the imposed ideas of a self-help book, but on the reality of your own achievement.

And I can tell you that this realisation is a very significant moment.

The horizontal axis on the following diagram shows that if something is harder to do it requires a higher level of motivation to create the conditions that will allow the activation of the routine. There is a point where despite very high motivation we are not able to initiate the behavior. For example, if you were motivated to do a marathon, you still could not run one right now because your physical fitness would make it impossible. But if you could break the marathon challenge down into a series of microHabits of Health you absolutely could do it in the future. On the vertical axis, you can see the motivation level to do easy things does not need to be very high. We can reach a point where we are not motivated because the behavior is not desirable. If I asked you to touch your nose, you would be able to do it but you would probably have no desire to do it repeatedly to make it a habit.

microHabit Installation Diagram

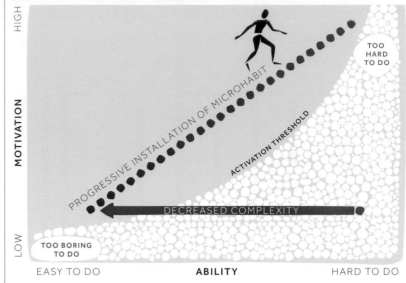

The diagram shows that when you take a more complex behavior and make it into a microHabit you move it above the activation threshold (beige area). This means that the level of motivation is sufficient so all you need is a cue to activate. Remember to install a certain behavior you only need enough motivation, ability, and a cue or reminder to do it everyday. By using microHabits we ensure motivation is never lower than the threshold. And you can see that as we build momentum and progressively increase the amount we do, we increase our ability and motivation to be able to do more.

This increase in self-efficacy occurs because of the design model of the microHabit, which builds both ability and motivation.

MICROHABITS OF HEALTH ARE NOT ENOUGH

Hopefully you are convinced that the microHabit of Health model allows the necessary repetition to install the new habit. All the same, you may be asking whether a small microHabit can really make a difference. If that's the case, let's get to the heart of why small baby steps actually create powerful transformations.

You might not have expected this, but I need to reassure you about the effectiveness of small steps by referencing Newton's first law of motion, sometimes referred to as the law of inertia. It states that an object at rest stays at rest and an object in motion stays in motion.

If we now look at the microHabits, we need to understand that once the cue has activated the micro-behavior and you are in motion, the conditions are favorable to do more repetitions or repeat the action. Often, it is the getting ready to perform the action that keeps us from doing what we have said we will do. Once you get going, you may feel like doing more.

I have a timer on my desk that reminds me to get up and do a squat every hour while I am writing. When I was writing this part, I actually did five instead of the microHabit of one. An additional five squats isn't that many, but during the week I averaged 20 a day, and I'll remember those additional squats when they drop me at 10,000 feet from a helicopter to powder ski with a bunch of 30-year-olds.

The big picture is that by getting up and moving as one of my own microHabits, I am offsetting the deadly effects of sitting for prolonged periods.[8]

The extra repetitions that you do are what we call plus activity, bonus reps, or extra credit. They are very helpful because we know that the more you do a health activity the more successful you will be in terms of installation, depth of improvement, and the level of skill you create. The idea is you install everyday and as you build your self-efficacy the progressive plus activity grows until you are able to do way more than just the microHabit and you will be able to climb the habit loop with more ability and higher motivation as you successfully install the habit (see the microHabit Installation diagram).

microHabit of Health

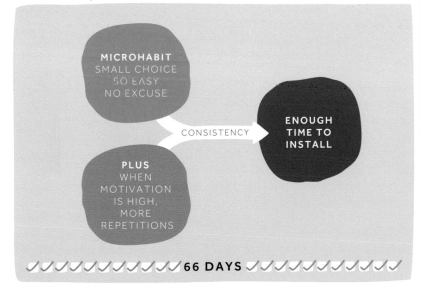

There is one other important benefit that we want to track as you install your new habit. We want to track your daily installation to start creating a chain of consistency. We know that in order to improve we need to measure our results. By tracking your daily victories, you can now hold yourself accountable for building your habit and ticking it off can serve as an additional reward for doing the behavior.

The Habits of Health App can track this for you, but a simple wall calendar (see Continuity Calender in sidebar) will also suffice (it just won't be as dynamic or as useful at being able to track things wherever you are).

mHoH Routine: Greater Progress by Adding More Plus Reps Over Time

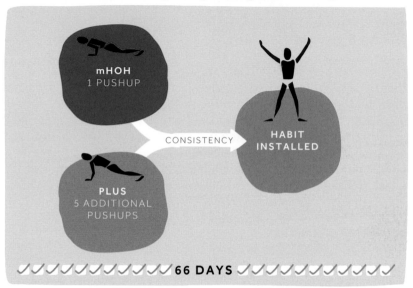

Continuity Calendar

The most important part of microHabit installation is not to miss a day. Even on difficult days, the simplicity and small amount of time required for your habits should always allow you to be able do it.

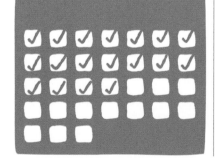

The most important part of microHabit installation is not to miss a day. Even on difficult days, the simplicity and small amount of time required for your habits should always allow you to be able to do it. And if you do miss a day (which will happen), it is super-important not to miss two in a row. The App will remind you at the end of the day, but if this happens you need to make performing the habit the next day your number one priority. If you miss three days in a row, then I am afraid you are going to have to start over! As the old saying goes: "Inch by inch, everything's a cinch."

An additional benefit of not breaking the chain is the positive feedback that you are developing and a new level of discipline, which is a habit in itself. And as you get better and build your self-efficacy and momentum the amount of reps you do every day will increase as you progressively build the ability to install the habit.

You now have a powerful tool that we will use throughout the book in tandem with the Habits of Health App and *Your LifeBook*. In the next part, we will prepare you to begin optimizing your surroundings in preparation for your journey.

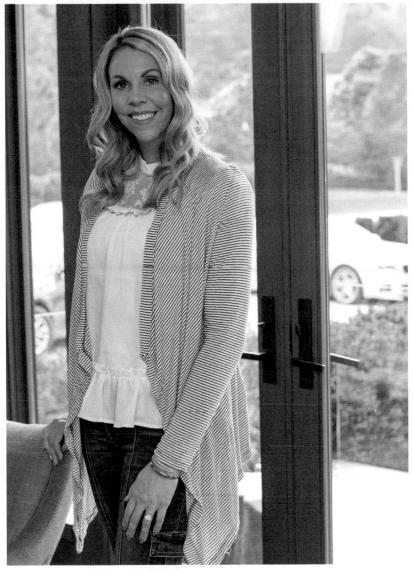

TRANSFORMATION: AMBER SMITHSON

I was overweight, had high cholesterol, and was prediabetic. I knew my health was going in the wrong direction. My two little boys would say, "Momma, let's go to the park. Let's go on the swings. Let's run." And I would say, "Let's watch a movie," and I knew that this wasn't the type of mom I wanted to be. So, I decided to lose weight and lower my cholesterol.

I found the Habits of Health later, but the cool thing was when I read that book; it was everything that I did. It was eating every two to three hours, getting proper sleep, lowering my stress level, and protein/carb balancing. It just jived right with everything that I believed in.

A few years ago, I found out that I had a brain tumor, I was in good health and with the support of my Habits of Health family surrounding me, had the tumor removed. The doctor was amazed at my recovery and said keep doing what you are doing.

"

I would say, "Let's watch a movie," and I knew that this wasn't the type of mom I wanted to be.

"

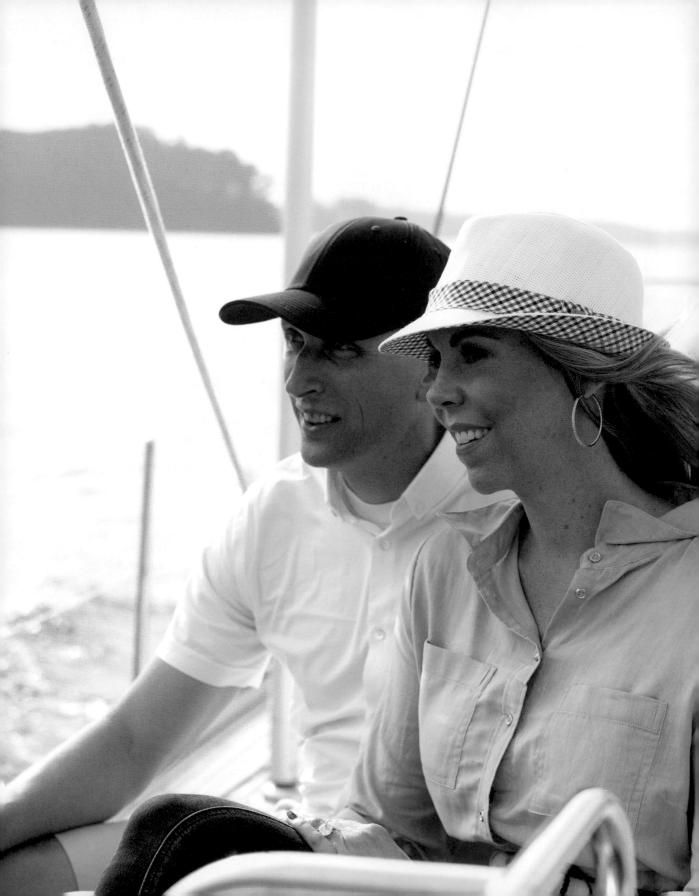

YOU IN CHARGE OF YOURSELF: SETTING UP FOR SUCCESS

In Part 1.5, The Bedrock of Transformation: Succesful Habit Installation, we discussed the role proper habit formation plays in helping you create sustainable transformations. The purpose of this segment is to align how you are going to approach this journey. Imagine if you and the world around you are working for and with you rather than against you. Although the ascent from your current reality to your desired outcome will take some effort, we want you and your world to be ready for the journey to optimal health and wellbeing.

Have you noticed in the past when you would set out to improve your health by making better choices and you feel confident that you are making progress?

You're eating healthier, started a walking program and things are beginning to change. In fact, you're rocking it and feeling pretty good about yourself. Then one Friday afternoon, you're planning on leaving early for a long weekend out in the country and your boss walks into your office, dumps extra work on your desk, and says he needs it right away.

You stomp down to the breakroom, grab some coffee and, before you know it, wolf down three doughnuts. In an instant your good intentions and hard work evaporate. You walk back to your office lamenting your weakness. Once again you have succumbed to temptation.

Needless to say, the weekend turns from hikes and salads to generous helpings of cheese and wine by the fireside, all while feeling a little bit depressed. Why do things like this happen so often? It's simple. You came into this world with an ancient mind that's being asked to function in a modern world.

In Part 1.1, *It's Not Your Fault That You're Struggling*, we talked a lot about our 10,000-year-old design versus living in our high-tech world. The fact is that your design and your surroundings are a complete mismatch.

You were engineered to be a highly responsive being with rapid detection and response programming to survive in the present moment. Your ancient brain focused on immediate concerns. If you were hungry you foraged. If the weather threatened you would seek shelter. If a dangerous predator attacked, you ran away. Your Cue—Routine—Reward went something like this:

Hungry—Eat—Full
Snows—Cave—Warm
Tiger—Run—Safe (or dead!)

You didn't think much about your future because you didn't own much and you were usually dead by 30. Life was about immediate gratification. Today, our world is all about delayed gratification and delayed return.

It's an ability to slow down our life and take the time to respond to our surroundings rather than react immediately to any stimulus that is presented to us. We are asked to go to school, to eat healthy, to exercise, reach a healthy weight, and save money, and yet there is no immediate return. There is no instant feedback to reinforce why we should continue these behaviours.

We are faced with an "immediate return" brain attempting to function in a "delayed return" society. When your ancient brain is reacting to an unreasonable boss and in all out emotional turmoil, it is asking too much of your ancient brain to have you rationalize any future benefit bequeathed to you. There is no instinct that will deny your overwhelming impulse to immediately devour the doughnuts. I'm sorry to say it, but you never stood a chance.

The last minute drop-in by your boss is just one of many examples of how life can get in the way when you start your journey towards

"A famous study known as the "Marshmallow Experiment" found that children who could resist the urge to immediately eat a marshmallow went on to be more successful in life than their peers who chose to eat the marshmallow right away.[1]

better health and wellbeing. Even equipped with your best intentions, there will be daily threats to your progress. Be prepared. Together, we'll look at your surroundings and reinforce the things that can help you either eliminate the pitfalls or at least have a contingency plan if elimination is not possible. By helping you be more aware of how and why you respond the way you do, we can help provide more effective assistance to learn to manage rather than fight your modern surroundings.

Our goal will be to optimize your brain and your mind for modern life. We will begin by widening your perspective of how you view yourself over time. Then I will explain how you can better manage your response time to threats, and finally we will discuss how we can create a microenvironment of health: a protective bubble to protect you from the daily threats and temptations to your future health and wellbeing.

PRESENT SELF VS. FUTURE SELF

How we think about our self in the present moment and how we think about our self in the future is very different. We can look to the advances in neuroscience to explain those differences. How we think and act in the present and the relationship with our future self becomes better understood when a person is placed in an FMRI brain scan—a machine that measures blood flow to the specific region in the brain that is activated by thoughts or emotions.

There is a particular area in the brain that has been mapped and shown to be devoted to self-reflection. When a subject is asked to think about themselves in the present tense, that precise area of the brain lights up. When they are asked to think about a stranger (non-self) the scan lights up a very different area in the brain.

Here is where it gets interesting. If volunteers are asked to think about themselves in the future and how they will perceive themselves five years from now, there is a wide range of responses. Most of the subjects' FMRI scans light up the same area that previously became more active when they were asked to think about a stranger and just a few activate the area that is associated with present self.

It gets better. Those that see themselves more as strangers when asked to think about the future also demonstrated a different profile. When compared to those that connected well to the future, the "stranger" brain group were more likely to struggle with delayed gratification, more likely to have poor habits, and have more difficulty saving money and dealing with the challenges of modern life such as when we are asked to delay actions to a future time.

Psychologists call the phenomena temporal discounting. It explains the tendency for your ancient brain to want to value immediate reward and devalue the importance of delaying gratification for a distant future benefit.

This is why it is so easy to get hooked on bad habits. It's the way your brain is wired. Immediate concerns driven by actual need or impulse fit very nicely into the "immediate return" brain that you were equipped with 10,000 years ago. You get instant feedback and reward and this becomes a bad habit quite easily. But when you attempt to adopt a good habit that will give you some future benefit—but the immediate reward or feedback is weak or missing—it seems harder to do.

Our brain treats time differently, especially when thinking about things in the moment versus things in the future. This observation and the supporting research gives us insights into why we behave the way we do. It also gives us a better understanding of how we can transform ourselves by bringing these two selves into closer proximity.

Your Present-Self is you in the moment, concerned with your current state, needs, choices, and immediate actions. This self is highly influenced by impulse, urges, and pleasure-seeking behaviors.

Your Future-Self is the person you plan on becoming tomorrow, next week, next year, or five years from now. Since there is no immediate action required, it is easy to plan our ideal behaviors.

Our two selves value things very differently. Your future-self says you want to lose 60 lbs, get eight hours of sleep, and run a mile every day. It feels good to set those ambitious goals and it's easy for your brain and your mind to see and value the benefit of those long-term rewards in the future.

However, when it comes time to act on those long-term health goals (rewards), we have to choose between eating a salad and not eating the piece of chocolate cake that Mom baked, between going to sleep early or staying up and watching that movie you are enjoying, between putting on your running shoes and heading out even though you have a headache and are exhausted and just feel like resting. These dilemmas are examples of you dealing with your present-self. And your present-self values the immediate return. It has little regard for potential long-term rewards.

> *Our brains are wired to favor immediate rewards over long-term ones, which means that we have to train ourselves to think differently about the choices we make.*

1.6

> *Recognizing where you are and where you want to go helps to create structural tension, which is the catalyst for change that we have previously discussed.*

Building Your Future Health and Wellbeing

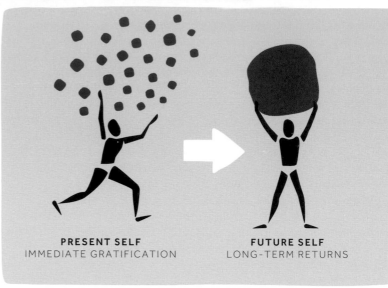

PRESENT SELF
IMMEDIATE GRATIFICATION

FUTURE SELF
LONG-TERM RETURNS

How can we overcome a natural tendency to discount the value of long-term health in order to help you avoid the daily temptations that are ever-present in our crazy lives? Simple. We have to narrow the gap between our future and present self.

If we tie future benefit into our present moment we can use our habit loop to help create new behaviors. We can even make the immediate rewards less attractive by adding a negative aspect that will help us be less likely to repeat bad habits. We are moving future rewards and punishments for specific behaviors into the present moment.

If we can design and identify immediate benefits and rewards into each of the Habits of Health, which we know are designed to provide long-term benefits, then we can connect your present self to your future self in more tangible ways.

In essence, if we can provide short-term incentives that are consistent with our long-term goals for health and wellbeing, then we can help keep our ancient brain in check.

There are a couple of ways we can do that. First, we can take an action that provides both immediate benefit and long-term benefit and connect them to create immediate and long-term reward thereby turning future consequences into present consequences.

We know that 20 minutes of activity provides long-term benefits in reducing the risk of disease and also allowing us to live longer. In addition, studies have shown that 20 minutes of activity have an immediate effect of boosting our mood for 12 hours. We can now connect a long-term benefit to immediate reward and establish a recipe for a new healthy habit installation.

This approach works equally well for eliminating an unwanted habit. We know eating a cheeseburger and fries is a Habit of Disease and will, therefore, create disease in the future. We know also that after consuming fast food we develop a high-fat hangover that ruins how we feel and perform the rest of the day. Tying the short-term negative or present effect on us to the long-term negative effect gives us a powerful reason to discontinue a negative behavior.

We can also make the long-term consequences of not doing a certain behavior more immediate by tying them into immediate pain or by creating the sense that we will pay the costs sooner if we do not perform them. As an example, let's take committing to run every morning with a friend; the morning comes, it is time to start, and the pain of disappointing your friend ties the routine to immediate feedback.

This also addresses another of the most limiting factors of our present self that prevents us from starting new habits—procrastination. We can use this same principle to get beyond the pain of procrastination and into action. We all procrastinate and we know that the shame, guilt, and anxiety of putting off the action is more painful than the actual energy and effort required to do the action. We can overcome this by taking the many things we love to do all the time and combining them with actions that we would rather not do but which have long-term future benefits.

It's called temptation bundling: you connect things you love to do with things you have a tendency not to do that are important for your health or wellbeing. You can watch your favorite TV show only while you are working out or listen to an audiobook only for the duration you are on an exercise machine. Or, you decide that you can only go to your favorite restaurant with your family (no smartphones) as a reward for reaching a previously determined health goal.

Another way to connect our present and future self is through commitment devices. These are ways to predetermine our future behavior by designing the conditions. We can use predetermined meal size by purchasing portion control packaged food in advance. This then has an influence on our future actions. We can have someone hide the TV remote to prevent mindless couch potato behavior.

We will spend more time later in this segment on the many ways we can modify our environment to influence our present behavior and satisfy our ancient brain.

We have already discussed the importance of increasing someone's ability by making it easier to move into action, despite the level of motivation on a day-to-day basis. This is important when considering ways to start future beneficial behaviors in your present state. Health behaviors do not usually have a sense of urgency because the consequences are not immediate.

If we can make them easier in terms of the amount of time needed and the degree of effort required, then it can help overcome the resistance and procrastination which we all have. If we can set a goal to be able to complete them in a very short period of time, maybe even less than two minutes, they become very useful especially when they are small and easily doable actions.

Use temptation bundling to move you closer to change. If you find a way to make a challenging activity enjoyable, you can make installing a new habit easier and perhaps even make it fun!

Those brief easy to do actions are perfectly supported by our microHabits of Health model. The model of small habit installation works well in your habit loops. It will work equally well as small additional actions that support health when stacked into an existing behavior.

Before moving to the next section, I think it is important that we take a moment and summarize the strategy, tools, and methods we have assembled to help you prepare for your journey.

You now have a robust understanding and a toolkit to install your new habits, facilitate positive actions, and help you increase the intensity and duration of what your successful behaviors are.

It's a simple four-step process which you will be able to use for the rest of your life to help guide you in building and maintaining the Habits of Health. This will allow you to command and take control of your health and wellbeing. We will use an example of some of the things it takes to reach a healthy weight to illustrate how it works.

STEP ONE: STRUCTURAL TENSION

We start by picking the primary choice you are focusing on and what secondary choices support the transformation in that category. Each of the six MacroHabit categories have a series of primary choices that are essential for mastering that area of transformation. The secondary choices are the Habits of Health actions that support reaching the desired outcome.

Structural Tension

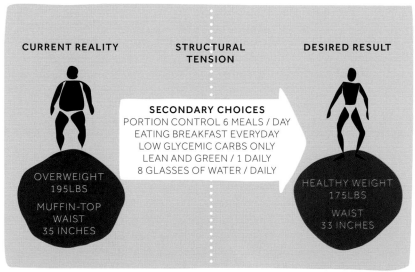

STEP TWO: SET UP HABIT LOOP FOR SPECIFIC HABITS OF HEALTH

These habit loops are normally the secondary choices which we set up into a habit loop. We find a new cue, or, anchor it to an already functioning behavior. We then outline the action or routine and provide an immediate reward or benefit to reinforce your installation of the behavior.

Habit Loop: Fueling Every Three Hours

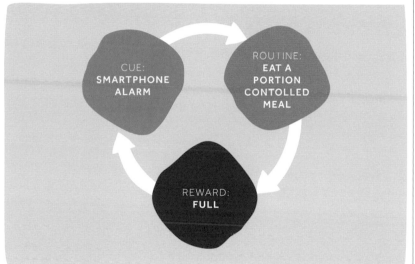

Many times you will only need the first two steps to install simple Habits of Health but, when needed, Step Three helps to simplify the routine (if necessary) into a microHabit. Step Four decides the immediate and long-term feedback or reward and then we create the transformational cycle which connects the immediate and long-term benefit into a long-term feedback accountability tool. This will allow us to track and create a chain to make sure we have consistency needed to install the new habit.

STEP THREE: IDENTIFY THE MICROHABIT TO INSTALL

Once you have set up the Habit Loop, there may even be smaller microHabits that come out of these secondary choices to ensure the installation can occur consistently and daily. See Element 03 in *Your LifeBook, How Do You Create What You Want?*, to learn why I picked chewing slowly as a microHabit for reaching a healthy weight.

mHoH

At the end of a day, reflect back and identify the cues that triggered a Habit of Disease loop. Taking the time to recognize these moments can help you to make healthier choices the next time you face a similar situation.

mHOH Routine, Chewing Slowly

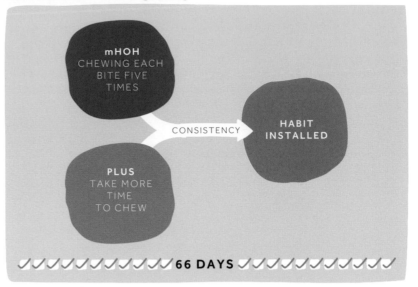

STEP FOUR: CONNECT PRESENT ACTION TO IMMEDIATE AND LONG-TERM REWARD

To ensure proper habit installation we will want to connect the daily action to immediate positive feedback. At all levels, using the Habit loops with cue, routine, and reward are crucial to the sustainable transformation necessary for creating optimal health and wellbeing. Here, we are connecting the immediate benefits of more energy and feeling better to the long-term reward of reaching a healthy weight.

Rewarding Present and Future

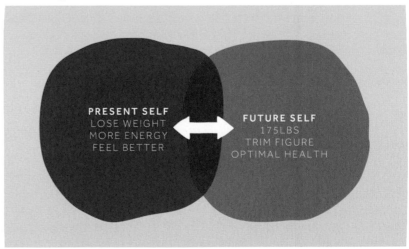

CREATE A TRANSFORMATIONAL CYCLE

Here is a model of how a transformational cycle can be used to connect all of the components of habit installation in one approach. This is the overriding summation of the process: We have picked the habit we are installing. We have decided the cue to activate the habit or action we're ingraining: the immediate reward to reinforce and give immediate feedback and the long-term investment that is being made. In the long-term investment, we have a chain which shows the daily deposit and also the overall benefit of creating this Habit of Health.

Habit of Health Transformation Cycle

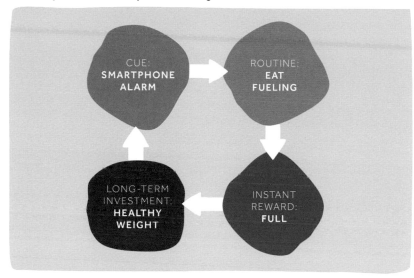

> *Developing new habits takes time. Break your Habits of Health into smaller microHabits to make the process more manageable and more gradual.*

1.6

Now that you know how to connect your present and your future self and how to develop powerful transformational habits, let's explore how to help you make the necessary adjustments so that your encounter with an insensitive boss doesn't trigger emotions that can throw you off track. Let's eliminate the comfort doughnuts permanently.

REACTIVE VS. RESPONSIVE MINDSET

The ability to put your mind where you want, whenever you want, for as long as you want, is one of the most powerful skills you can master in your lifebuilding process. It's an amazing skill to possess; nothing else can even come close when it comes to being able to really take control of your life.

When you can create a quiet mind and you can respond in a

measured fashion to whatever the world throws at you and you choose and command the actions that build your health and wellbeing, you have a powerful tool and a keystone habit.

It is the master habit that sets up unlimited possibilities not only for creating optimal health but also for creating the kind of state of wellbeing that is currently experienced by very few people. It is truly mastering the MacroHabit of a Healthy Mind.

Is it possible? It is. If you are willing to invest time, focus, and discipline, then we can transform your ability to become the dominant force in your life. Despite what many people think, how we respond to the world around us is not fixed.

It is going to require you to go to the mental gym on a daily basis, to learn, grow, practice, and master the critical skills of self-awareness and self-management.

In a future part, we will unpack the Habits of a Healthy Mind and explore the fascinating inner workings of your brain, mind, and relationships.

For now, I want to elaborate on a powerful tool which you will want to utilize right away as you begin installing your new habits in the next part.

Our brain is the most complex object in the universe. Yet in many ways its design is quite simple, particularly if we think of it in terms of what is important to re-program it to help you on your journey to create health and wellbeing. In simplistic terms, we have three brains nestled inside our skull—each of which developed over eons—which are all designed to serve us in very different ways.

The oldest—which we will call the automatic or lizard brain—takes care of our automatic functions like breathing, moving, seeing, and basic instincts like hunger, thirst, and survival. It also includes the basal ganglia or a concentrated group of neurons that aid habit formation which you will be using to make your habits automatic. Anatomically this area in the base of the skull is known as the brainstem.

The next area that sits on top of the brainstem is called the limbic system but it is better known as the emotional center or the Labrador brain. This region allows us to have emotions, and much richer experiences. If you have ever been around a Labrador (I have two of my own), they experience loyalty, fear, flight, fight, and a love for food and family. These primary behaviors are always fully present, ready to instantaneously react to any situations.

The last area to develop is the neocortex—more specifically the prefrontal cortex. This is the human brain—the thinking, willpower, or discipline brain. This is the area where we think about creating health and wellbeing and put together plans to make it a reality. This is the region where we think and act on our future self.

This human brain is functionally semi-independent from the lizard and lab brains. That is why our experiences in life, and our understanding of how our brain and mind works seem so odd. It's odd that language lies in the human brain, but emotions lie within the separate dog and lizard brains. So, emotions are in an entirely different world from language. Not only that, reason lives in the new human brain while emotions live in the older brain.

The lizard and dog brains are running their emotional reactive programs while the human brain is running its thinking programs. They don't have too much to do with each other. The older brains cannot speak and act; they can only feel and act. And because the information comes up through the lower areas before it hits the higher area (where our thinking brain lives) we need to have a tool to help us take back control of our actions so we can develop the new automated healthy habits we so desperately desire.

If we don't we will continue to grab the doughnuts every time the neural tripwire in our limbic brain (the amygdala) is activated by our boss. Your thinking brain will just be left to lament about what the heck just happened.

Our Three Brains

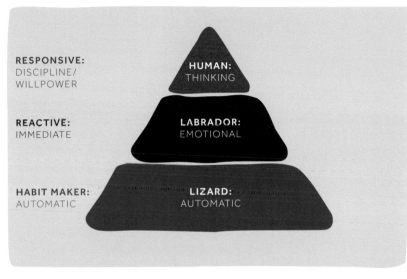

RESPONSIVE:
DISCIPLINE/
WILLPOWER

HUMAN:
THINKING

REACTIVE:
IMMEDIATE

LABRADOR:
EMOTIONAL

HABIT MAKER:
AUTOMATIC

LIZARD:
AUTOMATIC

STOP. CHALLENGE. CHOOSE.™

When we are not self-aware and something happens, a stimulus enters our brain stem and travels up to the Labrador brain. Your lower brain elicits emotion that creates an immediate action without consulting your thinking brain. This was imperative 10,000 years ago to respond immediately to avoid a threat or act on another survival need. This explains our impulsive nature and why we often get in trouble by doing or saying something without thinking about it.

The following illustration demonstrates that the emotional brain hijacks the stimulus and your thinking brain never has a chance to exert its influence and help make a decision which might better serve

This is an oversimplification of how the brain is integrated and its multiple connections but it demonstrates which brain is in charge of what and this will allow us to help control our impulsivity.

The lizard brain evolved first—it is very small and just controls the basics. Then came the Labrador brain (limbic system) which grew on top of the lizard brain and which controls the basic functions and adds emotions. Finally, the human brain (prefrontal/neo-cortex) emerged, and with it all the sophistication which goes with language. It is necessary to make us aware at a conscious level of healthy choices until our behaviors are automated through the Habits of Health. Our discipline and willpower resides here.

With that brief introduction to your brain, let's now describe how we can awaken your thinking brain and tame your lower brains so they do not sabotage your best intentions and throw in roadblocks on your journey towards optimal health.

Since we know that the unconscious, emotional, and reactive brains will hijack our best intentions we need to create a way that you can stop the automated stimulus response and create a chance for your thinking brain to make a choice that supports your new Habits of Health.

"

Stop. Challenge. Choose.™ was so successful in the field that we developed a free e-book on the process so that more people could incorporate it into their lives. The free e-book is still available at HabitsofHealth. com!

"

you in our modern world. Without awareness you remain a slave to the ancient brain that thinks only about immediate needs and return.

Our Lower Brains

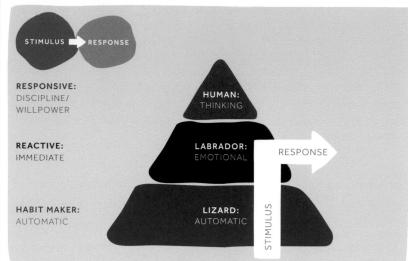

STIMULUS → RESPONSE

RESPONSIVE: DISCIPLINE/ WILLPOWER

HUMAN: THINKING

REACTIVE: IMMEDIATE

LABRADOR: EMOTIONAL

RESPONSE

HABIT MAKER: AUTOMATIC

LIZARD: AUTOMATIC

STIMULUS

How do we break this stimulus response that triggers reactive behavior and gains control over our automated brain and subconscious mind?

It is all about becoming fully aware in the moment when the stimulus or event happens and then voluntarily delaying the immediate response from being triggered by engaging our thinking brain.

Self-awareness is the first key step in changing your previous programming. It will be one of the most important Habits of Health you will learn for daily use and continue to develop along your journey.

There are many ways to work on being more aware, including a focus on your breath and the importance of meditating. For now, I am going to give you some cues your body serves up when it's about to go "prehistoric" on you. These will give you ways to start breaking the stimulus-response behavior instantly.

It starts by becoming more aware of your body and detecting the signals coming up out of your unconsciousness to the surface.

Anytime you feel that something isn't quite right, you sense your breathing change, your heart rate increase, a lump forming in your throat, a queasiness sitting in the pit of your stomach—all signals that make you stop before saying or doing anything.

In a later part of the book, we will get into much more detail of how to detect and manage your emotions. For the moment, once you have stopped the immediate response there are some things you can do to cool off. Usually the negative feelings are generated when our ego and

YOUR MIND AND BODY ARE TIGHTLY LINKED. PHYSICAL SENSATIONS, SUCH AS A GUT FEELING, ARE CUES THAT SIGNAL YOU TO IMMEDIATELY TAKE OVER CONTROL OF YOUR CURRENT CONDITIONS.

STOP

1.6

CHALLENGE

BY GETTING GOOD AT STOPPING, YOU ARE PUTTING YOURSELF IN A POSITION TO KNOW HOW TO CONTROL YOUR RESPONSE TO A NEGATIVE FEELING OR EMOTION.

CHOOSE

THIS BOOK NOW IS MAKING YOU AWARE AND TEACHING YOU THE PRINCIPLED HABITS OF HEALTH SO YOU WILL HAVE A GROWING REPERTOIRE OF BETTER CHOICES TO MAKE IN EVERY CIRCUMSTANCE. LIKE ALL OTHER HABIT INSTALLATIONS, USING STOP. CHALLENGE. CHOOSE.™ WILL TAKE PRACTICE TO LEARN AND INSTALL BUT IT WILL BECOME AUTOMATED IN TIME.

identity are somehow threatened. It takes about two minutes max for the emotion to pass (once you recognize it).

I find if I drink a glass of water before talking or take a deep breath before acting, I can then fully engage my rational brain and decide what is the action that will move me forward in my health, my relationships, and my overall wellbeing. If your immediate urge has been brain candy, such as sugar, chocolate, salty snacks, or another Habit of Disease, you can now control your subconscious mind to send out similar signals and prevent mindless eating etc.

If you think about it, your detected feeling is the Cue which signals you to stop whatever you are doing, and the Routine is your thinking challenge of sorting out what is going on, and Reward is you making the right choice by choosing an action that turns a potential negative action into a positive choice, thereby giving you a sense of accomplishment.

Below, we show the ability of Stop. Challenge. Choose.™ (scc) to delay the stimulus response by creating a pause and by activating the thinking brain to choose a Habit of Health rather than a Habit of Disease.

Engage Our Thinking Brain:
Creating the Gap Between Stimulus and Response

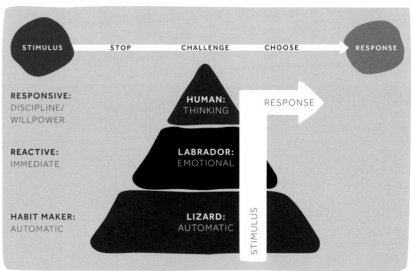

I think you will find Stop. Challenge. Choose.™ a powerful tool to help you start to gain more control over your world. You will find now that you are no longer competing with the people around you and, instead, you are looking within to continue to get better at being in control of your inner world. In the next part, we will move from within you and take a look at your surroundings and see how we can recruit the people, modify the places, and change the things that touch your world.

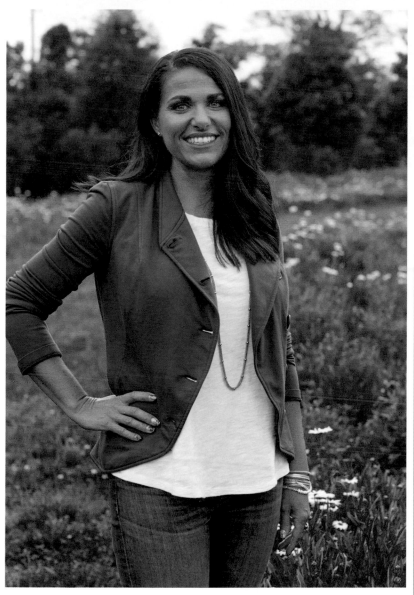

TRANSFORMATION:
GINA ECHOLS

I came to the program about seven and a half years ago. I was very, very sick and actually had two aneurysms requiring brain surgery. I came out of that alive, and knew that I needed to do something different for my health.

I really dove deep into the Habits of Health for myself, but honestly, it was also more about my children. If I just look at this one bad thing and how I can break it, or if I can work on this habit, then it's really going to change the dynamic and the trajectory of my family, and that was really, really important to me.

What makes it most sustainable for us is that we don't take every habit and overhaul our whole life. I had a lifetime of bad habits that needed to be cleaned up, but if I had tried to overhaul my life in one fell swoop, it wouldn't have stuck. But because I took it one baby step at a time and one habit at a time, that's really what helped us stick to this. Long-term health is possible, but it is only possible through choosing healthy habits: one habit at a time.

1.6

> "
> *Long-term health is possible, but only through choosing healthy habits: one habit at a time.*
> "

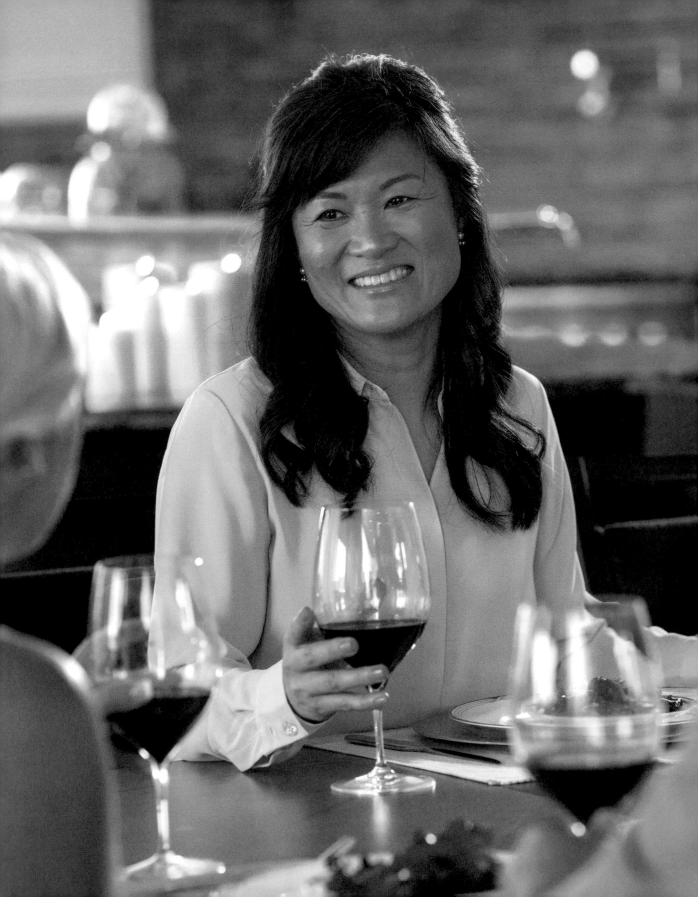

OPTIMIZING YOUR SURROUNDINGS: CREATING YOUR MICROENVIRONMENT OF HEALTH

The world we live in has a tremendous influence on our behavior. We have a tendency to blame the people, places, and things that we are exposed to when something goes wrong. If we can consistently change our surroundings and optimize their conditions, then we can help create and sustain our Habits of Health. Our behavior is extremely dependent on our surroundings. How do the people you surround yourself with, the places you live and work in, and the things that you are exposed to affect your daily behavior?

PEOPLE

Who surrounds you and how do their actions and habits affect your habits and daily behaviors?

Our family, friends, and co-workers have a tremendous impact on how we act and their influence is a powerful contributor to how we eat, move, sleep, handle stress, spend our free time, and enjoy our occupations. I mentioned earlier that studies have shown that if we radically change our surroundings then we can radically change our behavior.[1]

As you begin your journey you may not have the ability to make radical changes in who you actually spend time with but you will want to be aware of the effect of those living the Habits of Disease are having on your health and wellbeing. The most memorable events, experiences and times in your life—as well as the most agonizing—are rooted in our relationships.

A huge longitudinal Harvard study by Nicholas Christakis et al. showed the direct impact that an individual's total social network has on health, weight, fitness, happiness, and overall wellbeing. If a friend of yours becomes obese, it increases your probability of becoming obese by 57%. If it is your sibling who has become heavy there is a 40% probability of you doing likewise and if it is your spouse, it drops to 37%.[2]

If your best friend exercises regularly and is really active, it triples your chances of also being physically very active. If your best friend eats really healthily, you are five times more likely to also have a healthy dietary pattern. Your friend's habits are more important than the eating pattern in your family history. It extends well beyond moving and eating habits.

How likely you are to get colds, heal, and even die of cardiovascular disease is related to the frequency and quality of our interactions with others. The takeaway message is that it is recommended that you avoid those in your life whose current actions and behaviors are not leading them to health and wellbeing and if you cannot do this, at least ask them to support you on your journey. And if you can change your culture to be surrounded by people whose normal behavior is mirrored by your desired behavior, then that can be extremely helpful.

There are many ways to make that a reality, including exercising with a friend, walking your dog with a neighbor, joining some type of healthy living organization, developing health enhancing hobbies, and other ways to engage friends, colleagues, and relatives to help provide emotional, practical support, listening ears, or even partnering with a group on the Habits of Health.

Throughout the book, I will refer to a robust community that I have helped design and build to provide an amazing support network of people who have developed a culture of optimal health and wellbeing. This dynamic social structure has already positively affected over a million people.

The social motivation of having like-minded people around you is a powerful motivator. Whether you are best served by a drill sergeant,

> *Joining a healthy community, such as a group fitness class, can help you to meet and engage with people who prioritize their health.*

1.7

A health coach is a direct line to the behavioral support and best practices that we know, from research and field experience, to help drive lasting, vibrant transformation.

a cheerleader, or just an encouraging word from a friend, it is nice to be around people who desire to improve their health and their lives.

And you definitely want to get away from accomplices. Friends will help you, and your accomplices will help you get into trouble. Beyond your associates, you can acquire a coach, mentor, trainer, or counselor that can actually help you increase your social ability to create optimal health and wellbeing. We will talk more about what options are available but feel free to jump ahead and explore if you want some professional help as you get started.

It's a good idea to preemptively stack the deck with people that can assist you on your journey to a healthier you but you will still have to connect with people that will try to draw you down into the drama of an emotionally toxic world. Let's talk about some ways you can rise above the line and keep your thinking brain in charge.

THE DRAMA TRIANGLE

I have been helping people transform their lives for almost 20 years. There are so many lessons that I have learned about the influence, both positive and negative, that others can have on our health and wellbeing when they intersect into our lives.

Let's now discuss how others can lead us below the line, where we move from being fully responsible for our life to feeling like a victim, or even feeling like we must come in and save the day. When this happens we can become closed to new ideas, defensive in how we respond to others, and have our ego come in and have us needing to be right.

Let's use a structural tension chart to show how we can decide to move back above the line when we drift and focus on being open to growing, as well as curious about what we can do to develop and improve in our mission to create optimal health and wellbeing.

Taking Responsibility

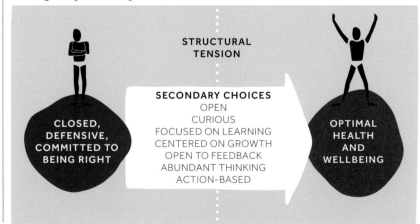

Now how can we use our decision to take personal responsibility to help us function in a fully responsible way when we are negotiating and dealing with difficult people that come into our lives daily? Stephen Karpman described a social model of human interaction 40 years ago in order to help explain how, in relational interactions and behaviors of people drifting below the line, they can take different positions in what has become known as the drama triangle.

The Victim: The victim's stance is "Poor me!" The victim feels victimized, oppressed, helpless, hopeless, powerless, ashamed, and seems unable to make decisions, solve problems, take pleasure in life, or achieve insight. The victim, if not being persecuted, will seek out a persecutor or villain and also a rescuer or hero who will save the day but also perpetuate the victim's negative feelings.

The Hero: The hero's line is "Let me help you." A classic enabler, the hero or rescuer feels guilty if he/she doesn't go to the rescue. Yet his/her rescuing has negative effects: It keeps the victim dependent and gives the victim permission to fail. The rewards derived from this rescue role are that the focus is taken away from the rescuer. When he/she focuses their energy on someone else, it enables them to ignore their own anxiety and issues. This rescue role is also very pivotal because their actual primary interest is really an avoidance of their own problems disguised as concern for the victim's needs.

The Villain: The villain, sometimes referred to as the persecutor, insists "It's all your fault." The villain is controlling, blaming, critical, oppressive, angry, authoritative, rigid, and superior.

We can put it into a visual model:

The Drama Triangle

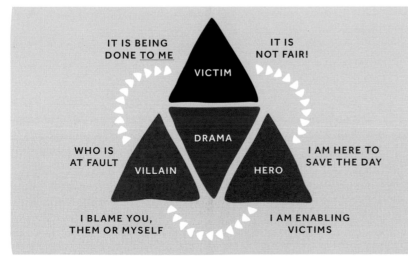

Apply the Stop. Challenge. Choose.™ method when identifying and reacting to the drama triangles in your own life.

Want Better Health?

Health creation professionals help people utilize the relatively new science of health creation by teaching key behavioral, physiologic, and lifestyle changes. Through instruction and motivation, health creation experts help those who've made the fundamental choice of optimal health reach and maintain the highest degree of health possible.

Initially a drama triangle arises when a person takes on the role of a victim or a villain. The person then feels the need to bring others into the conflict. A hero will often come to the rescue and the roles may change. The motivations of each person are to have their needs met without taking responsibility.

You may have family, friends, or colleagues that respond to your decision to change your life in one of these roles. If they are still in pre-contemplation or contemplation it may better serve them to blame you or want you to feel sorry for them. I am not asking you to figure them out but just to warn you that entropy and your relationships are not necessarily on the same path as you. This will happen:

The Drift Shift Model

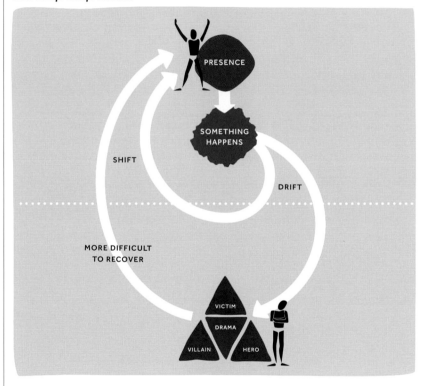

All you have to do if you sense that you are drifting below the line is to become self-aware just like we did before and pull out and use your new friend: the approach that is to Stop. Challenge. Choose.™ It will help get you back above the line, make the choices that your new Habits of Health support, and avoid the common descent into the drama triangle. Also in Element 04 of *YourLifeBook, Building a Healthy Mindset,* you can see how you can create an empowerment triangle as you are building stronger emotional agility. For now if you use Stop. Challenge. Choose.™ it will help pull you back up.

Healthy Mind Shifts

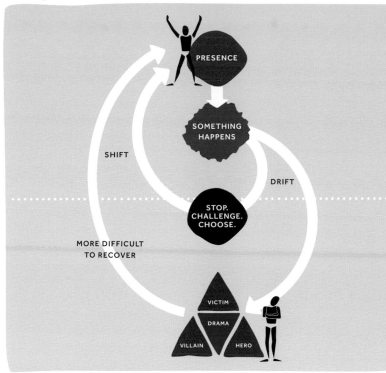

Studying the Habits of Health doesn't mean anything if you don't carry them out. Fortunately, modeling the optimally healthy people you admire can help motivate you to stay on course. However, I'm from the school of thought that believes you can never get enough help, so I highly recommend you consider exploring additional means of support.

1.7

So, we've talked about the people that can help you on your journey and why it makes sense to recruit them. We have also discussed how to manage those who don't understand what you're trying to do, and those who actively drag you back into Habits of Disease.

You have tools to help you understand and manage their position. But if we zoom out and look at the networks we are a part of, we can discover new opportunities for our health and wellbeing. Instead of being trapped inside a vortex of drama triangles, we can thrive inside a support network of people who are also working to be above the line in every choice they make.

SUPPORT SYSTEMS

What kind of support system works best? Everyone needs something different, from working on your own (if you have the discipline!), to sharing the experience with others in a group, to utilizing the guidance of a professional coach or health professional, to a comprehensive support system that combines aspects of all of the above.

OPTIMIZING YOUR SURROUNDINGS: CREATING YOUR MICROENVIRONMENT OF HEALTH

145

YOU ON YOUR OWN

For some of you, working on your own with a user-friendly, sensible system like _Dr. A's Habits of Health Transformational System_ is enough. In this second completely revised edition, I have coordinated all three essential elements to provide you with a complete system that can be self-instructed.

And because I've written this text in the same style and with the same methods that I use when I'm coaching, you have the benefit of my support when you use this book, _Your LifeBook,_ the Habits of Health App, and my website (www.HabitsofHealth.com). If you can overcome the logistical issues of today's complex lifestyle and have discipline, you can succeed with these sources alone.

But I wouldn't recommend going it alone when you have help nearby, especially if you have tried to create health in the past and were frustrated by a lack of progress.

YOU IN A GROUP

Whether it's a friend, co-worker, family members, or a larger, more organized group, working with others can make all the difference. When two or more people share similar goals and values, people create synergy. Along with encouragement, you'll have someone to walk with, eat with, and build healthy habits with. And research says you are much more likely to be successful and happier as a result.[3]

This collective journey to optimal health can take place:

- In informal group settings, such as family or social gatherings, where you surround yourself with likeminded people.
- In formal settings, such as behavioral groups or programs led by health professionals who offer guidance and foster a supportive community of people, like you, who are at various stages of their health journeys.
- Online, using internet-based programs, like social media groups and web conferences, to keep you connected and immersed in healthy support.

In the end, I believe that having someone to work with is the most powerful form of support there is, and it can come in any combination of the settings described above. For weight loss, and creating optimal health and wellbeing it's invaluable. For that, you need a coach.

YOU WITH A COACH

Personal health coaching is a growing specialty because it fills a huge demand for personal instruction. I believe in personal coaching so much that we have created an entire network of coaches who model the *Habits of Health Transformational System* and are trained to support them.

Your coach helps you stay accountable by holding up the mirror to make sure you're clear and honest about your current reality and progress. Working together, you and your coach can devise a customized plan using *Your LifeBook* to guide you. It will be a plan that focuses on the healthy habits you need to work on the most, at an appropriate pace. If you have the services of a certified trainer, you can also get instruction on how to exercise properly.

What I love about this system is that we have positively affected over a million lives already. Also, it's comprehensive and built on all that experience.

Unlike our system, some clinical and commercial coaches can be expensive and time consuming. After all, it only works if you keep going and trekking to a group meeting or a clinical facility every week for the rest of your life, which may not be the answer for you. So when you select a coach, make sure that you find one that fits your personality and budget, and that you'll be able to work with for the long term. The logistics will only work if their services are convenient to your lifestyle.

My recommendation? If you have difficulty starting or need some help staying on track until your new Habits of Health have become automatic, a personal coach may be your answer. For more information about OPTAVIA™, visit Optavia.com or HabitsofHealth.com.

" *Modeling works! Studies show that by associating with others who have the qualities you desire— optimal health, for example— you're more likely to develop those qualities yourself.*[4] "

1.7

Your Ideal Support System: Microenvironment of Health

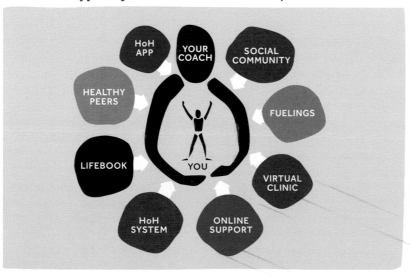

> "
> *Apply the power of choice architecture to your own life. For example, bring a big refillable bottle of water with you to work and keep it at your desk.*
> "

Let's switch gears now and talk about the places you travel through and to on a daily basis and how the triggers, exposures, and environments you are exposed to can influence your behavior and habits.

PLACES

The hidden forces that surround us and the structures we find ourselves in have a major impact on our tendencies and our ability to change and create new behaviors and habits. We make many of our choices by what is presented to us rather than from a conscious choice.

As an example, a study was done at a hospital cafeteria where they simply rearranged the position and amount of bottled water available to their patrons and moved the soda machines to a more remote position. In a three-month period, they increased the consumption of water by almost 25% and decreased unhealthy soda selection dramatically without any other intervention. When they interviewed the individuals, they made up many reasons why they were consuming more water but in reality they were not even aware of the real reason—someone had just moved the soda further away.

This is an example of the power of choice architecture. It's used by grocery stores, restaurants, and fast food restaurants and the result is poor health choices.[5]

We know that we tend to behave to the defaults we set in our lives. When interviewed, fewer than one in 10 individuals even claimed to be able to be good at resisting the temptation of unhealthy options on the menu. It is better to pick a healthy restaurant in advance than try to eat healthy once you have entered the front door.

And if you have a cocktail before ordering your meal (immediately putting those health-seeking thinking brain neurons on hold) you are much more likely to order unhealthy options. If we enter a fast food joint with the intention of ordering a salad, we are three times more likely to select an unhealthy option.[6] It is imperative that we get out in front of our immediate impulses before we are in an environment where we have to make a choice.

So we want to look at the places you live, work, and play and make sure we modify the spaces to support your daily choices and make it easier to avoid triggered temptations.

What can you do right now to get prepared as you start your journey? As far as food goes, it starts with the healthy choices you make at the supermarket. These choices will determine your home food environment. First, make sure you are well rested and also make sure you have eaten a healthy meal before you step into the grocery store. If you are tired and/or hungry you will have a tendency to be attracted to the sugary, sweet, and brightly designed foods most of the time.

And the choice architecture at the supermarket is designed to get you to the high profit shelves and draw you into the colorful middle aisles filled with processed food. The more you shop in the perimeter with healthy fruit, vegetables, and whole foods the more you'll stock your refrigerator and pantry with healthy choices.

A good start to this is to put your house on a diet by taking all of the processed food in your refrigerator, freezer, and pantry and dumping it into a large garbage bag. Then place it in the garbage can as a rite of passage and symbol that you are starting your journey. It is a powerful gesture as well as an immediate radical change in your environment. It will also have immediate and significant behavioral implications. If you have others in your household that have not decided to join you, ask them if it is all right if you position their items on the lower shelves, hidden away in cupboards, and far from view.

The same applies to making adjustments to your office space and other areas where you spend time. In addition to food items, there are many other modifications that you can make to your surroundings which will affect such things as your movement, sleep, stress, and your overall sense of wellbeing.

We will explore and unpack each of these in the corresponding segments and give you plenty of ideas to create a healthy choice architecture in your life.

A few simple things you can start now: you can make immediate changes to move more at work by using the stairs, the washroom at the other end of the building, or working while standing using a standing desk or even a rubber ball seat when you need to sit. Improving your surroundings to decrease the noise, distractions, temperature, and lighting can all affect (and benefit) your mood and stress level. This is particularly important in your bedroom where dark, quiet, cool conditions can immediately affect your sleep quality and increase your relaxation.

The goal will always be to keep a lookout on how making choices in advance will make it easier to do the Habits of Health and harder to do things which are unhealthy for us. Let's take a brief look at some of the things that we can change or modify to serve our long-term goals.

THINGS

Since the earliest times, we've had to be sensitive to our surroundings to survive. We've had an innate awareness of our environment and looked for environments with certain qualities—for safety and security—and physical comfort, like an environment with the right temperature.

In addition, we look for places that are psychologically comfortable: for example, environments that are familiar but with the right amount of stimulus. What I want to help you do is create a baseline condition that minimizes your stress, give you a sense of wellbeing and reconnects you to your surroundings.

> *Later in the book, we will learn how seemingly small changes in behavior, like standing to take phone calls, can aggregate to form powerful Habits of Healthy Motion.*

1.7

OPTIMIZING YOUR SURROUNDINGS: CREATING YOUR MICROENVIRONMENT OF HEALTH

Modern life has turned us into an indoor species. Our children spend as little as seven minutes a day outside.[7] This indoor biome is made of structures, HVAC systems, artificial light, controlled temperature, and digital stimulus, all of which has a direct effect on our health and wellbeing. We no longer experience the warmth of the sun, the splendor of the night sky, or our connections to nature.

As you start on your journey please spend the time to reconnect on a daily basis in a safe, comforting way to things like these.

At the same time. take off your electronic leash and disconnect from your smartphone, computer, and television. The input from these devices is not only distracting but unhealthy unless consumed in moderation. The triggers embedded into these devices are capable of sabotaging your best intentions.

In addition, the mere presence of a smartphone decreases the depth of meaning of conversations between people.[8] The psychological connection we have with these devices has raised our level of stress so that we are constantly in the sympathetic state in our autonomic nervous system that further isolates us from each other. The parasympathetic state of quiet, alert, slow breathing and heart rate, which was always our default for empathy, compassion, and real connection is rare today unless we move to that state with slow, deep, intentional breathing and by turning off these devices.

This illustration shows that as our environmental stress goes up so does our personal stress.

Personal Stress / Environmental Stress

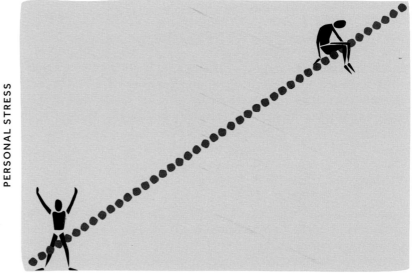

PERSONAL STRESS

ENVIRONMENTAL STRESS

To unplug during your day and create tranquil conditions will be very helpful to you as you begin this journey. Creating an infrastructure for success starts by modifying your surroundings so you make small improvements every day. It means planning for where and when you do this and making sure you have the things that will help you be successful.

Get rid of things that can slow you down. Wear comfortable shoes to work that you can walk in, rather than choosing the trendy pointed ones that kill your toes.

You need to identify the things in your life that are Kryptonite and throw you off. Identify them now and make a conscious decision to eliminate their presence to avoid future roadblocks. Make simple plans, make sure you have the time and resources, and don't make reasons why you cannot do something (because your brain thinks reasons make it okay). Use the power of observation to note when you are most likely to mess up and decide on a contingency so that if that happens then you know what to do to preemptively avoid a bad behavior.

And have multiple options and not just one way to get it done. You should always do something, even when the weather is too bad for a run or you don't have enough time. Do something so that there is never an excuse to do nothing. As you improve on your path you will find that the most successful people in your position *never have a zero-sum day*.

There are so many little things you can do or not do that will start making a difference over time. I'm going to end this section with an amazing story about the British cycling team. I saw an interview with Sir Dave Brailsford—a sporting guru who was hired in 2003 to improve the Team Sky professional cycling team who, up to that point, had never been very good. They were so bad in fact that manufacturers were refusing to sell them bikes because it would damage their reputations.

Brailsford initiated a new strategy and started looking at all the little ways they could improve their performance. He looked at tire pressure, uniforms, the air resistance of their helmets, what they were eating, how they were training, and how much sleep they got.

He also started looking at things that you might not think would make a difference. The laundry detergent they washed uniforms in. The massage gels they used post-race. He even tested different pillows to see which one each rider used to get the best night's sleep and then transported it to the next night's hotel.

He transformed them into what many consider the best sports team in the world, winning three Tour de France victories in the last four years. He attributed it to these simple methods which he called the aggregation of marginal gains. If you go after all these incremental gains and aggregate them together, you can do just about anything.

I know as you turn the page and start your journey you may feel the idea of optimal health and wellbeing seems so far away it's almost a dream. Like Sir Dave Brailsford, I believe in giving you all-embracing ownership over your journey and I believe that you can become the

"
Small victories add up. New uniforms and better pillows might not be enough to win a race in isolation, but a series of small changes can become a big transformation.
"

1.7

best possible version of you that you can possibly be if you are willing to approach your days one at time. And like Brailsford's team, if you're committed to getting a little bit better every day, together we will find so many ways to improve, a little bit here and a little bit there.

We will differentiate between your vision of optimal health and wellbeing and the small targets that we can work on every day.

The microHabits of Health will allow you to make small daily incremental steps of improvement until one day you will be living healthy and thriving in your life. Let's take that first step.

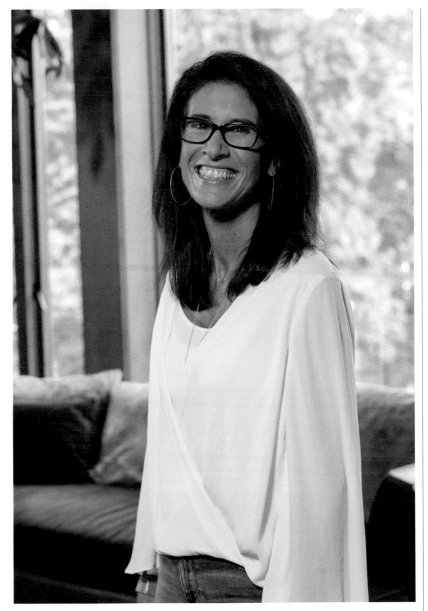

TRANSFORMATION: MICHELLE HEYMAN

Four years ago, I was probably a serial yo-yo dieter: really good at losing weight, but never had the habits to keep it off. I would just diet to lose weight and then go back to my old ways. This program really has taught me how to adopt those microHabits where I can learn to create a healthy lifestyle that I can implement every single day.

I think the picture of what I was trying to create before was just too big. When I wasn't finding success and I felt like a failure, I would just go back to my old ways. But then when I would create these small little habits that I could feel successful with, I could just move forward in my health and have more success to get me to my ultimate goal.

Learning from Dr. A has been crucial to my health journey because he almost knows what we're thinking, and he really covers so many aspects of our life that often we don't even think of as part of our health. I never really thought of how a community could help me on my health journey, or how sleep or even reading a book and changing my mindset could positively affect my life.

"
This program really has taught me how to adopt those microHabits.
"

YOUR JOURNEY TO OPTIMAL HEALTH AND WELLBEING

In Part One, Preparing for Your Journey, we explained how our ancient biological and mental programming is failing to perform effectively against advancing technology. This mismatch shows up for so many as a progressive deterioration in our physical, mental, social, and spiritual lives.

For you, it may show up as weight gain, unwanted fat accumulation around your waist, lack of energy, lower enthusiasm, poor sleep, or feeling like you're just getting by in many or all aspects of your life.

It doesn't have to be that way. Let's explore a path focused on taking responsibility, organizing your choices and making your decisions in a very different way.

It moves away from the problem solving the zero-sum game taken by so many and instead moves to the transformational creative process of the Habits of Health.

We investigated your readiness to make the necessary changes to create optimal health and wellbeing in your life. We dove into the six key MacroHabits and how their installation will update your 10,000 year old software to help you adapt to a rapidly changing world.

We then discussed the power of habits as the master lever in transforming your health and life, including how habits are formed, how we build new ones, and how we use the creative process to methodically install your new Habits of Health, one microHabit at a time.

A deep dive into you, and how you think, feel, and act has equipped you with a new way of taking back control of your decisions and choices. You took your place in the driving seat of this system and are ready for the journey. And we discussed how you can influence the people, places, and things in your surroundings to support you on a journey which is really going to be a lifetime's adventure.

In this edition, we are going to organize your journey around learning, understanding, assimilating, installing, and becoming the six MacroHabits which we discussed earlier.

I want to set the stage for you with a story...

Let me retell a story I have heard many times since I was a young man. It's the story of rocks, pebbles, sand, and a mason jar.

A teacher comes into a classroom and places a mason jar filled with rocks before the class and asks them if the jar is full. "Yes" they respond. "Not so" says the teacher, and he reaches for a pail of smaller pebbles. He pours them into the jar, shaking it until they fill the spaces between the rocks.

He asks the class if the jar is full? "Yes" they say again. "Not yet", says the teacher, and he adds a scoop of sand to the jar. He tilts the jar until the sand has run all the way through the gaps to the bottom.

Once again, he asks the class if the mason jar is full. The class inspects the jar. They conclude there is no more room for anything else. Smiling, the teacher grabs a pitcher of water and proceeds to fill the jar to the brim.

As he places the jar back on the desk, he explains how the jar is an analogy for our lives. The jar is your life. The rocks are the big things in your life: family, spouse, health, hopes, and dreams. The pebbles are the things that give life meaning: friendships, work, hobbies. And the sand and water represent the small stuff that fills the rest of your time.

The point? If you fill your life with small stuff, how will you ever be able to find space for the big, important stuff?

The Habit of Health system is like the mason jar, creating a micro-environment of health to protect you against your unhealthy surroundings.

I love this story for lots of reasons. Its principle lesson is the building block of the *Habits of Health Transformational System.* Life is a series of choices and some of them are more important than others. It's the prioritization of those choices that creates the proper motivation to drive everything you can accomplish.

Since the origin of the story is unknown, I am going to adopt this strong visual analogy because it's a wonderful way of explaining and describing our system. It is a perfect structure that we can use to empower your new story and your journey.

The Habit of Health system is like the mason jar, creating a microenvironment of health to protect you against your unhealthy surroundings.

The six MacroHabits of Health are the foundations of optimal health and wellbeing. These are the rocks that must be placed in the jar in order to create lifelong transformation and protect you from the modern world's negative side effects. They are the foundations.

It is critical that we address all six MacroHabits of Health. We have to take time to focus and place these rocks in our jar to create the foundations necessary for long-term success. If we fail to tackle each of these keystones of our microenvironment of health, then the structure will be weakened and our chances of withstanding the effects of our modern world will be decreased.

Next come the primary and secondary habits that are derived from the six MacroHabits. These primary and secondary habits are the pebbles that now surround, reinforce, and actually arise from the foundational rocks.

These Habits of Health can be further broken down into the sand—the microHabits of Health. These are the thousands of small choices that are part of our daily life—the positive actions that are so small that we can always do them.

If you consider that we make over 200 food decisions every day, each microaction either adds to our health and life or detracts from it. The sand represents what appears to be insignificant choices when made on their own but when placed in the jar and mixed with water, they become the concrete that makes the jar a formidable force against any external challenges to your health and wellbeing.

We live in an obesigenic world where we are surrounded with so many things that can have a negative effect on our weight and our health. As we describe in Part 1.1, *It's Not Your Fault That You're Struggling,* of this book, it is clear that it really isn't your fault that you are struggling with your weight, your health, and your wellbeing.

And this chaotic, unhealthy, stressful world full of unhealthy food is not going to change in the near future. So, it makes sense to start this journey by addressing how we help you overcome the effects of this obesigenic world and put you in charge of your weight management system. Our focus on you becoming your own boss and empowering you with the capability to reach and sustain a healthy weight will place the first keystone in the jar and set a platform for all the others.

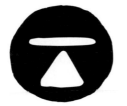

**HABITS OF HEALTHY
WEIGHT MANAGEMENT**

**HABITS OF HEALTHY
EATING AND
HYDRATION**

**HABITS OF
HEALTHY MOTION**

**HABITS OF
HEALTHY SLEEP**

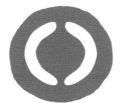

**HABITS OF A
HEALTHY MIND**

**HABITS OF HEALTHY
SURROUNDINGS**

THE ROCK, PEBBLE, AND SAND

It is important to note that the installation of each of these six MacroHabits will be accomplished most successfully by utilizing all the parts of the *Habits of Health Transformational System*.

Dr. A's Habits of Health is the compendium for health and wellbeing. It is the definitive guide to accompany you for the rest of your life and it will give you what is necessary to optimize your health and wellbeing. It will provide you with the evidence, science, and detailed explanation to help you really understand what it takes to create optimal health and wellbeing. It's the book you're holding at this very moment.

Your LifeBook is a personal journal and modular system to make sure that you are hitting the milestones on your health and wellbeing journey. It is the practical companion to this book and it will help you with your application of the system. It is the documentation of your new and developing story. I know you may not have used a journal before but there's evidence to suggest that those who write down their goals and use a journal to monitor their own progress are more successful.[1]

This hybrid personal piece also contains a series of Elements that contain critical building blocks that you will want to master. If you work with a coach, as I suggest you should, they will help guide you through this succession of important Elements at a pace that works for you.

The Habits of Health App is a companion to the system, designed to act as a habit installer—a way to set day to day reminders to help make sure you are consistently building the microHabits that over time will change everything. It becomes available to you once you join our health community and, along with your own personal coach, will become an important asset in building your new life and story.

We will unpack the six MacroHabits in Part Two as you progress on your journey to optimal health and wellbeing. Many of the parts will include more than one of the MacroHabits and we will do an extensive review of each one. The parts build and are designed to be read in sequence (though reading them independently will also be of benefit). The sixth MacroHabit—Habits of Healthy Surroundings—will be embedded throughout because the modification of what is around you will be uniquely applied to each area you are working on. We will pull valuable information from each MacroHabit when necessary to support the area you are focusing on at the present moment.

You will note that in Part Two, *Your Journey to Optimal Health and Wellbeing,* we will build a progressive path to better health and wellbeing focusing on and then placing each of the keystone MacroHabits in your jar.

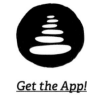

Get the App!

Download the Habits of Health App now to help install your habits on your journey to optimal health.

We spent Part One teaching you the why, how, and what of building a new transformational life. In Part Two we have first outlined the importance of addressing all six of the MacroHabits and how you will want to use the book, *Your LifeBook*, and App as powerful tools on this journey to optimal health and wellbeing. We will start with the first keystone MacroHabit of Healthy Weight Management, which is a habit that eludes so many because it is interdependent on so many factors, all of which we will unpack in the upcoming segments.

So, turn the page and let's demystify this crazy world of nutritional pollution, diets, and fat accumulation, and instead lay out a simple, effective way to help you not only reach but also maintain a healthy weight in this obesigenic world.

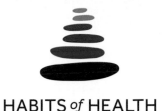

HABITS *of* HEALTH

The Habits of Health logo is designed to represent the path to optimal health and wellbeing. It is built on the six MacroHabits as six progressive solid walking stones. In addition, the design depicts a cairn, with the six MacroHabits stack designating the support and balance to each other in a powerful interdependency. And as a cairn in nature indicates a trail head; our logo designates the adventure awaiting you as you ascend on the path to optimal health and wellbeing.

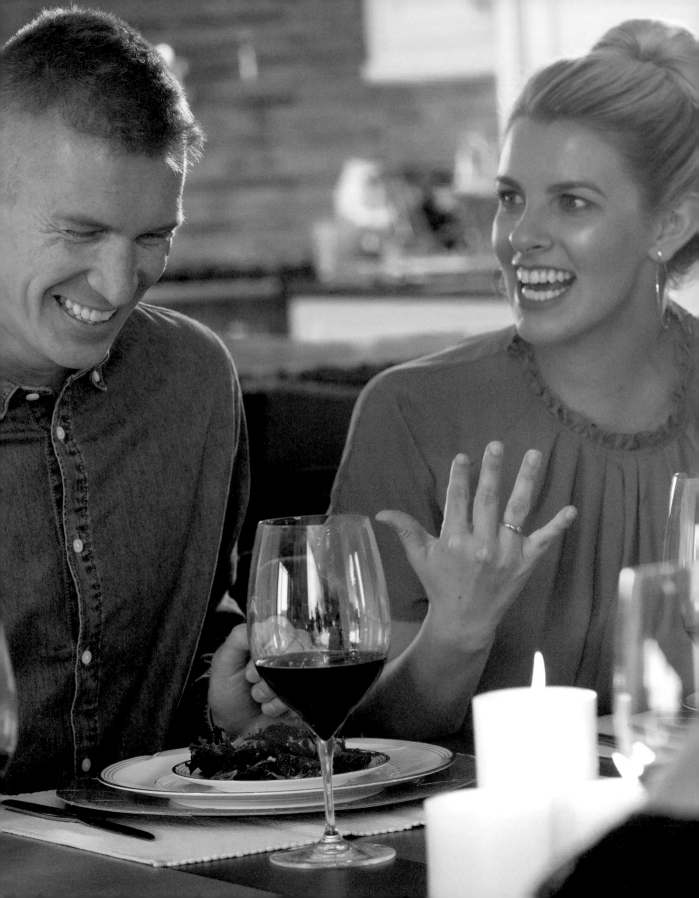

PART 2.1

HABITS OF HEALTHY WEIGHT MANAGEMENT

**HABITS OF
HEALTHY WEIGHT
MANAGEMENT**

Reaching and maintaining a healthy weight is the most important gift you can give yourself and those you love and care about. It is the foundation of optimal health and wellbeing and without it the mason jar cannot support long-term health.

So why is it so important? Well for starters, it can:

- Help you live longer
- Improve the quality of your life
- Slow down the aging process
- Give you more energy and vitality
- Improve your mental outlook and increase your happiness
- Improve your work performance
- Improve your sleep
- Lower your blood pressure, cholesterol (especially bad cholesterol), and triglycerides
- Lower your risk for heart attack or stroke
- Lower your blood sugar
- Eliminate insulin resistance
- Reverse and possibly eliminate metabolic syndrome
- Dramatically lower your risk of developing diabetes or, if you have diabetes, arrest and even reverse its progression
- Lower your risk for liver and gallbladder disease
- Lower your risk for varicose veins, deep vein thrombosis, and blood clots
- Help you breathe better
- Eliminate sleep apnea
- Lessen or eliminate asthma, bronchitis, and other lung problems
- Lower your risk of getting arthritis or, if you have arthritis, relieve your pain
- Reduce or eliminate the amount of medication you use
- Increase your chances of becoming pregnant
- Improve the health of you and your baby during pregnancy
- Markedly lower your risk for many types of cancers[1]

Just a 10% reduction in your weight lowers your risk of disease by over 50% and that risk continues to drop as you reduce your BMI (body mass index) below 25.[2] In fact, the only drawback to weight loss that I've ever encountered is that you'll have to spend money on a new wardrobe!

Let's start by finding out where you are currently and then go to work in installing the new habits that will help you reach and sustain lifelong weight control. The following diagram shows this new energy path as the linear progression you will take over time:

> *In Phase I, we're going to give you a jumpstart to help you reach a healthy weight.*

Your New Energy Path to Optimal Health and Longevity

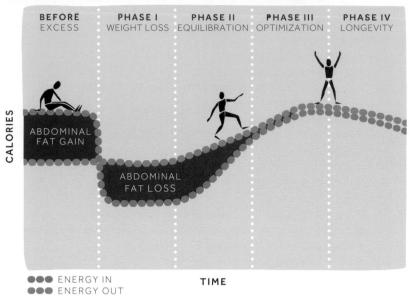

WHAT PHASE ARE YOU IN NOW IN TERMS OF YOUR WEIGHT MANAGEMENT?

This is where we put the tools you learned in Part One, *Preparing for Your Journey*, to use. In each of the MacroHabits, we will set your current level. Because this will be your starting point or current reality, it will inform you where you are now and how we can focus on what you should be doing and what phase you are in. You will want to track your current location in *Your Lifebook* as well.

Throughout the book we will address your weight management in a continuum of progressive mastery. To make this easier, I have designed four progressive phases to our weight management program. The usual starting point is the state we find almost 70% of our adult population in, which is an energy excess state of being overweight or obese.

The phases are dynamic states of active intervention to create progressively healthier states of being. It's important to know your current reality as we begin your journey.

Your Weight Management Phases

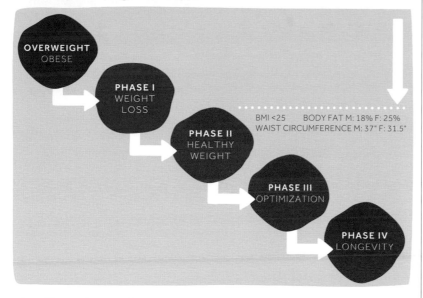

BMI <25   BODY FAT M: 18% F: 25%
WAIST CIRCUMFERENCE M: 37" F: 31.5"

Just a 10% reduction in your weight lowers your risk of disease by 50%.[3]

We will use three different measurements to assess your current phase in your weight management.

Body Mass Index:

This is the gold standard because of its simplicity. When combined with your waist circumference it provides an accurate assessment of whether we are at a healthy weight. The following chart can help you quickly calculate your current BMI. You can also use one of our online calculators.

WEIGHT (LBS)

HEIGHT	100	110	120	130	140	150	160	170	180	190	200	210	220	230	240	250	260	270	280	290	300	310	320
4'5"	25	28	30	33	35	38	40	43	45	48	50	53	55	58	60	63	65	68	70	73	75	78	80
4'6"	24	27	29	31	34	35	39	41	43	46	48	51	53	55	58	60	53	65	68	70	72	78	80
4'7"	23	26	28	30	33	35	37	40	42	44	46	49	51	53	56	58	60	53	65	67	70	72	74
4'8"	22	25	27	29	31	34	36	38	40	43	45	47	49	52	54	56	58	61	63	65	67	69	72
4'9"	22	24	26	28	30	32	35	37	39	41	43	45	48	50	52	54	56	58	61	63	65	67	69
4'10"	21	23	25	27	29	31	33	36	38	40	42	44	46	48	50	52	54	56	59	61	63	65	67
4'11"	20	22	24	26	28	30	32	34	36	38	40	42	44	46	48	50	53	55	57	59	61	63	65
5'0"	20	21	23	25	27	29	31	33	35	37	39	41	45	45	47	49	51	53	55	57	59	61	62
5'1"	19	21	23	25	26	28	30	32	34	36	38	40	42	43	45	47	49	51	53	55	57	59	60
5'2"	18	20	22	24	26	27	29	31	33	35	37	38	40	42	44	46	48	49	51	53	55	57	59
5'3"	18	19	21	23	25	27	28	30	32	34	35	37	39	41	43	44	46	48	50	51	53	55	57
5'4"	17	19	21	22	24	26	27	29	31	33	34	36	38	39	41	43	45	46	48	50	51	53	55
5'5"	17	18	20	22	23	25	27	28	30	32	33	35	37	38	40	42	43	45	47	48	50	52	53
5'6"	16	18	19	21	23	24	26	27	29	31	32	34	36	37	39	40	42	44	45	47	48	50	52
5'7"	16	17	19	20	22	23	25	27	28	30	31	33	34	36	38	39	41	42	44	45	47	49	50
5'8"	15	17	18	20	21	23	24	26	27	29	30	32	33	35	36	38	40	41	43	44	46	47	49
5'9"	15	16	18	19	21	22	24	25	27	28	30	31	32	34	35	37	38	40	41	43	44	46	47
5'10"	14	16	17	19	20	22	23	24	26	27	29	30	32	33	34	36	37	39	40	42	43	44	46
5'11"	14	15	17	18	20	21	22	24	25	26	28	29	31	32	33	35	36	38	39	40	42	43	45
6'0"	14	15	16	18	19	20	22	23	24	26	27	28	30	31	33	34	35	37	38	39	341	42	43
6'1"	13	15	16	17	18	20	21	22	24	25	26	28	29	30	32	33	34	36	37	38	40	41	42
6'2"	13	14	15	17	18	19	21	22	23	24	26	27	28	30	31	32	33	35	36	37	39	40	41
6'3"	12	14	15	16	17	19	20	21	22	24	25	26	27	29	30	31	32	34	35	36	37	39	40
6'4"	12	13	15	16	17	18	19	21	22	23	24	26	27	28	29	30	32	33	34	35	37	38	39
6'5"	12	13	14	15	17	18	19	20	21	23	24	25	26	27	28	30	31	32	33	34	36	37	37
6'6"	12	13	14	15	16	17	18	20	21	22	23	24	25	27	28	29	30	31	32	33	34	35	37

■ UNDERWEIGHT   ■ HEALTHY   ■ OVERWEIGHT   ■ OBESE

HABITS OF HEALTHY WEIGHT MANAGEMENT

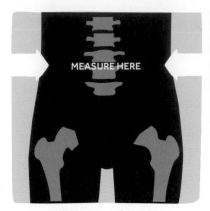

To correctly measure waist circumference:

- Stand and place a tape measure around your middle, just above your hip bones
- Make sure the tape is horizontal around the waist
- Keep the tape snug around the waist, but not compressing the skin
- Measure your waist just after you breathe out

Waist Circumference:

This allows us to evaluate the visceral or organ fat accumulation, which is a very good indicator of whether your extra fat poses a health challenge. Your health is at risk if your waist size is

- Men: Over 94 cm (about 37 inches)
- Women: Over 80 cm (about 31.5 inches)

Body Fat (Optional):

Tracking body fat (if you have an accurate source available) can offer a third source of measurement to assess your current weight management. It helps show that you are losing fat and not muscle. Our Habits of Health programs are designed to minimize muscle loss. In Phase II, III, and IV body composition becomes important to make sure you are building muscle and not just adding fat! For now if you have access to a Bod Pod, DEXA, or someone who can help you use a set of skin calipers you can also use these numbers to determine your current phase.

Note: Most electrical impedance devices are not very accurate but may give you a trending option.

Body Fat Chart

SEX	FATNESS	BODY FAT% AGE 20 – 39	BODY FAT% AGE 40 – 59	BODY FAT% AGE 60 – 79
MALE	UNDERFAT	<8%	<11%	<13%
	NORMAL	8 – 20%	11 – 20%	13 – 25%
	OVERFAT	20 – 25%	22 – 25%	25 – 28%
	OBESE	>25%	>28%	>30%
FEMALE	UNDERFAT	<21%	<23%	<24%
	NORMAL	21 – 33%	23 – 34%	24 – 36%
	OVERFAT	33 – 39%	34 – 40%	36 – 42%
	OBESE	>39%	>40%	>42%

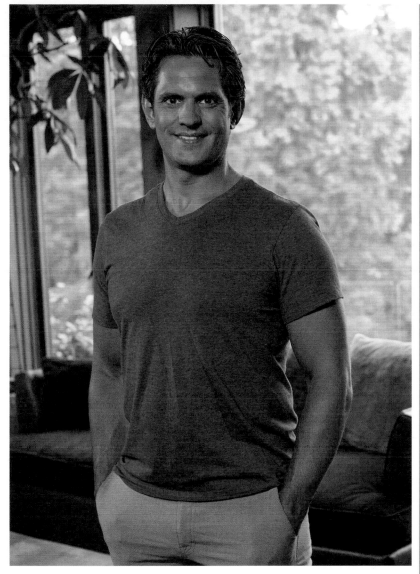

TRANSFORMATION: KEVIN TINTER

My Habits of Health journey started just over seven years ago. I was kind of in that "middle-aged guy" phase where my gut was starting to get a little bit bigger than I wanted.

My wife started her own journey and, for a couple months, I honestly wasn't ready. I was still eating all the junk food that I was addicted to at the time, but also starting to notice my wife's transformation and realizing that at some point in the near future, I was going to be ready to get healthy myself.

One of the great things about the Habits of Health is that it's a tool to help us get to a healthy weight. But you're not saying "no" to anything for the rest of your life. I still do occasionally enjoy some sweets and junk food, but the frequency and the serving sizes have gone down significantly.

I had back surgery about six months before I started our program. I lost 35 lbs* initially, and not a single healthcare practitioner suggested that I lose weight to try to avoid surgery. My back is as good today as it ever has been. I'm so grateful for the weight loss that has allowed my back to really thrive over the last seven years.

> ❝
> *I was kind of in that "middle-aged guy" phase where my gut was starting to get a little bit bigger than I wanted.*
> ❞

*Average weight loss on the Optimal Weight 5 & 1 Plan® is 12 lbs.

WHICH PHASE ARE YOU IN CURRENTLY?

CURRENT REALITY

PHASE I

OVERWEIGHT/OBESE

BMI >24.9
Waist circumference:
Male >40"
Female >35"
Body fat (optional):
Male >18%
Female >25%

This is the current state most people find themselves in. If you are like two-thirds of Americans then this will be the current starting point for your journey.

We will start with a quick review of why you are here and then dive right into our weight-loss phase. Start Part 2.1, *The Habits of Healthy Weight Management.*

WEIGHT LOSS

BMI <25
Until Waist Circumference:
Male <37"
Female <31.5"
Until Body Fat (optional):
Male <18%
Female <25%

We will provide a couple of options to choose from to guide your weight loss journey. Start Parts 2.1–2.8.

PHASE II	PHASE III	PHASE IV
HEALTHY WEIGHT	**OPTIMIZATION**	**LONGEVITY**

BMI <25	*BMI <25*	*BMI 21–24.9[5]*
Waist Circumference:	*Waist Circumference:*	*Waist Circumference:*
Male <37"	Male <35"	Male <32"
Female <31.5"	Female <31"	Female <29"
Body Fat(optional):[4]	*Body Fat (optional)*	*Body Fat (optional)*
Male <18%	Male <18%	Male <12%
Female <25%	Female <25%	Female 17–22%

The general guidelines for healthy weight is a body mass index (BMI) of 24.9 and a waist circumference of 31.5 inches for a woman, 37 inches for a man. Having a healthy fat composition is also important. It is age dependent but as a general guideline we will want to lower your body fat to less than 25% for women and 18% for men.

We will move you into eating healthy for life. This will lead you into the second MacroHabit: Healthy Eating and Hydration.

This is an exciting phase, as it is when we are modifying your food intake and energy expenditure to optimize your health and wellbeing for your age and lifestyle. We are also adding healthy motion, sleep, stress reduction, and other Habits of Health that support optimization.

In Part Three of the book, once you have optimized your health, we'll explore the things you can do to create Ultrahealth™ and potentially live a longer healthier life.

Let's get rid of some unhealthy fat and start bringing back your vibrancy and wellbeing!

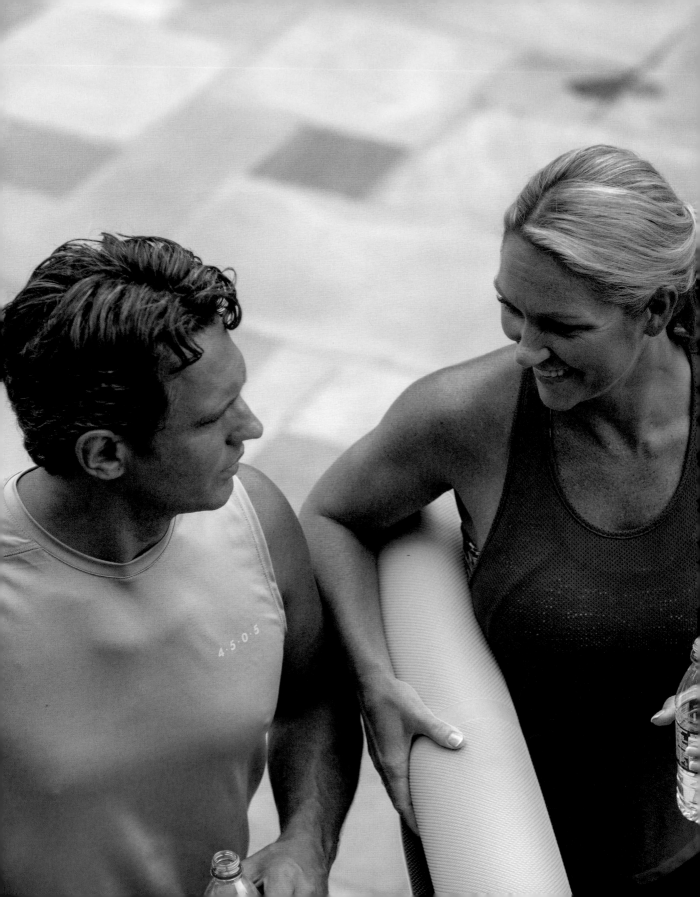

YOUR BLUEPRINT: SAFE WEIGHT LOSS AND HEALTH GAINS

If you've tried more than a few weight loss plans, you already know there are lots of suggestions on how to lose weight.

Many plans view weight loss as an end in itself. Any number of methods—low-carb or low-fat diets, medication, colonics, exercise boot camps—will sometimes get you to your destination and then drop you off. The problem with plans like these is that even if you do get through the deprivation involved and manage to lose weight, you almost immediately meander back to your old ways— like when a golf course tries to get rid of a flock of Canada Geese by moving them a few miles down the way. Sooner or later, they'll be back.

Other plans take a more conservative approach, advising you to eat sensibly and be more active. Well, that's great advice if you're already healthy and in shape. But the problem here is that the sort of subtle changes these programs recommend just don't make enough of a difference in the short term to give you the positive reinforcement you need to continue with them. The lure of fast food and a weekend on the couch are just too strong!

I've spent 17 years studying why most diets don't work on their own, and why most people never change. And as a result, I ask a very different question than most people do—not just "What is the most effective way to reach a healthy weight?" but "How can I go beyond weight loss to achieve optimal health and stay healthy for the rest of my life?"

I believe that the answer lies within our own bodies. After 38 years of medical practice, I still marvel at the human body's incredible ability to adapt to a wide range of physical, mental, and social conditions. Unfortunately, today's world is challenging these adaptations—overwhelming our defenses, eroding our health, and moving us down the path toward non-sickness—or worse. But one amazing human attribute can help us change direction: resiliency.

No matter how much we abuse our bodies, if we stop the assault of unhealthy habits and put ourselves back into position to function as we were designed, we can tap into the body's inherent capacity to heal itself. And what's the best tool we have for doing that? The food we eat! All the medicines and treatments in the world pale in comparison to the impact of a healthy eating strategy.

The healthy eating system you're about to learn is built around Habits of Health that give you the ability to control the quantity and quality of your food intake. Most people aren't able to master this most fundamental principle, even after a lifetime of struggle, because they're relying on their internal programming to select their food choices.

But as we've discussed, that programming—which was optimal for a time when we needed to grab and hoard every calorie—is no longer helping us. Today, unlike 10,000 years ago, we are surrounded with cheap, great tasting, energy dense but nutrient poor food. This highly processed food is flipping metabolic switches and creating an almost continuous state of fat accumulation.

And we lack the activity we need to dispose of all that excess energy. So, if we consume more than we need, which is almost always the case, the extra calories get stored away as fat. That fat around your middle is a symptom of an imbalance between your energy intake and energy output, with your intake set higher than it should be.

In this segment, we will first review why we have accumulated so much additional weight and then you will learn the fundamentals behind our healthy eating system—a system that was strategically developed to change your health rapidly, but with long-term health as the goal. And we're going to start by focusing on the central principles that will enable you to reach a healthy weight and set the stage for eating healthy for life.

> "Modern research has found that weight loss is more complicated than a simple energy in/energy out formula. The number of calories you consume plays a key role, but the quality of your fuelings is also important, and the Habits of Health Transformational System covers both ends of that spectrum."

HOW DO WE HELP YOU REACH A HEALTHY WEIGHT EFFECTIVELY?

As your body's boss, you need to fire your old energy management system. It's not working!

Eating a little healthier or walking a little more isn't going to get you to a healthy weight. The evil forces out there—tempting you with too many unhealthy calories and offering convenient ways to move that rob you of exercise—are just too powerful. We live in an instant-gratification society. If our pizza is not here in 30 minutes, it's free! If we have to wait more than five minutes for our Uber, we go crazy!

Nope. The steady-as-you-go approach just isn't going to work for most of us. It's certainly never worked for me. So instead, let's use your biological design to advantage and revamp your energy management system. We'll start by giving you a new simple eating strategy that will help you reach a healthy weight.

The strategy we are going to use will allow you to lose weight while keeping you from being hungry and eliminating your cravings for carbohydrates.

You will start losing weight safely and effectively and soon enough you will feel better and have more energy. Only then, once you are on your way to a healthier weight and you have some momentum will we start adding additional habits to assist you on your journey.

Now that the most efficient way for you to lose weight safely is to take advantage of the actual way your body manages its use of the food you consume on a daily basis.

And the operating principle of the *Habits of Health Transformational System* is always to use new habit formation so that every effort we make is designed to help you install a new habit so that it only has to be programmed once! The crazy thing about diets and other gimmicks is they want you to do something difficult for a restricted period of time. It's not sustainable.

And then when you cannot sustain this Spartan-like existence long term and your willpower lets you down, you find yourself quitting without leaving any lasting behavioral change. Remember in Part 1.5, *The Bedrock of Transformation: Successful Habit Installation*, we discussed that as we increase the degree of effort necessary it becomes much harder to sustain the behavior. We want to use microHabits so that you can incorporate these new behaviors consistently to transform how you act automatically.

Your experience is going to be very different. Unlike the yo-yo structure of dieting with its dismal track record, we will build a structure that supports every step of your journey.

The creative process and structural tension we learned earlier will advance you towards a healthy weight because we are going to build a series of small habits that, once installed, will serve you from now on. This all starts with you setting your goal that has reaching a healthy weight as your desired outcome.

Healthy weight is different for each and every one of us but here are some general guidelines to help you picture what that will look like for most. A healthy weight is a body mass index (BMI) of 24.9 and a waist circumference of under 31.5 inches for a female and 37 inches for a male. A healthy fat composition is also important. It is age dependent but, as a general guideline, we want to lower your body fat to less than 25% for women and 18% for men.

That may seem like a daunting task from where you sit (unless you're reading this standing up) but I have helped people lose as much as 700 lbs on their journey to optimal health and wellbeing. What we need to do is pay attention to what and how much you are eating and how it affects your body's storage and metabolic processes.

But don't worry because based on my experience of helping thousands of people through this process, you'll still have plenty of energy to carry you through the day. How is that possible? Well, we're going to use the abundant stores of energy in that extra fat around your tummy to turn you into a fat-burning machine! And to do that, we're going to alter your food intake to create a stable energy source. It's a process that taps into two core principles of energy management:

- Controlling your energy intake
- Managing your insulin pump

These principles form the basis of the healthy eating strategies we'll be learning in this weight-loss phase, and mastering them is, quite simply, the key to long-term success. Unless you can take control of how much, how often, and the quality of your food intake you will struggle to reach and sustain a healthy weight and body, as well as improving your overall wellbeing.

Let's take a look at a typical Western eating pattern and see what happens when these core principles are ignored.

Modern Life's Disease Path

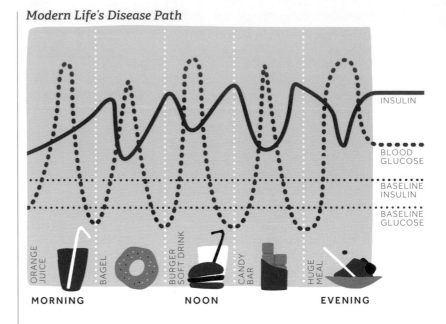

As you can see above, the typical Western diet of highly processed, high-glycemic foods—soft drinks, candy bars, bagels—causes blood sugar (also called blood glucose) to rise dramatically. And that makes the level of insulin rise. This elevated insulin level actually then causes blood sugar to plummet, creating the rapid rise and fall you see in the chart.

As blood sugar falls below normal, the brain sets off a series of messages that cause cravings and soon you're scrambling for something sweet and full of calories. And so the cycle of high and low blood sugar levels continues, thereby reinforcing eating patterns that lead to poor health and obesity.

When insulin levels stay elevated this way, the body continuously uses glucose for fuel, rather than both glucose and fat. And when it's not needed as fuel, all that extra energy—saturated excess sugar and saturated fat—is laid down in fat cells. In short, you become a fat-storage factory. That huge meal right before bed keeps your body in fat-storage mode through the night and disrupts your sleep, leading to even poorer eating habits and even more weight gain.

Let me build a visual model to illustrate the central role the management of your fat cells plays in all of this.

Your fat cells are called adipocytes—they are the body's energy depot. The other sources of energy that are in food, protein, and carbohydrates are not as efficient at storing energy.

So the ability to store fat was critical to our ability to survive and thrive 10,000 years ago. We evolved 40 billion fat cells that served us well in times of famine, and when we were carrying heavy workloads.

Because of the constant accessibility of excess calories, especially in processed food full of sugar, flour, fats, and salt, we have created a gross imbalance in the normal balance of energy management.

Ask yourself these questions to see if your body is currently getting its energy by burning fat or by using quick carbohydrates:

1. *Do you eat a lot of refined, processed foods and drinks?*
2. *Do you have a hard time concentrating or staying focused?*
3. *Do you skip meals and end up eating only one or two a day?*
4. *Do you struggle with cravings and low blood sugar?*
5. *Are you irritable if meals are missed or delayed?*
6. *Do you struggle with mid-morning or afternoon slumps?*
7. *Do you have difficulty staying asleep?*

If you answered yes to more than a couple, you probably have a high level of insulin that's keeping you in fat-storage mode and creating weight gain. The following illustration demonstrates what is happening inside your body:

Habits of Disease Weight Gain State: Expanding Waistline

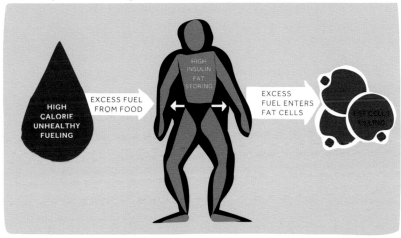

As you can see, the unhealthy fuelings of the American diet are adding excess calories from poor quality nutrients such as sugar, flour, saturated fats, and other high glycemic carbohydrates, while also raising your blood sugar and increase insulin production. The higher insulin production drives energy into the fat cells and the normal balance is disrupted and it is difficult to obtain energy when needed from the fat cells between meals.

Dr. David Ludwig from Harvard, described as an "obesity warrior", has gone as far as stating that the fat cells in this high-insulin state are hoarding energy and, in effect, creating a one-way turnstile where the insulin is ushering calories into fat cells but restricting the passage back out. Consequently, the body runs low on accessible energy within a few hours of eating. When the brain senses a lack of available energy, it transmits a call for help, setting up a cycle

Our bodies are efficient fat storage machines because food sources were difficult to find for our ancestors. Where we can easily open the refrigerator for a snack, our ancestors may have had to go long intervals between meals, so our bodies adapted to the challenge by saving up energy to be used during these lean times.

of constant hunger. Inactivity, lack of sleep, and stress make the situation worse and further demonstrate why the Habits of Health are so interdependent.

How can you break that cycle? Let's look at a study that offers some clues to a new, better way of eating that also happens to be a core Habit of Health.

THE MYTH OF THREE SQUARES

A study by David Jenkins, MD, PhD— the University of Toronto pioneer in low-glycemic eating—demonstrates that eating small portions at frequent intervals is good for your health in a number of important, and even remarkable, ways.[1, 2]

The researchers divided their subjects into two groups. Both ate exactly the same food with the exact same number of calories. But one group ate their food divided into the usual three meals a day. The other ate more often, consuming lots of little meals.

Surprisingly, the group that ate small meals throughout the day lost more weight. It wasn't that they were less hungry (although, in fact, they were less hungry). They lost weight because their blood sugar didn't continually spike and then dip down to an even lower level, the way it does after a big meal. Their glycemic levels—the amount of sugar in their blood—remained steady and their cravings for sweet foods went down.

That's not all. After only two weeks, they found that the people who ate every three hours reduced their blood cholesterol by over 15% and their blood insulin by almost 28%. That's key because, in addition to regulating your blood sugar level, insulin plays a pivotal role in fat metabolism, inflammation, and the progression to metabolic syndrome. When your body produces less insulin, you're much less likely to convert dietary calories into body fat. Your body begins to work differently, and you're no longer the fat factory you once were.

So what does this study tell us? That it's not just what you eat, it's also when you eat it. Small amounts of nourishment throughout the day are better than the same amount of food concentrated into three big hits. If we feed the body at regular intervals, we send a signal to the body that it doesn't have to store calories.[3]

Conversely, when we skip meals, we send just the opposite signal for the body to store calories, thereby creating a negative effect on our metabolism.

Eating satisfies our ancient programming, prevents activating the alarms of starvation, and turns off fat storage. It's our modern-day version of hunting and gathering! And by adding low-glycemic foods to meals, and making them more like our ancient diet, we do even more to control blood sugar and turn off the insulin pump that leads to fat storage—fat that's crippling our health and leading directly to disease.

We pioneered the use of the glycemic index as a practical method of helping turning off insulin and shifting the body away from fat storage over 10 years ago. Ludwig's—a leading researcher and nutritional expert from Harvard Medical School—published a book two years ago, *Always Hungry*, that reinforces the power of glycemic index. It's the principle index he uses to help people lose weight without hunger.

Now we know that eating smaller, low-glycemic meals is a great way to turn off insulin and provide healthier fuel for our body, what else can help us achieve long-term weight loss?

PATTERNS OF SUCCESS

In the introduction, you learned that over 85% of people who go on a diet without other behavioral support fail.[4,5] By some estimates, more than 80% of people who have lost weight regained all of it, or more, after two years. Researchers at the University of California at Los Angeles analyzed 31 long-term diet studies and found that about two-thirds of dieters regained more weight within four or five years than they initially lost.

On the flipside, that means that just under 15% succeed. What can we learn from them? Studies provide some intriguing answers. In one of the most impressive, led by Dr. James Hill and Dr. Rena Wing from the National Weight Control Registry, researchers gathered data from over 10,000 individuals, many of whom lost over 65 lbs and kept the weight off for at least five years. The weight-loss methods varied, but what these individuals had in common were certain core practices that have proven critical to successfully and safely maintaining a healthy weight. Here's what they did:

- They ate breakfast.
- They ate a balanced diet, paying close attention to the amount of dietary fat and calories.
- They increased their physical activity quite a bit.
- They monitored their weight regularly.[6]

So we want to add breakfast, lower the fat content of our food, make sure it is nutrient dense, become more physically active, and monitor ourselves for early warnings of weight regain. These scientifically proven fundamentals are crucial components of our weight-loss and long-term optimal eating strategy. Let's put these healthy behaviors all together and see how that strategy looks.

THE KEY TO HEALTHY WEIGHT LOSS

What's the key to successful mastery of both weight loss and long-term health? There are really two main food intake components:

The Science of Six Fuelings

What are the benefits of eating a small amount of food more often? Preliminary research supports the idea that when the typical "three squares" diet is replaced by smaller, more frequent meals. It can:

- Help you lose weight
- Control hunger
- Reduce blood insulin (a factor in fat storage and inflammation)
- Lower total cholesterol levels
- Reduce LDL ("bad") cholesterol
- Reduce levels of apolipo-protein B (the "very bad" stuff!)
- depress glucose levels
- Increase bile acid secretion
- Suppress free fatty acids levels
- Reduce serum uric acid levels, a common risk factor for coronary artery disease
- Increase uric acid excretion
- Reduce adipose tissue enzyme levels
- Reduce fluctuations in satiety (fullness)[7-10]

Why Exercise Alone Won't Help You Lose Weight

Trying to fight fat with exercise? You may want to rethink your strategy.

When you take in more calories than you expend, especially if they are from highly processed junk foods the excess gets stored as fat. There are 3,500 calories in one pound. Eating just 100 extra calories a day—a bagel, a candy bar, a soda—translates to 36,500 calories of excess energy over the course of a year. Even if your body stores only half of that, the result is over five extra pounds of fat a year!

You could try burning those excess calories through exercise alone. But in order to burn just one pound, you'd have to run 33.8 miles. Just for one pound! And nearly one-third of us have an extra 30 lbs of fat. To burn that much, you'd have to run 1,040 miles or 40 marathons.

1. The ability to master the amount of fuel you take in
2. The quality of that fuel

If we can devise a plan that delivers lower-calorie, nutrient-dense foods in the proper proportions, we have a recipe for success.

How does it work? Well, portion size is key. When you eat healthy foods—low-glycemic carbohydrates, healthy fats, and high-quality protein—in smaller portions than your body is used to, a magical transformation occurs. As you lower your total calories and turn off insulin by avoiding high sugar, flour, and other high glycemic foods your body turns to plan "B" and begins to utilize the unhealthy fat around your middle to make up the deficit. Remember that 10,000-year-old programming we discussed? That storage system of fat begins to be used as it was intended, providing your body with a constant source of calories while signaling it to turn off insulin, hunger, and cravings for carbohydrates.

And there's another great benefit. By providing your body with these nutrient-dense, protein-rich fuelings in small portions throughout the day, you protect your muscles from being cannibalized, unlike in some low-calorie weight-loss programs. But that doesn't mean you won't see results. In fact, you can expect to lose weight safely and may reduce hunger and cravings.

This efficient, safe platform not only carries you through your initial weight-loss phase, it also sets the stage for a whole new pattern of healthy eating for life. Let's see how your body's going to respond to this new healthy fueling strategy.

Your New Eating Pattern for Weight Loss and Health

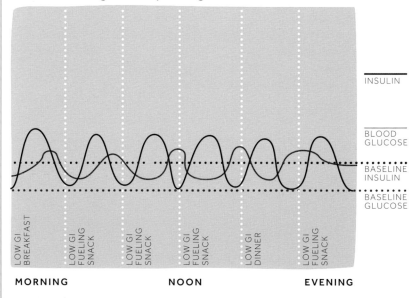

That's a whole different picture than before (see Modern Life's Disease

Path, page 180). First, we've reduced your total energy intake by introducing smaller, portion-controlled meals and snacks. Second, we've switched to low-glycemic meals that keep your blood sugar and insulin levels from spiking. This constant, stable energy source means no more wild swings in blood sugar. You've turned off your insulin pump and taken control of cravings.

The next illustration shows the shift in energy now *flowing out* of the fat cells. Your fat cells will be in this state for the amount of time it takes to reach your healthy weight. Hopefully you can see why your waist circumference will become smaller and your percentage of body fat will decrease as we empty your fat cells and eliminate this unhealthy condition.

Leptogenic:
Your Brave New World

Leptogenic comes from the Latin word "lepto", meaning thin or slender. It's the opposite of the obesigenic world we've been living in!

Habits of Health Weight Loss State: Shrinking Waistline

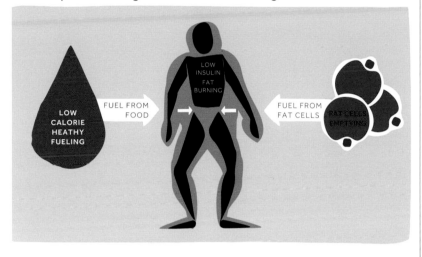

Eating this way—every three hours, starting with a healthy breakfast—helps you build a whole new energy management system that disperses energy throughout the day in accordance with your body's natural design. And once you begin to use energy more efficiently, your body quickly starts to offload excess calories, producing the perfect internal environment for hunger control and weight loss.

That's the science behind our plan, but how will this translate to your daily life?

THE LOGISTICS OF HEALTHY EATING

Can you eat every three hours? If so, you can change your life. Let me help you figure out how to fit this meal schedule easily into your day. This is the schedule you'll use during the weight-loss phase. If you are using our fueling system already, all of the times represent a fueling, except your dinner which is your lean and green meal. We will unpack this in the next part.

First, eat a healthy breakfast within 30 minutes of rising, say at 7:00 in the morning. Three hours later, eat a little something else. And so on, throughout the day:

- 7:00 breakfast
- 10:00 nourishment
- 1:00 nourishment (or small lunch)
- 4:00 nourishment
- 7:00 dinner
- 9:30–10:00 small nourishment

You'll see that our plan includes a healthy evening meal. It may be smaller than the standard American dinner of enough meat and potatoes to feed an army. But the good news is that your body won't want a big meal. You'll be satisfied with a modest amount of healthy food because your body's desires will have changed. And this is where your App will be extremely helpful as a reminder and to keep track.

Like many of our patients and clients, you may think you don't have time. It takes too much effort to prepare meals. It's inconvenient. It doesn't fit your lifestyle. Don't worry as I've got you covered. In the next part, you'll learn about an amazing technology that's going to help. In my many years of practice, I have yet to encounter a single person who wasn't able to make this plan work once I showed them how.

By planning your meals in advance and making sure to have healthy fuelings with you wherever you go, the program is actually quite easy to manage logistically. More importantly, it's easy to manage biologically and that's the point. You want your body to cooperate with you, which won't happen if it's starving.

In our plan, you won't feel hunger pangs. You won't feel the lack of anything. You'll feel satisfied. You'll feel in control again. And, as a bonus, you'll begin to restore your sense of taste and learn to experience the flavors of food in new and exciting ways. And all this while losing weight.

CREATING A MICROENVIRONMENT OF HEALTH: YOUR NEW LEPTOGENIC SURROUNDINGS

In Parts 1.3–1.6, you learned how to develop an internal framework focused on the motivation and choices that support your goal

mHoH

The color blue has been shown to decrease appetite, while red and yellow increase it. If you introduce more blues into your kitchen, perhaps with a fresh coat of paint, you can influence your appetite in a positive way.

of optimal health. Now we're going to begin supplementing that healthy internal environment with the healthy environment we talked about in Part 1.7, *Optimizing Your Surroundings: Creating Your Microenvironment of Health*. This brave new world—what I call a leptogenic world—supports optimally healthy, fit individuals.

> **Leptogenic:** *Adjective. (comparative more leptogenic, superlative most leptogenic) Causing weight loss or creating thinness.*

Here's how we're going to start building it. From the moment we get up in the morning until the time we hit the pillow at night, somebody or something is tempting us to eat. This world of nutritional pollution is hard to ignore.

It all goes back to our development as a species. Over the course of many thousands of years, our brains perfected a system that rewards behavior it deems essential to our survival. Food gives us sensations of pleasure, which we've learned to anticipate and seek out. In fact, food—especially high-calorie junk food filled with fat and sugar—affects our brain receptors in just the same way that drugs and alcohol do. Back in our ancestors' day, this was an important survival mechanism.

High-density foods were rare, and it was always in our best interest to eat as much of them as possible. But even today, this conditioning is so strong that we're stimulated by the mere hint of food—just by being in certain environments or around smells that we associate with eating.

What's the take-home message? In your kitchen, you have a 100% chance of finding food. But today, unlike in the past, it's not helping you survive. In fact, it's harming you.

You need to change the inventory, bring in the Hazmat team, detoxify, and outwit your ancient hardwiring, especially in the beginning when your new Habits of Health aren't yet automatic. In essence, you need to build a microenvironment that gives you the best chance of success—a protective bubble of health.

As we proceed, I'll teach you additional techniques to support your new healthy world. By the time you've reached your target weight, you'll be armed inside and out with the motivation, structure, and daily choices you need to maintain optimal health.

There is a tremendous discrepancy and confusion on what is healthy to eat—low-carb, high-carb, low-fat, high-fat—as well as all kinds of theories and conflicting information. Exhausting debates on calories are not the same, and the same goes for the battle between saturated versus unsaturated fat and it goes on and on.

Let me touch on the quality and types of food that are supported by current science as being healthy.

Do Low Fat Diets Cause Weight-Gain?
Absolutely not. What causes weight-gain is the consumption of a highly processed Western diet. Over the last three decades in an attempt to decrease the epidemic of obesity, the emphasis on lowering fat in our diet guided conventional wisdom. A gram of fat is more

than twice as many calories than carbohydrate and protein. The food industry—which is always looking to capitalize on the emotions of consumers and make greater profits (see Part 1.1, *It's Not Your Fault That You're Struggling*)—took the fat out of processed foods.

To replace it, they had two choices: to add protein or to add carbs. Since carbs are dirt cheap and readily available, they loaded up with sugary, starchy fat-free products, like Snackwell's, and the low-fat craze was born. As you now know, excessive calories from refined sugar and flours turned us into fat factories and weight gain and chronic disease are the result.

The point is macronutrient manipulation has no meaningful affect on weight management. We thought that we reduced the amount of fat ingestion but we didnt, we kept that the same, we just increased the amount of unhealthy carbohydrates.

Are Carbohydrates the Enemy?

Low glycemic carbohydrates from plants in their natural state are an amazing source of all kinds of nutrients. Fruits, vegetables, legumes, nuts, seeds, dairy, and some grains are part of some of the healthiest diets on earth. It is the processing that refines the sugar and flour and fills the shelves with massive amounts of unhealthy calories that creates a weight management nightmare. This industrialization, and the creation of food science, has moved us from whole, complex food into refined, simple, and disease-inducing foods that are slowly killing us.

So is Higher Fat Now Recommended?

Only if you do not want to lose weight and be healthy! Yes, we do want to consume a reasonable amount of healthy fats. Olive oil, coconut oil (now recommended), medium chain triglycerides, avocado, nuts, seeds, and of course the oil from healthy fish in moderation are all wonderful. But they still have nine calories per gram and if eaten in large quantities you will probably gain weight!

Stay away from partially hydrogenated fats, and lower your consumption of vegetable and seed oils, such as soybean, sunflower, corn, and canola oil.

Do the Amount of Calories I Consume Matter?

I wish I could give you a hall pass, but as your Dad told you when you were a kid, if it sounds too good to be true it probably is!

Unlike the zealots who would like to discard the First Law of Thermodynamics, your total calorie intake still affects your weight management system.

Yes, it does matter where you get your calories from. A large leafy salad with a drizzle of olive oil and balsamic vinegar is better than a Snickers bar. But you already knew that.

I assure you that both during the weight loss and the Healthy Eating MacroHabit installations, you will have a variety of tasty, filling, diverse, easy to prepare choices that you will be able to eat for the rest of your healthy days.

And we are going to help you naturally increase your daily motion so you can offset any extra calories you do consume.

There's much more to come! But for now, let's set you up for success by giving your house a health makeover. This is helping build the Habit of Healthy Surroundings.

Note: These are general guidelines for converting to healthy surroundings for long-term health, which address all of the concerns expressed above. Depending on which plan you select to use during your weight-loss phase we will have more specific guidelines.

REDUCE YOUR REFRIGERATOR AND FREEZER

Begin by bringing a trash can over to the refrigerator. Get ready to dump the following foods, take them to the local food bank, or give them to your neighbors, depending how much you like them!

Here's what needs to go from freezer:

- frozen fruit with added sugar
- frozen vegetables with seasoning that contain sugar
- orange juice, lemonade, other fruit concentrates
- bread, rolls, etc.
- frozen entrees containing rice and pasta
- frozen pizza
- frozen desserts, ice cream, sorbets, cakes, cookies

Now fill your freezer back up with:

- frozen vegetables like broccoli, spinach, cauliflower, green beans
- unsweetened fruits like blueberries, peaches, raspberries, strawberries
- frozen shrimp, fish, seafood without sauces/sugar
- lean beef, poultry
- veggie burgers from soy, beans, no refined grains, potatoes, or sugar products

Here's what needs to go from the fridge:

- whole-fat dairy products such as milk, cheese, yogurt, butter, cottage cheese, and mayonnaise
- processed deli meats, bacon, hot dogs
- sugary sodas and juices
- beer and wine
- foods high in calories, fat, or sugar, including peanut butter, jellies, and salad dressings (except low fat and low calorie)
- sweet pickles, relish, ketchup
- puddings, applesauce

"Now that you are cleaning out the pantry and stocking up on healthy snacks, it's a great time to teach your kids to eat healthy too."

Now fill your fridge back up with:

- fat-free or low-fat dairy products such as skim or soy milk, low-fat cottage cheese, and low-fat yogurt
- low-fat protein sources such as lean chicken and meats, tofu, hummus, and eggs
- fresh fruits and vegetables (and frozen fruits and vegetables for the freezer)
- condiments such as mustards, pickles, and vinegars
- mineral water, sparkling water, unsweetened ice tea
- olives, capers,
- herbs and spices, hummus

PERK UP YOUR PANTRY

Get rid of the tempting foods that could sabotage your healthy eating choices (and don't use this time to finish off that bag of cookies you find!) If you have children or teenagers, this is a great chance to help them eat healthier too. But if you must keep foods for them in the house that don't fit your plan, put them in a low, out-of-the-way cupboard, and don't go near them!

Start by getting rid of:

- white rice, white flour, and white bread, crackers, rice cakes, croutons, and breadcrumbs
- hydrogenated vegetable oils, including hard or semi-soft margarine and shortenings (such as Crisco), partially hydrogenated oils
- white potato, potato mix, cornmeal, and corn grits,
- refined cereals (whole-grain is okay) and flavored oatmeal
- cookies, candy, cakes, and muffins
- chips, crackers, pretzels, and popcorn

Now fill your pantry back up with:

- brown rice
- canola and olive oil
- natural, non-flavored oatmeal
- whole-grain, high-fiber breads, and pitas
- whole-wheat flour
- walnuts, almonds, and beans
- a variety of spices and herbs
- tea, coffee, and unsweetened cocoa
- seeds (chia, flax, and sunflower)
- oils (avocado, olive, safflower, coconut, and sesame)

CLEAN UP YOUR KITCHEN AND YOUR KITCHEN BEHAVIORS

As well as the food in your freezer, refrigerator, and the food you keep in your pantry, there are other simple actions you can take to create healthier surroundings in your kitchen and at the dinner table. Apart from banning smartphones at mealtimes, here are some other good behaviors:

- Put away any cookie jars or food triggers that are sitting out on the counter.
- Smaller plates support smaller portions. Put your regular dinner plates in the back of your cupboard and bring out the six to nine-inch salad plates.
- Never stand or walk while you're eating. Take the time to sit down at the table.
- Buy some blue placemats and plates. The color blue has been proven to decrease appetite, while yellow and red increase it. Guess where the inspiration for the golden arches came from, and why the interiors of many fast food restaurants are yellow, gold, or red. It's because they make you salivate, increase your appetite, and tempt you to buy their fat and grease-laden food!
- Never use serving bowls on the table. Plate your meals in the kitchen (using nine-inch plates).
- Turn up the wattage! Bright lights have been shown to make us eat less.
- Read in Element 07 of *Your Lifebook, Creating a New Leptogenic World,* many more things you can do such as:
  - Colored plates: When your plate color contrasts with your food the size of the portions sticks out and we sense we are eating more. When they blend in the amount does not register and we eat more. Buying green plates makes sense as its okay to eat bigger portions of green vegetables.
  - During the weight-loss phase filling half your plate with vegetables can help create fullness.

HEALTHY SURROUNDINGS: READY YOUR BEDROOM

Creating an environment that optimizes sleep quality is critical to good health. In fact, several studies confirm that poor sleep directly contributes to poor eating habits. We'll spend considerable time in Phase II on this MacroHabit and I will give you some tips but, for right now, here are a few simple steps to make your bedroom more conducive to healthy sleeping:

This system sets you up for a lifetime of healthy eating, with all of the knowledge and strategies you need for success.

- Organize your bedroom and put away clutter.
- If you have a TV in your bedroom, remove or unplug it.
- Choose a bedtime that means you get eight hours of sleep and stick with it.
- Keep your room cool while you sleep.
- Never eat in bed.

See Element 19 of *Your LifeBook, How Do You Create Healthy Sleep and Unlimited Energy?*, if sleeping is a current issue for you.

CREATE A JOURNAL: USE YOUR LIFEBOOK AS YOUR DAILY COMPANION

I designed *Your LifeBook* as the instrument to use as a daily companion for the next 12 months and beyond to document and progress with your new optimal health and wellbeing story. Many people, including myself, have just never been into keeping a journal. *Your LifeBook* is a great start to writing down things that you learn about yourself along the way to better life. It has lots of stuff that will help you as you get started and makes it easy to track things that you find specifically important for you.

In addition, it has a daily and monthly tracker that you can use to create your own journal.

Keeping a journal of everything you eat can give you further insight into your current behaviors and eating habits. You can also get one when you're out buying your new groceries and you can download the daily and monthly tracker at our website, www.HabitsofHealth.com.

YOUR WEIGHT-LOSS STRATEGY

My years of experience as a physician helping people who have previously struggled with losing and maintaining a healthy weight have taught me what works in the real world. I'm not going to teach you theory based on some laboratory findings, or marketing department hype. The specific eating strategy I'm about to describe works because it's practical, cost-effective, and it provides consistent weight loss. It delivers the simplicity of a turnkey system that helps you get results quickly, and it's easy to learn. It allows you to lose weight as you build a practical plan to eat healthy for life.

There are actually two approaches which I'm about to describe that differ in the time, effort, and skills they require to master. Combining them into an overall strategy allows you the time necessary to learn the Habits of Health while you reach your healthy weight. I want to bring you along at a pace that relates to your level of cooking experience and your understanding of healthy food choices.

Learning both of these strategies will arm you with the best possible preparation to create the outcome we want—long-term success. You'll be able to pick and choose from a compendium of tools that provide you with several options based on your current weight, time availability, and even personality.

Both components of our overall eating strategy work in synergy and share these important features:

- They're based on two core principles of energy management for safe weight loss.
- They both set the stage for all the other Habits of Health.
- They contain important techniques you can incorporate into your daily habits as you build the tools, skills, and techniques for long-term success.
- Both approaches have been studied extensively at major universities around the world and have extensive research to support their efficacy and safety.
- They offer simple, straightforward ways to fuel your body efficiently, lower your energy intake, turn off your insulin pump, and put you in fat-burning state.
- Both allow you to choose from diverse, satisfying, and balanced foods for sustainable weight loss.
- Both focus on foods that are low glycemic and which contain healthy carbohydrates, healthy fats, and healthy proteins.
- With each method, you'll eat breakfast every morning and continue to eat every three hours throughout the day.
- They provide the versatility to customize a plan that fits your lifestyle.

Let's spend a little time discussing both of these approaches to our overall strategy and see how they apply directly to you.

THE CATALYST TO REACHING A HEALTHY WEIGHT: PACKAGED FUELINGS

For quick, effective weight loss without a lot of preparation, scientifically formulated, low-calorie portion-controlled meals offer a convenient, ready-to-use food system in the form of prepackaged, low-glycemic meals. In fact, the success of these systems is well documented in the medical literature.

As I mentioned previously, I have considerable experience using packaged fuelings to help people lose weight. I've found them to be a powerful tool that consistently delivers predictable weight loss by relying on a specific nutritional footprint. Because they're so easy to use and fit so nicely into a busy lifestyle, I highly recommend them. In fact, for people who need to lose more than a few pounds, this is the tool I use to ensure that they get a strong start as they begin their journey on the road to optimal health.

How Does it Work?

The nutritional footprint of prepackaged portion-controlled meals provide a low-glycemic, healthy-protein mixture that enables you to safely and comfortably lower your caloric intake when you eat them in place of traditional meals. They're also fortified with vitamins and minerals. Once a day, at a time that works for you, you'll have a prepared meal with a healthy portion of lean meat, poultry, or fish, along with a salad or your choice of vegetable. This combination allows your body to rapidly enter a reliable mild fat-burning state that produces safe, effective weight loss.

In Short...

Prepackaged fuelings are convenient and effective. As you're learning to eat healthy for the first time, the ease and fast results of this ready-to-go approach are very appealing. As you learn the fundamentals of healthy eating, they enable you to grasp the principles of low-glycemic eating and menu choice gradually in bite-sized pieces. We'll also use them as a convenient, high-quality (and tasty) portable fuel as part of our long-term healthy eating strategy.

DR. A'S HEALTHY EATING SYSTEM: A LOW-GLYCEMIC PORTION-CONTROL APPROACH TO SUPPORT OPTIMAL HEALTH

This simple, straightforward approach to shopping, preparing, and cooking healthy meals makes nourishing your body every three hours easy and convenient. I will teach you everything you need to develop an eating strategy that will last a lifetime. If you have only a few pounds to lose or are already at a healthy weight, this easy system will help you maintain your weight and can be used with the scientifically formulated, low-calorie fuelings to give you the best of both worlds.

How Does it Work?

You'll utilize the principle of low-glycemic eating to shut off excess insulin secretion and turn off fat storage as we discussed earlier that is key to releasing stored fat and it will turn you from a fat storage to a fat burning machine.

This plan gives you everything you need to control portion size and lower your intake of calories, including a unique color-coded system to make shopping for healthy foods stress free. You'll find information on selecting acceptable carbohydrates, proper fats, and proteins that work together to promote weight loss, as well as flexible menu choices that make meals fun. I'll even teach you to use a portable cooker to prepare delicious, easy meals wherever your busy day takes you!

In Short...

This healthy eating system teaches you how to make good choices and prepare healthy meals from day one. It's going to take a little practice, but, once you have it mastered, you'll have a complete eating strategy for life. If you take the time to learn this system while you're losing weight on the prepackaged fuelings, you'll be in perfect position to transition into my permanent healthy eating strategy once you reach a healthy weight. If you're already close to your goal weight, you can simply adopt my healthy eating system, which includes prepackaged fuelings right out of the gate.

THE TEACHABLE MOMENT

Now that we've described your weight-loss strategy, I encourage you to jump right in! In just a week or so, as you start to lose weight, you'll see substantial improvement in your physical and mental health. You'll feel better, have more energy, sleep better, and may begin to reduce medications for certain weight-related health conditions. Soon, you may also notice an improvement in your thinking, your memory, and your desire to learn more. It's the period I call the teachable moment, and it's the best building block I've found for long-term success. It's the moment when the Habits of Health truly begin to take root!

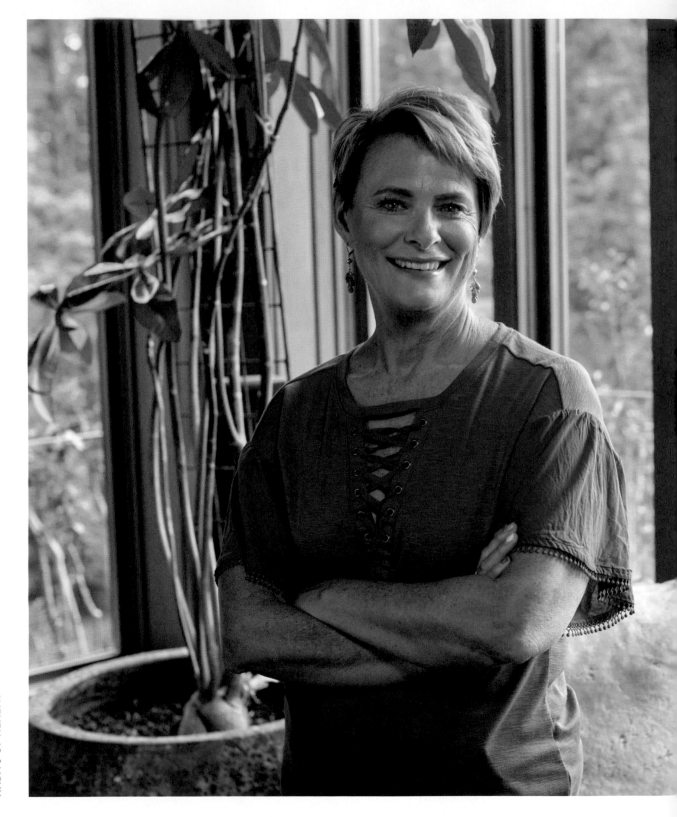

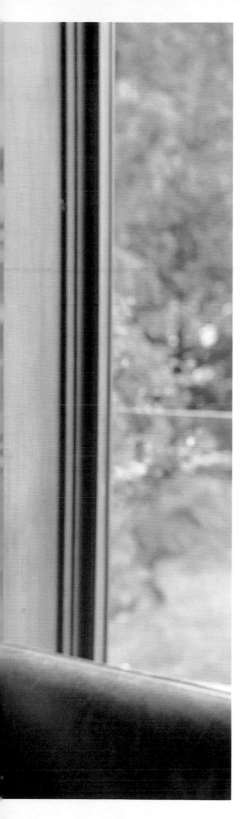

TRANSFORMATION: PATTI GLICK

I actually started my health journey back in June of 2008. I wasn't the example to my patients that I wanted to be, and I couldn't create the health that I wanted to create for myself. So how could I even have the tools to be able to help my patients? I've been struggling with my weight and my health for about 19 years, and it seems that no matter what I did, something always happened where I just hit a wall and quit, and I couldn't figure out why.

Then I found the Habits of Health, and all of a sudden, the pieces of the puzzle came together. My husband and I did our journey together. We lost a combined 99 lbs.* And more importantly, we really developed a change of mindset. We learned a different way of thinking, a different way of being, a different way of making choices, and a different way of living.

I learned what healthy eating looked like. I learned how to hydrate my body and why that was important. I learned that I didn't have to be crazy at the gym in order to incorporate healthy motion in my life, but that I could do the things that gave me joy: hike with my family, water ski, snow ski, do the things that really involved motion. And when I started doing that and actually having fun doing that, it made me want more.

For me, the Habits of Health made a difference because I wasn't on the journey alone. Having that coach, which I was a little bit resistant to in the beginning, helped me to look at things differently. When you partner with someone who shows you a different way, it opens up a whole new world. I learned different ways to find out where my struggle areas and unhealthy habits were. Once I could identify them and had the support of my coach and all of the education and support pieces that went along, that made all the difference in the world.

When you change the way you look at things, the things you look at change. And that's what the Habits of Health Transformational System gave me. It's the opportunity to change the way I looked at things, and the choices that I made in my life really changed where my outcome was going to be.

> " *I wasn't the example to my patients that I wanted to be, and I couldn't create the health that I wanted to create for myself.* "

*Average weight loss on the Optimal Weight 5 & 1 Plan® is 12 lbs.

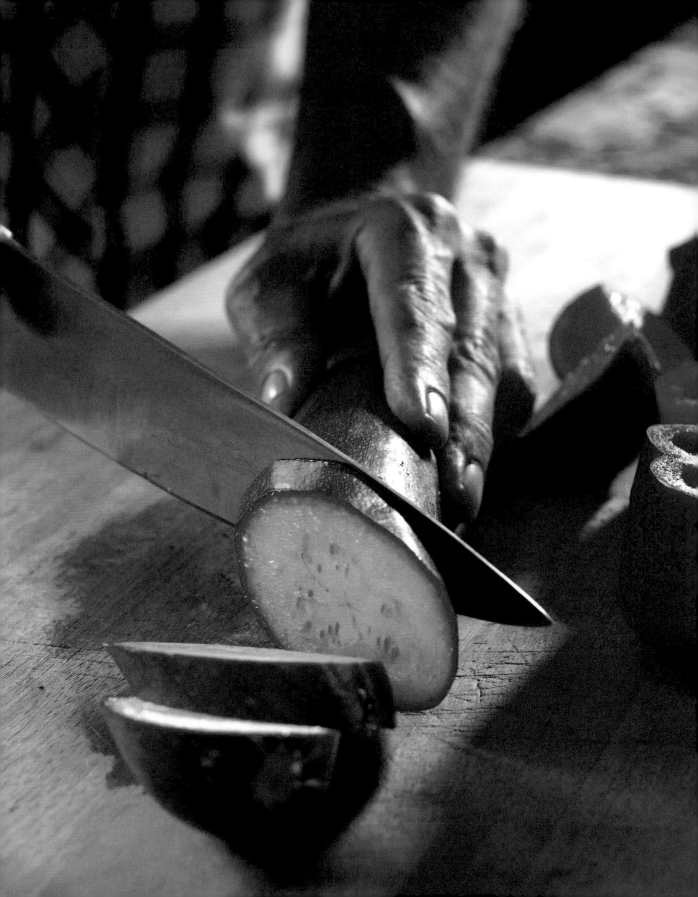

THE CATALYST TO REACHING A HEALTHY WEIGHT: HEALTHY FUELINGS

In this part, I am going to outline the system I have found most effective to help people who need to lose a lot of weight. This plan will get you results right out of the gate and give me time to teach you my healthy eating system.

We'll use this incredible tool to help you lose weight and begin your journey toward optimal health. Then, in Part 2.4, Dr. A's Healthy Eating System, I'll outline my healthy eating plan, which will empower you to have complete command over your eating environment. You will learn a comprehensive approach that provides the techniques, shopping methods, and a meal plan that will deliver your body a full array of healthy food. But first, let me describe this tool that I use daily to help people start their journey to optimal health. If you're still a little skeptical, keep reading and you'll learn how easy it is to get going.

HEALTHY FUELINGS: CATALYST TO SUCCESS

A lot has changed since portion-controlled meal replacements (PCMRS) were first developed in the 1970s. Originally created to spur weight loss in extremely obese, high-risk patients, PCMRS provide specific combinations of nutrients in small dose-controlled portions that protect lean muscle while burning fat.

Patients in those days received all their nutrients from these packets, often taking in as few as 300 calories a day. PCMRS were extremely efficient at helping patients lose weight, but they were also criticised especially when used long term. Medical experts complained that those early PCMRS didn't teach people healthy eating habits. Patients also found PCMRS expensive and restrictive.

Fast forward to today. Medically proven low-calorie portion-controlled meal replacements have undergone significant improvements in the last few decades. In fact, I truly believe that they're on the verge of becoming an overnight sensation, or at least an integral part of many of our lives. Why? Because they're a powerful tool—not as a complete diet in and of themselves, but as part of a comprehensive approach to healthy eating. And one that's coming just in the nick of time.

Our fast-paced society puts tremendous demands on us. As a result, we're facing a deterioration of our health that's just not sustainable. We need a breakthrough!

Now, I realize that meal replacements alone can't do the trick. As I've already discussed, isolated weight-control strategies that don't address the whole person and their unhealthy lifestyle are universally unsuccessful. In fact, there's not one documented case of a stand-alone diet, drug, or dietary supplement that has brought about consistent, sustained weight control over the long term by itself. A well-orchestrated comprehensive approach that includes lifestyle change and proper support is extremely effective in sustaining long-term health.

The *Habits of Health Transformational System* is such an approach. One of the most critical components of the Habits of Health is eating small, healthy meals throughout the day that are portion-controlled and low glycemic. But, for many of us, finding the time and energy to prepare these meals can be daunting. And then there's the learning curve. Teaching you to fix healthy, low-glycemic meals is one of my most important goals, but I'm also a realist. I know, for example, that most of you have never programmed your microwave, and that the LED clock is probably still blinking. We just have too much on our plates—no pun intended!

Today, more than ever, we need an easy, straightforward approach to healthy eating and energy management—a catalyst to get the ball rolling. Think of yourself as a jet on the runway. Takeoff requires a huge amount of energy, but once you've reached your cruising altitude you can settle down into a comfortable rhythm. Healthy fuelings will help you get to altitude by minimizing the effort of planning meals

"Healthy fuelings are a powerful tool as part of a comprehensive approach to healthy eating."

2.3

and making a lot of choices at the beginning. And before you know it, you'll be cruising toward health.

I know this from experience because I could never seem to find the time to eat healthy. I was standing still, getting heavier and heavier, until one day I started looking for answers and found the technology of fuelings. And that made all the difference!

MY OWN JOURNEY WITH FUELINGS

As a critical care physician working as many as 110 hours some weeks, I was eating and living the Habits of Disease. Up at 5:00 a.m., grab a glass of high- glycemic orange juice (like many of you, I thought that was a healthy start to my day!), and off to the hospital. By 10:00 a.m. I was ravenous from hypoglycemia as a result of my sugar-laden OJ, so I'd satisfy those cravings by sneaking a piece of candy from a patient's nightstand. I was never short on high-glycemic ways to elevate my blood sugar enough to get through the next surgery. Add in long hours, 10:00 p.m. dinners, poor sleep, not enough exercise, and soon enough I started gaining weight—27 lbs, nicely concealed by the drawstring of my scrubs.

I was heading down the path to disease. So, I decided to do something about it. But I realized that I had no idea how to change my bad habits to healthy ones. I didn't really understand how to eat healthy and, besides, I had no time to cook. That's when I discovered prepackaged low-calorie meals. And thankfully, they helped me lose that accumulated weight in a relatively short period of time.

Now I've enjoyed 17 years at a healthy weight, I get eight hours sleep a night, and I have plenty of time to spend with family and friends. Whether in the format of healthy fuelings or whole foods, I eat a low-glycemic menu every day. I've gotten pretty good at picking healthy foods both at home and when I'm out to eat. I am actually getting great at fixing a large salad now that the lettuce comes prewashed, already cut, and I just throw in some cut veggies, walnuts, and drizzle a little extra virgin olive oil and vinegar and I am good to go.

It is the prepackaged low-calorie fuelings that have made all the difference. These fuelings are especially helpful when I'm busy, on the road, or just feeling lazy. Grabbing a prepackaged low-calorie meal that has a nutritional footprint, which ensures my body is getting a healthy fueling, without having to think about it, helps me to eat a little something every three hours. And eating every three hours is a key Habit of Health.

Best of all, my professional focus has gone from keeping unhealthy people alive to creating healthy lives. I spend my days finding better ways to help people reach a healthy weight and learn habits that support great health.

The fuelings that I've helped others experience with success for many years are made by Medifast®. I picked them as my partner and

I served as their medical director for almost 15 years. I also chose them because their products and programs set the gold standard, with more than 35 years of efficacy and safety. They are backed by studies and recommended by over 20,000 healthcare providers since their founding. And to top it off, Medifast® has gathered a medical advisory board and research team committed to keeping these scientifically formulated meals at the forefront of science and technology.

A lot has changed since I made that choice so many years ago. I have helped create a growing community of coaches called OPTAVIA® that uses my *Habits of Health System* and which has helped over a million people impact their health over the last decade and half. The fuelings have evolved considerably and are best in class. In fact, they still play a central role as one of the core components as we help people transform their health and wellbeing. I am also Scholar in Residence at Mount Saint Mary's University in LA and help teach college wellness advocates the power of the Habits of Health.

We are changing the way we define success beyond academia to help the next generation prioritize their health and wellbeing. My desire is always to lead from the future, thereby advancing the idea of health and wellbeing as a priority. I want to foster new ways of thinking and begin to convert our unhealthy world into a new type of health community. But it starts with what we are putting in our body!

HEALTHY FUELINGS: HEALTHY FAST FOOD FOR THE TWENTY-FIRST CENTURY

In our chaotic world, we rarely find time to plan meals. Most of us don't even think about fueling our bodies until we're hungry and hypoglycemic. That's the mentality that's given rise to the fast food phenomenon, now a $208 billion a year business.[1]

If you were driving across the desert, you would fuel your car before you started, and you'd probably give at least some thought to where the next gas station was. But I'll bet you start your day in a hurry by skipping breakfast or, worse, grabbing a doughnut and coffee. Then, just at the moment your body is screaming for food, the fast food industry steps in with the sights, smells, and convenience that lead to bad decisions. As we discussed in Part 1.6, *You in Charge of Yourself: Setting Up for Success,* you are designed to make decisions in the moment and the fast food industry has the playbook on immediate gratification. Bright signs, flashy colors, alluring photos, and convenient drive thrus are hard to resist especially when you just sensed the smell of French fries being wafted out of the local burger joint by an exhaust fan.

Sadly, those unhealthy fast food fueling stations aren't going away any time soon, so it's all the more important to find healthy alternatives that are convenient, readily available, and support the Habits of Health. So, I'd like you to think of healthy fuelings as high-quality fast food and a "safety net" to protect you from nutritional pollution.

Fuelings give you what you need to feed your body when hunger strikes and you don't have time for a sit-down, prepared meal. They're completely portable for convenience. They're sealed for safety. They're individually packaged for reliable portion control. And they taste good whether they're for breakfast, lunch, or dinner.

Most importantly, the fuelings provide a balance of high-quality protein, complex carbohydrates, and added probiotic, along with 24 vitamins and minerals, to protect your body and help you feel full and satisfied. And because they give you a scientifically determined dose of energy—between 90 and 110 calories—you'll find it much easier to control your energy intake. Soon you'll be turning on your fat-burning machine and starting to lose weight safely and effectively.

I believe that fuelings are the easiest way to enter the path to optimal health. In time, I'll help you develop a complete healthy eating strategy to support you for the rest of your life, including advice on how to choose groceries, select from a restaurant menu, and cook a quick, low-glycemic meal. Fuelings can give you just the boost you need to get started on your journey to permanent weight loss and optimal health—just as I did.

ARE YOU READY?

If you are ready to get started, then there is no time like the present. The Habits of Health is a journey and you are going to be working on your health and wellbeing for the rest of your days.

If you have some weight to lose I cannot think of a better place to start. Remember in the last section, when I asked if you could eat every three hours? If you answered yes, you're going to find using fuelings a breeze.

You can, of course, wait and read about the healthy complete eating system I will be describing in the coming parts to support your journey but if you want to get started immediately you will have a plan you can begin this week! By the end of this segment, you will have everything you need to start your weight loss journey.

If I am making prepackaged fuelings sound like the way to go, I do have a bias toward the system. It's an extremely versatile, clinically effective tool. On top of that, we've worked to keep fuelings affordable and attainable to you without the additional costs associated with companies that produce comparable scientifically formulated products. In fact, the parent company has recently adopted the shared vision that, in order for the fuelings to create lifelong transformation, they need to be part of a comprehensive approach. They will help you start losing weight but, in order for you to have lasting success, the fueling plans need to be supported by a coach, who can guide you on installing the *Habits of Health Transformational System*.

Eat a healthy meal every three hours to help push your body into a state of fat-burning.

If you are ready and do not already have a coach you can go online and order the fuelings and you will be assigned a coach at no additional cost. It's an amazing offer and, as I've already said, having the support of a coach and especially one who is using the Habits of Health is a powerful combination in helping you on your journey. Go to optavia.com for more information.

YOUR WEIGHT LOSS EATING PATTERN USING FUELINGS

Remember our old friend, the *Glucose-Insulin Response Curve*? Let's take another look to see your eating plan using fuelings.

Your Weight-Loss and Health Plan

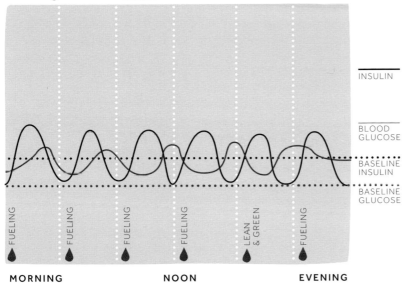

You'll note from the graph above that a steady dose of low-glycemic fuelings helps you stabilize your blood sugar and keep your insulin level in control. With the fuelings, you'll fuel your body throughout the day—every three hours, supplemented by a healthy meal in the evening, or whenever it fits best into your schedule. As you lower your total energy intake and enter a mild fat-burning state—one of our core principles—you'll start losing weight almost immediately.

Your weight-loss results may be a little slower if you have hypothyroidism, polycystic disease, or are on medications, such as hormone replacement therapy. Consult with your healthcare provider if you have such a condition.

Before you start your journey, I suggest you schedule a visit to see your healthcare provider.

No doubt your healthcare provider will be excited that you've decided to lose weight and create health in your life. After all, it makes their job easier! In the appendix, you'll find a sheet of information to give your physician that explains this "health makeover" you're doing. It's also available for download at the website at www.HabitsofHealth.com.

A special note for those with type 2 diabetes: Checking in with your healthcare provider before you change your diet is particularly important if you have type 2 diabetes. As you switch to a low-calorie, low-glycemic way of eating, your blood sugar will lower immediately, and your level of medication may need to be reduced accordingly.

The great news is that this is a signal of your body's initial step toward health. Your disease progression is being arrested! But do remember to watch your blood sugar closely in the beginning to make sure your medications are properly adjusted.

The calorie state you'll enter during your weight loss phase may be lower when compared to what you're eating now, but within three days you'll turn on your fat stores as your energy source. Soon you'll feel great and have plenty of energy, and you won't be tired or hungry.

GETTING STARTED

Before you start using your fuelings for Phase I, there are a few things you should think about. Remember, you'll need five fuelings on hand each day. I suggest you purchase a month's supply of fuelings right off the bat for the sake of variety, economy, and to ensure you don't run out.

Choosing a system designed like OPTAVIA® has a number of benefits, including the diversity of menu choices it offers. Choosing from over 60 different varieties of fuelings helps minimize "taste fatigue", a condition that occurs when an individual tires of the same monotonous tastes, textures, and flavors. But because all of those varieties are part of a carefully designed system, they work together using the same building blocks to support your health and burn fat. So, while you're enjoying your oatmeal, brownie, or biscuit fueling for breakfast, you have the backing of ingenious food technologists who've kept the nutritional footprint of all these various meals nearly identical. The OPTAVIA® fuelings contain no colors, flavors, or sweeteners from artificial sources. Each product contains probiotic cultures which help support digestive health, as part of a balanced diet and healthy lifestyle.

Best of all, with a scientific based system such as this, you can choose your shakes, chili, soups, bars, and whatever else appeals to you without having to think about calories, nutritional content, or glycemic index. It's an intelligent system that provides the nutritional footprint, portion control, low-glycemic ingredients, and reduced calories you need to optimize your body, thereby creating a safe, healthy environment for fat burning while protecting precious muscle mass.

In the following pages, with permission from OPTAVIA®, I will use our sample menus, charts, and plan to demonstrate an efficient system of rapid, safe weight loss using OPTAVIA® fuelings.

YOUR WEIGHT LOSS EATING STRATEGY USING FUELINGS

Your eating strategy is simple: just select any five fuelings and one healthy, low-glycemic meal each day. It is called the Optimal Weight 5&1 Plan® and it is a critical habit to your success. As you begin your journey eating every three hours is the first Habit of Health installation.

Ideally, you'll have your first fueling within 30 minutes of waking, and then choose another every three hours. You'll also eat one healthy, low-glycemic meal a day, at whatever three-hour interval you prefer. Most people choose to have this healthy meal—what we call "lean and green"—in the evening, to coincide with their family dinner. It's designed to give you your necessary fats, natural enzymes, and phytonutrients, while maintaining the low-calorie, low- glycemic requirements that keep you in a mild fat-burning state. During the weight-loss phase, your lean and green meal includes lean meat, fish, or poultry and a green vegetable or salad.

So, depending what time you wake up, your day should look something like this:

SAMPLE MEAL PLAN

7:00 a.m.	**Breakfast** *Choose one Fueling:* *oatmeal, hot cereal, or cinnamon swirl cake*
10:00 a.m.	**Fueling** *Choose one Fueling:* *shake, yogurt smoothie, or chai latte*
1:00 p.m.	**Lunch** *Choose one Fueling: herb penne, vegetable chili, or smashed potatoes*
4:00 p.m.	**Fueling** *Choose one Fueling: oatmeal raisin bar or vanilla pudding*
7:00 p.m.	**Dinner** *Prepare or order: Lean and Green meal* *For example:* • *5-ounce steak; green salad with low-fat dressing* • *6-ounce grilled chicken breast; 1½ cups cooked asparagus with one teaspoon olive oil* • *5-ounce portion grilled salmon; salad (two cups mixed salad greens, ½ cup total of diced tomatoes, cucumbers, and celery with two tablespoons low-carb salad dressing)*
10:00 p.m.	**Fueling** *Choose one Fueling: brownie or minty soft serve*

"

One serving of fish a week can reduce your risk of fatal heart attack by 40%.[2-12]

"

SHOPPING FOR YOUR LEAN AND GREEN

One thing that's great about this eating strategy is that there's actually very little you need to do in terms of preparation. The fueling system you choose will include simple instructions on preparing and using the products, and getting ready for your lean and green meal involves little more than clearing out your pantry (as detailed in Part 2.2, *Your Blueprint: Safe Weight Loss and Health Gain*) and making a quick trip to the market.

If you haven't had much experience selecting healthy protein and vegetables, you may want to take a bit of time to ask the butcher or produce department for help. I learned a great amount simply by asking store employees which items were fresh, healthy, and locally produced. Once you have it down, you should be able to get your weekly shopping done in no more than 15 minutes.

Your shopping list should include selections from these four major groups:

1. *Lean protein*
2. *Healthy fats and oils*
3. *Green vegetables and salad*
4. *Healthy snacks and condiments*

Let's take a closer look at each.

1. LEAN PROTEIN

Shopping for protein is a great opportunity to try out new food sources, flavors, and recipes, and to learn a very specific Habit of Health. By choosing the leanest meats, experimenting with meat alternatives, and increasing your variety of fish and seafood, you're lowering and even eliminating unhealthy fats, while adding healthy omegas to create a powerful, nutritious meal. To keep that fat content low, you'll be grilling, baking, broiling, or poaching your selections. And to make it easier for you to choose the leanest options, I've devised a color-coded system that takes you from lean (light green) to leanest (dark green). Here's a rundown of your lean and green protein sources.

Seafood
When you eat fish, you're choosing a great protein source and significantly reducing your risk of disease. Eating fish one to three times a week is an important Habit of Health that can have a profound impact on your wellbeing over time. In fact, one serving of fish a week may reduce your risk of fatal heart attack by 40%![3-12]

Seafood Choices

LEAN (>9g FAT) 5 OZ PORTION; NO ADDITIONAL FAT SERVINGS	LEANER (6 – 9g FAT) 6 OZ PORTION; ADD ONE ADDITIONAL FAT SERVINGS	LEANEST (6g FAT) 7 OZ PORTION; ADD TWO ADDITIONAL FAT SERVINGS
• Salmon • Tuna (bluefin steak) • Farmed catfish • Mackerel, herring	• Swordfish • Trout • Halibut	• Cod, flounder, haddock, orange roughy, wild halibut, grouper, tilapia, mahi mahi • Tuna (yellowfin) canned in water • Wild catfish • Crab, scallops, shrimp, lobster

Meat and Poultry

I was brought up in a family where meat was part of daily life, and although I eat much less now, I still enjoy an occasional steak for dinner. It's important to lower your consumption of meat and eat more fish, white-meat poultry (skinless), legumes (such as beans), and low-fat or nonfat dairy. But if you're like me, and once in a while need that savory taste of meat, just minimize the amount of saturated fat so you can enjoy this great protein source and still stay healthy.

Did you know that wild meat—the kind our ancestors ate 10,000 years ago—contains much less saturated fat than farm-raised meat? Our cattle are fed on high-glycemic foods and as a result they suffer from the same fate that we do when we eat carbs that turn on fat storage. Our meat contains an unhealthy amount of fat, growth hormones, and antibiotics. By eating meat, we concentrate our ingestion of fat and calories, and have a high level of omega-6 which can cause inflammation!

However, wild meats, such as buffalo and elk, contain very little fat and it is mostly omega-3 which is anti-inflammatory. I've found both of these very enjoyable, as well as venison (deer). Venison might taste a bit "gamey", but it's delicious if prepared properly. Many of these wild meats are available in grocery stores such as Whole Foods Market®. But even traditional American beef can be a fine choice if you select cuts such as fillets and sirloin, rather than those that contain excess marbling from fat.

Meat and Poultry Choices

LEAN (>9g FAT) 5 OZ PORTION: NO ADDITIONAL FAT SERVINGS	LEANER (6 – 9g FAT) 6 OZ PORTION: ADD ONE ADDITIONAL FAT SERVINGS	LEANEST (6g FAT) 7 OZ PORTION: ADD TWO ADDITIONAL FAT SERVINGS
• Lean beef, beef steak, roast and ground beef • Lamb • Pork chop or tenderloin • Ground turkey or other 80 – 88% lean meat	• Breast or white-meat turkey or chicken without skin • Ground turkey or other 95 – 97% lean meat	• Buffalo, elk, deer • Ground turkey or other 98% or more lean meat.

Meat Alternatives

If you'd like to eliminate meat from your diet, or just reduce the amount you eat, there are some great meatless options available. I recommend that you stick with just the choices on the list, but if you do find an additional alternative you'd like to try, please make sure it contains no added sugar.

Meatless Choices

LEAN (>9g FAT) 5 OZ PORTION: NO ADDITIONAL FAT SERVINGS	LEANER (6 – 9g FAT) 6 OZ PORTION: ADD ONE ADDITIONAL FAT SERVINGS	LEANEST (6g FAT) ADD TWO ADDITIONAL FAT SERVINGS
• 3 whole eggs (limit to once per week) • 15 oz tofu, firm or soft variety	• 15 oz tofu, extra firm • 2 whole eggs plus 4 egg whites • Add 1 additional fat serving	• 14 egg whites • 2 cups egg beaters

2. HEALTHY FATS AND OILS

One of the important modern improvements in today's meal fueling systems is that they now ensure that users get the right amount of healthy fats. An adequate supply of fat helps your body absorb fat-soluble vitamins such as A, D, E, and K, and contributes to gall bladder health. Fats also help you lose weight by giving you a sense of fullness and adding texture to your meals.

Our focus in the weight-loss phase will be on eliminating unhealthy fats while supplementing your diet with healthy omegas that can accelerate your journey toward optimal health. Having a good supply of omega-rich antioxidants is particularly smart during the weight-loss phase, when your body is unloading fat cells and unhealthy fat-soluble substances. A Healthy Fat serving should contain about five grams of fat and less than five grams of carbohydrate. Add up to two healthy fat servings daily based on your Lean choices.

Fat and Oil Choices

EACH =1 FAT SERVING

- 1 teaspoon of canola, flaxseed, walnut, or olive oil
- Up to 2 tablespoons of low-carbohydrate salad dressing
- 5 – 10 black or green olives
- 1 tablespoon of reduced-fat margarine
- 1 ½ oz of avocado

3. GREEN VEGETABLES AND SALAD

I love vegetables and salads. As you'll discover in the following sections, I believe you just can't eat too many healthy fruits and vegetables (with very few exceptions) once you reach your healthy weight. During the weight-loss phase, however, I'm going to ask that you avoid fruit, which can be extremely high in carbohydrates, and really focus on selecting moderate amounts of vegetables from the green areas.

When we talk about the vegetables you will eat during this phase, we're referring to nutrient-dense, low-glycemic carbohydrates that support your health while you lose weight. Some popular diets reduce carbohydrates to such a low level that they bring about a profound state of ketosis, accompanied by dehydration and metallic-tasting breath. I don't advocate that. Rather, this plan will create an efficient physiological state of mild dietary ketosis or what I like to call a fat-burning state. This allows you to burn fat while providing enough carbohydrates to maintain muscle and brain health— around 80 – 85 g per day. The list on page 212 is designed to create this ideal state for optimal weight loss.

As you'll see, your choices are color-coded, this time based on the amount of carbohydrates they contain. Darker green selections give you fewer carbohydrate calories. So if you're having trouble getting into a fat-burning state or if your weight loss slows down, it's probably a good idea to confine your choices to the dark green group, while also reducing or eliminating condiments and making sure your salad dressings are low fat and very low carb.

From the following list, select any combination of three servings each day.

Green Vegetables and Salad

HIGHEST CARBOHYDRATE SERVING SIZE = ½ CUP UNLESS OTHERWISE SPECIFIED	MODERATE CARBOHYDRATE SERVING SIZE = ½ CUP UNLESS OTHERWISE SPECIFIED	LOWEST CARBOHYDRATE SERVING SIZE = ½ CUP UNLESS OTHERWISE SPECIFIED
• Broccoli • Cabbage, red • Collards or mustard greens, cooked • Green or wax beans • Kohlrabi • Okra • Peppers, green/red/yellow • Scallions • Summer squash, crookneck/straightneck • Tomato, red ripe/canned • Turnips • Winter squash	• Asparagus • Cabbage • Cauliflower • Eggplant • Fennel • Kale • Mushrooms, portabello • Spinach, cooked • Summer squash (scallop or zucchini)	• Mustard greens (1 cup) • Collards, fresh / raw (1 cup) • Romaine lettuce (1 cup) • Endive (1 cup) • Lettuce, butter head (1 cup) • Celery • Cucumber • Mushrooms / white • Radishes • Sprouts, alfalfa or mung bean • Turnip greens

4. SNACKS AND CONDIMENTS

Use condiments to add flavor and zest to your meals, but just remember that they contribute to overall carbohydrate intake. We recommend reading food labels for carbohydrate information and controlling condiment portions for optimal results. A condiment serving should contain no more than one gram of carbohydrate per serving. You can enjoy up to three condiment servings per day.

Examples:
• ½ teaspoon most dried herbs and spices, pepper, ketchup, sauce, or cocktail sauce
• ¼ teaspoon salt

- 1 tablespoon minced onion, yellow mustard, salsa, soy sauce, low-fat or fat-free milk/soy milk
- 2 teaspoons lemon/lime juice
- 2 tablespoons sugar-free flavored syrup (Walden Farms, Inc.®, DaVinci®, Torani®, etc.)
- 1 packet zero-calorie sweetener
- 1 cup refrigerated, unsweetened original or vanilla almond or cashew milk

Healthy Snacks and Condiments

CONDIMENTS	OPTIONAL SNACKS
• ½ teaspoon of most dried herbs and spices	• 3 celery stalks
• 1 teaspoon balsamic vinegar	• 1 fruit flavored sugar free popsicle
• 1 teaspoon minced onion, lemon/lime juice, yellow mustard, salsa, soy sauce, low-fat or fat-free milk or soy milk	• ½ Cup serving sugar-free Jello® gelatin
• Up to 2 tablespoons sugar-free flavored syrup such as da vinci® or torani®	• Up to 3 pieces sugar-free gum or mints
• 1 packet artificial sweetener such as splenda®	• 2 dill pickle spears
• Tabasco® (or other hot) sauce and red, white, or cider vinegar (feel free to use liberally)	• ½ oz. of nuts: almonds (10 whole), walnuts (7 halves) or pistachios (20 kernels)
	Note: Nuts are a rich source of healthy fats and additional calories so choose this optional snack sparingly

So now you have your four-part grocery list and the entire inventory you need to restock your kitchen for Phase I using the fuelings. It couldn't be simpler but, remember, it's a precise eating strategy that works best exactly as outlined. That means to get results, you must confine yourself to only the foods on these lists.

Now let's spend a moment looking at a typical meal schedule.

Secrets to Success

- **Eat one fueling every three hours.** Don't skip meals even if you're not hungry. It's absolutely critical to fuel as scheduled and, in fact, your weight loss may be slower if you don't.
- **Get some extra rest.** You may feel a little tired during the first three days as your body switches on its fat-burning mechanism and gears up to use its stores of fat.
- **Drink at least eight (eight ounce) glasses of water every day.**
- **Eat slowly.**
- **Stay busy and avoid sights and smells that remind you of food,** especially during the first few days. Soon enough, your own energy stores will kick in and you'll feel more in control.
- **Use your support system.** Call your coach and if you don't have one yet, get one!
- **Limit caffeine to no more than three servings a day.** You may find that your body is more sensitive to the effects of caffeine, making this a great time to cut back on your daily consumption.
- **Avoid alcohol.** It causes dehydration, throws you out of the fat-burning state you've worked so hard to achieve, and it's a powerful appetite stimulant.
- **If you slip up, just get right back on track.** But remember, it will take about two to three days after a slip-up to get back into a fat-burning state. (For some extra motivation, review Parts 1.3 – 1.5 on making good choices.)

YOUR DAILY MEAL PLAN

Begin each day by having your first fueling within one hour— or better yet, 30 minutes—after you wake up. Your day should look like this:

Your Daily Meal Plan for Phase I Using Prepackaged Fuelings

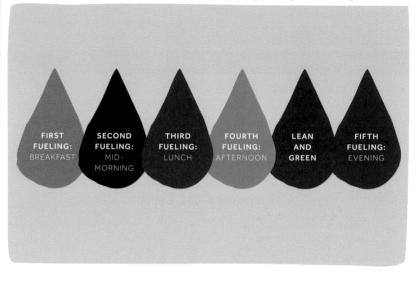

FIRST FUELING: BREAKFAST — SECOND FUELING: MID-MORNING — THIRD FUELING: LUNCH — FOURTH FUELING: AFTERNOON — LEAN AND GREEN — FIFTH FUELING: EVENING

YOUR DAILY HYDRATION PLAN

Water plays a key role in supporting health, particularly during weight loss because it helps remove toxins and other unhealthy substances stored in your fat cells. Being well-hydrated helps all your organs and systems function properly. In fact, every function in your body takes place in water. It's the solvent that moves nutrients, hormones, antibodies, and oxygen through your bloodstream and lymphatic system, and removes waste. And, of course, it's essential to your kidneys' ability to filter and eliminate metabolic byproducts and toxins. If you don't drink enough, your body is forced to recycle dirty water, diminishing the efficiency of every metabolic function.

During Phase I of your weight-loss plan, there are even more good reasons to make a conscious effort to drink your eight (eight ounces) glasses a day. Here are a few:

- It's calorie free, but helps you feel full and satisfied.
- It keeps you from overeating. Studies have shown that when we feel hungry some of the time our bodies are actually signaling for water.[13]
- It facilitates the removal of toxins, such as pesticides and preservatives from your cells.

- It prevents dehydration as your body eliminates excess salt and water from a diet full of too much processed food.
- It minimizes or eliminates fatigue, lack of energy, headaches, and unclear thinking.
- It speeds up metabolism. A recent study showed that drinking two eight-ounce glasses of cold water increased metabolic rate by 30% for 90 minutes.[14]
- It helps your liver convert fat to energy.
- It compensates for the loss of glycogen stores as you lose weight.

We will spend much more time talking about hydration in the Eating and Hydration MacroHabit Section.

OPTAVIA® has an amazing set of infusers that will allow you to purposefully hydrate by giving you cues on when and why to hydrate throughout your day.

- **Start using *Your LifeBook* and print off tracking sheets. This is a great way to monitor your progress and help you focus.**
- **Avoid exercise for the first three weeks. Or, if you do choose to exercise, reduce your usual amount by half.**

HABITS OF HEALTHY WEIGHT MANAGEMENT

So, there you have it—a very simple method to help you lose weight quickly and safely while introducing you to crucial dietary information, including:

- fueling every three hours
- eating breakfast
- making healthy food choices
- eating low-glycemic foods
- planning your meals
- drinking eight glasses of water a day

Once you have a handle on these habits, you'll have the framework for success— not only for weight loss, but for a lifetime of maintaining your healthy weight and optimal health.

CHECKLISTS FOR CHANGE

Before you begin your weight-loss plan, make sure you've taken these important first steps:

- You've created a microenvironment of health by changing your surroundings. See how we are changing our internal environment in Part 1.6, *You in Charge of Yourself: Setting Up for Success,* and our outer world in Part 1.7, *Optimizing Your Surroundings: Creating Your Microenvironment of Health.*
- You've gone shopping and replaced your pantry and refrigerator with foods from all four groups on the grocery list.

- You've purchased and received your fuelings. (For more information on ordering your fuelings, see the resource list in the appendix.)
- You've taken the wellbeing evaluation in the beginning of *Your LifeBook* and are beginning to write your new healthy story, and have started tracking your daily progress using the LifeBook Tracking Sheets.
- You are using your Habits of Health App to track your fuelings and daily water consumption.
- You've created a structural tension chart for your first goal of reaching a healthy weight. (For more information, see Parts 1.3–1.5 of this book and reference Element 03 of *Your LifeBook, How Do You Create What You Want?* as well.
- You are using *Your LifeBook* and have started journaling, writing, and are regularly recording your daily eating habits. (See tracking choices that support optimal weight and health in Element 13 of *Your LifeBook, Track Your Journey to a Healthy Weight and Beyond*).

Once you're on the move, here are some tips:

- Get through your first three days successfully.
- If you need some extra motivation, review Parts 1.3–1.5 on motivation for change, fundamental choice, and the discipline of daily choices.
- Look at your "3 x 5 Card" daily with your concrete statement of Why You are Doing This (See Element 01 of *Your LifeBook, Be Clear Why You Are Here*).
- Start Using Stop. Challenge. Choose.™ as described in Parts 1.6 and 1.7.
- By day four you'll enter a mild fat-burning state, characterized by lots of energy and the beginning of weight loss.
- After a week, if you're ready and feel good enough, start slowly increasing your daily activity. Avoid active exertion for the first three weeks.

HOW LONG WILL I BE IN PHASE I?

So now you have your fueling system to start your journey to a healthy weight and optimal health and wellbeing. So let's get started! What can you expect moving forward? And how long will you be in Phase I? This primarily depends on how much weight you have to lose and how long you take to lose it, as well as your target BMI. While your weight-loss goal can be whatever you've determined is healthy for you, there are some guidelines concerning body composition. Generally speaking, if your waist circumference is less than 37 inches (for men) or 31.5 inches (for women) and your BMI is less than 25, you're ready to transition to the healthy eating phase. In general, you should count on being in the weight loss phase until you meet your goals and are able to maintain them for at least two weeks. Here's what to expect:

- If you have just a small amount of weight to lose, you'll transition to Phase II fairly quickly. You should read the next sections on my healthy, low-glycemic portion-control system. In Parts 2.4–2.6 of this book. I also advise that you start progressing through *Your LifeBook* with your coach to help guide you before you begin transitioning (see Part 2.8, *Healthy Eating for Life: Your Transition to Permanent Health*, because you'll be using much of that information as you learn to eat healthy for life). After that, you'll begin the progressive movement plan outlined in Parts 2.9–2.12 and do the corresponding Elements 17–19 in *Your LifeBook*.

- If you have a lot of weight to lose, you'll be in Phase I for a while. When the time comes, and you've reached your healthy weight, Part 2.8, *Healthy Eating for Life: Your Transition to Permanent Health*, will teach you about transitioning to Phase II. In the meantime, you should read the parts on my healthy low-glycemic portion-control system (Parts 2.4–2.6) because you'll be using much of that information as you learn to eat healthy for life. In addition, once you've settled into a fat-burning state (after the first three weeks), you should start the progressive movement plan outlined in Parts 2.9–2.12.

   At this point you will be using your Habits of Health App to track your daily progress. In addition you will be using *Your LifeBook* to lay down the foundational Elements that will allow you to master your Habits of Weight Management. You will move into Phase II at the pace that is right for you. In the next part, I will start teaching you my healthy eating system which will prepare you for eating healthy for the rest of your days. That way transition will no longer be a scary time but instead a time to utilize all you have learned and installed.

You should lose weight fairly consistently. However, your weight loss can vary depending on your gender and certain medical conditions that may slow down your weight loss, such as hypothyroidism and polycystic ovarian syndrome (PCOS).

WHAT'S NEXT? TRANSITIONING TO PHASE II HEALTHY EATING FOR LIFE

Our first goal—reaching your healthy weight—is the underlying dynamic that unlocks all the possibilities to follow. It's also our signal that you're ready to begin transitioning into Phase II.

   In Phase I, we've laid the foundation for a more efficient energy management system. As you transition to Phase II, we'll boost both your energy intake and your energy expenditure. The thread that connects the phases is the relationship between energy in and energy out. Let's take another look at the energy diagram. Notice that the colored boxes in Phase II highlight our three key focal areas: a healthy body mass index, or BMI (white), increased activity and exercise (green), and increased caloric intake (red).

Energy Management in Phase II

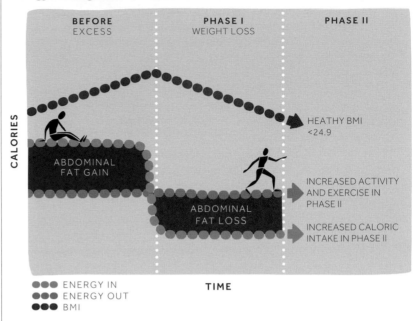

If we go back to your fat cell which is the key player in your long-term weight management we can look at what a healthy fat cell and an effective long-term weight management environment looks like.

Habits of Health Healthy Eating State: Healthy Waistline

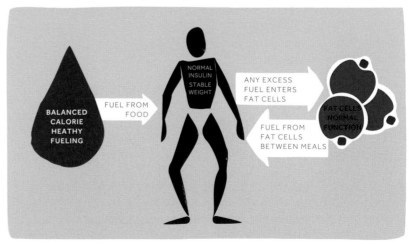

You can see in the illustration that Phase II, the healthy eating status that you are about to enter, is highlighted by three changing conditions.

> **First:** *as your* BMI *reaches being less than 25, your waist circumference being less than 37 as a male or less than 31.5 as a female, and as your body fat approaches a healthy composition, then we know that your fat cells are returning back to their healthy fat level.*

> **Second:** *you are eating from a low sugar, low glycemic index carbohydrates plan and your insulin level is low so the fuel you ingest is used for your bodies needs, meaning that between fuelings you have access to any additional energy that is needed and readily available from your fat cells.*

> **Third:** *you are about to start expanding your diet to include fruit, a full selection of vegetables, dairy, grains and, most importantly, more calories.*

As you add more calories and expand your food choices beyond the fuelings and your specific lean and green, it will be important to watch how your body responds. First, we want to keep your insulin level normal. How do we do that?

> **First:** *Make sure we are choosing correctly from the glycemic index chart's low and medium numbers.*

> **Remember:** *Stay in the green to stay lean.*

> **Second:** *Pay attention to your weight and waist circumference and body fat as you add calories by checking your weight and waist circumference daily. (Note: You will gain two to five pounds through transition as your body re-establishes its normal glycogen stores and redistributes water). Remember the extra weight you lost during the first week.*

> **Third:** *Continue to work on the habits of movement, sleep, and stress reductions as you can see they will help keep your insulin level lower.*

Before you move on to Phase II and learn how to maintain your new healthy weight, consider the following:

- Have you identified and started to develop the fundamental Habits of Health that will help you keep weight off, including proper motivation and choice?
- Have you reached your goal weight and BMI?
- Have you read and studied the healthy eating habits in Parts 2.4–2.6?
- If you've been in Phase I for more than three weeks, have you read Parts 2.9–2.12 on motion and started your movement plan?
- Are you progressing through *Your LifeBook?*

Your LifeBook is a powerful piece that will help solidify the necessary pieces and elements that will be part of your Habits of Health for your lifetime. So now you have your fueling system to start your journey to a healthy weight and optimal health and wellbeing

The beauty of the *Habits of Health Transformational System* is it allows you to go at your own pace. If you are going go be in Phase I for a few months using the prepackaged fuelings, as we have described in detail in this part, we have you covered. You can progress through the Elements, reinforcing all of the key Habits and Elements that support long-term weight management.

It isn't until Element 13 of *Your LifeBook, Track Your Journey to a Healthy Weight And Beyond,* that we start your transition to Phase II and beyond. By then, you will have mastered the skills to eat healthy and manage your weight for the rest of your life.

So, whether you are dialed in to our prepackaged fueling system getting into a fat burning state or you are already well on your way to a healthy weight, we are now going to start unpacking my healthy eating system. It will give a simple, yet effective, way to manage your weight and your eating for the rest of your days.

And if you are going to use the system à la carte and learn all of the things necessary to do it on your own, then let's get started.

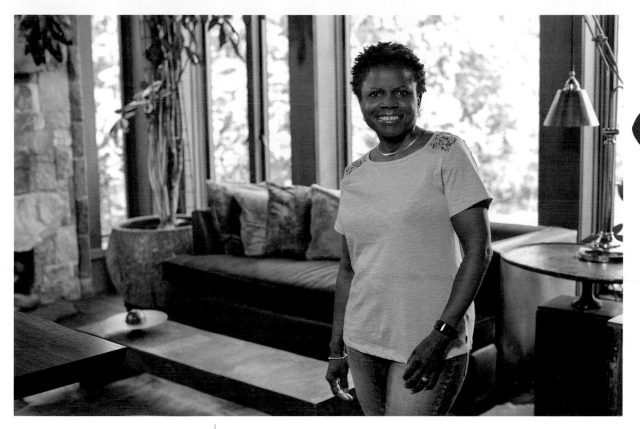

TRANSFORMATION: JEAN JEFFREYS

I started Dr. A's program about four months ago. The Habits of Health have just been incredible —healthy mind, healthy body, healthy weight. I've lost about 15 lbs* already while also helping other people to get healthy by focusing on my family and friends to encourage them to get healthy and live that optimal lifestyle.

The one thing that stuck out with the Habits of Health is how it really is scientifically based and has been proven to work. I wanted to try it myself so that I could really have something that I could stand behind. After talking to Dr. A and his love for people and wanting to get the world healthy, I really connected with that. It's been a wonderful experience, and I just know that there is so much more to come while I'm also helping others to get healthy.

The program has been helping me to move more, make healthier choices, and improve my diet. I realize now that I don't have to eat everything that's in front of me, but I have to eat to fuel my body. It's helped me to stay balanced, it's helped my energy, and it's helped me to create a lifestyle that is sustainable for myself and for others.

*Average weight loss on the Optimal Weight 5 & 1 Plan® is 12 lbs. Clients are in weight loss, on average, for 12 weeks.

> **"**
> *I've lost about 15 lbs* already while helping other people to get healthy.*
> **"**

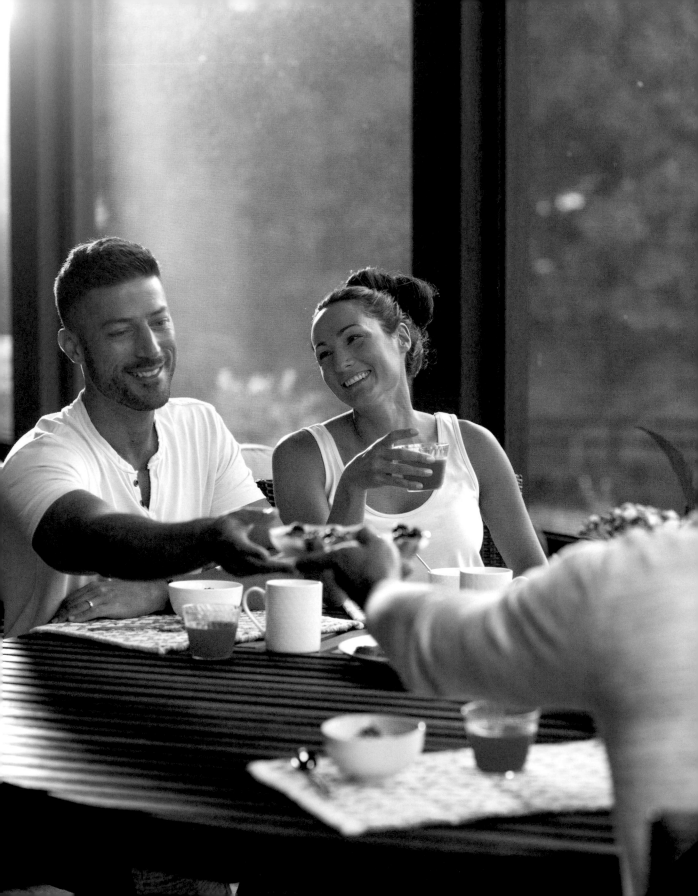

DR. A'S HEALTHY EATING SYSTEM: A LOW-GLYCEMIC, PORTION-CONTROL APPROACH TO SUPPORT OPTIMAL HEALTH

**HABITS OF
HEALTHY WEIGHT MANAGEMENT**

**THE HABITS OF
HEALTHY EATING AND HYDRATION**

"Tell me what you eat, and I will tell you what you are."
Jean Anthelme Brillat-Savarin

In the last part, I talked about the benefits of prepackaged low-calorie fuelings. Whilst this packaged system does provide an effective tool for weight loss as part of your long-term plan, it's critical to master eating healthy for life using a traditional approach with food as well.

Our next step is to give you the additional Habits of Health you will need to design and execute a comprehensive eating strategy to help reinforce long-term success.

If you're close to or at a healthy weight, Phase II in our weight management approach will be your entry point to your journey to optimal health and wellbeing. Taking the healthy food approach to weight loss doesn't just tell you how to lose a few pounds as it will also teach you how to build a permanent eating strategy for your health.

Over the next three parts, you will gain an in-depth understanding of how to make healthy selections with all your food choices. I designed this system to make the habits of healthy eating easy to learn. Over time, they will become automatic. You'll discover new ways to think about food, new ways to shop, prepare food, and eat. Our goal is to make healthy eating easy, portable, and so satisfying that you'll no longer be tempted by the tricks used by the food industry—like flashing yellow and red signs that stimulate appetite. The all-too-familiar golden arches will disappear!

You'll also set the foundation for new eating habits that will support healthy weight for the rest of your life. And, as a bonus, as you learn to eat healthy, you'll awaken sensations of taste, smell, sight, and texture that have been dulled by the illusionary satisfaction the food industry creates by their use of bulk, salt, fat, and sugar.

Important Note

The information presented here contains key Habits of Health that will prepare you for the permanent eating strategy you'll need for long-term success. However, if you have significant weight to lose, and you are still in Phase I, I would continue using the fuelings system outlined in the previous part. You will then add this whole food eating system once you've reached a healthy weight and have gone through transition as outlined in Part 2.1, *The Habits of Healthy Weight Management.*

THE USDA ADVANCEMENT FROM THE PYRAMID TO THE MY PLATE

In the early 1980s, the U.S. Department of Agriculture (USDA) began developing guidelines for healthy eating, eventually adding information on serving sizes and what's needed to maintain a healthy weight. You might remember the USDA pyramid, which divided foods into six major groups. It was the recommended guideline when I wrote the first edition of this book. The good news is the USDA has taken my lead and has abandoned the pyramid in favor of a plate system which bears an uncanny similarity to mine. They call it "My Plate" and there's no question it can be a valuable resource.

It is a major improvement in their recommendations and, like my own efforts, the goal is always to provide simpler and easier ways for people to eat healthy. So, in order to tap into this valuable resource I am going to make a couple of adjustments to my plate system so the two approaches are compatible.

First, I am going to separate fruits and vegetables so that instead of being one category they are now two. They will still be the same 50% total but by subdividing them into two 25% will make it easier to separate the percentage each contributes. This will also depend on whether you are in the weight-loss or healthy eating phase. I will also use the word "grains" instead of starch in the other quadrant to eliminate any confusion. This will make it easier to look at whole foods and separate them from ultra-refined starches.

A Habit of Health:

Learning to control your portions.

The good news is that these changes will make these guidelines compatible and you can go to www.choosemyplate.gov and receive materials and visuals free of charge that will work with my own healthy plate system.

While I applaud the USDA for its efforts, our rates of pre-obesity and obesity have continued to rise. So why aren't they working? Simply, because they are not that practical and don't fit today's habits and lifestyle.

It's also not easy to use, so the system I'm going to describe, which has been used by thousands of people, is very simple.

Our goal is to take all the information that's available—including parts of the USDA guidelines—and use them to build a practical eating strategy that supports both weight loss and optimal health.

My healthy eating system helps you monitor and manage your energy intake while ensuring that you get a healthy, balanced diet. It's a simple visual system that teaches you the basics of portion size and the correct proportion of foods from our designated four major food groups: vegetables, fruits, proteins, and grains. We will also address the current thinking on dairy, and we will make sure that you get the correct number of vitamins, minerals, and phytonutrients you need to support health without having to count calories. It's so easy you can even use it in restaurants.

With the system, you'll use a nine-inch plate to help you judge proper portion size and proportion. If you don't already have a nine-inch plate in your kitchen, now is as good a time as any to go out and buy a few. Ideally, the plate should be shallow with just a small lip to prevent you from heaping it with too much food.

If you go online you'll notice that nine-inch plate systems are all the rage which is pretty cool since they were non-existent when I wrote the first edition. The bottom line is that I want you to have the easiest possible way to judge your portions and how much of each food group you are eating without major disruption in your routine and culture. The harder it is, the less likely it is that you'll do it.

Take a look at the following diagram. I've simplified it into a four-component system that mirrors the way most people eat. Our typical meal is made up of:

- healthy vegetables
- healthy fruits
- healthy protein (meat, chicken, fish, dairy, nuts)
- healthy grains (wheat, rice, oats, cornmeal, barley, or another cereal grain)

DR. A'S FOUR-COMPONENT HEALTHY EATING SYSTEM

This breakdown gives you a healthy balance of nutrients in the right amounts to satisfy your hunger and burn fat. All you need to do is visualize this chart on your nine-inch plate, and plan your meals accordingly.

As long as you maintain this ratio of grain, protein, fruit, and vegetable, you can be sure that you're getting a healthy, balanced diet. In fact, we'll be using these proportions to build your long-term health plan, which is an important Habit of Health.

Dr. A's Low Glycemic Portion-Control Plate System

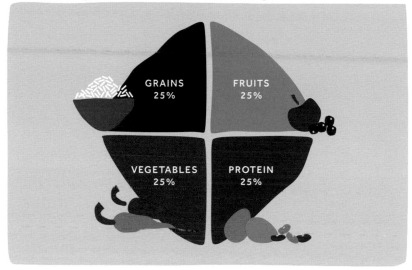

It's worth noting that although we designate 25–25% for the fruit and vegetable, as much as 50% can come from vegetables. As a general guideline I would avoid more than 25% coming from fruit category.

Phase I Weight Loss Using my Healthy Eating System Instead of Prepackaged Fuelings or in Combination With Them.

If you're at a healthy weight and are using this system to start eating healthier, or if you just want to get a little leaner by using my healthy eating system for your Phase I, you'll be preparing two meals a day until you have reached your goal. You'll have four more opportunities for smaller fueling breaks each day, using foods from the list in Part 2.6, *Building Healthy Meal Plans for Optimal Health*, or you can use prepackaged fuelings.

This customized meal plan will provide you with an average of 1,200–1,300 calories per day, through two 400-calorie meals (breakfast and dinner) and four 100-calorie fueling breaks. Here's a breakdown of what a combination of the healthy foods and small fueling snacks

For an even stronger visual cue, use a food-safe marker to draw these proportions right on your plate.

would look like for those that want to do it on their own. The list of 100 calorie snacks is in Sample Fueling Breaks and in Part 2.6, *Building Healthy Meal Plans for Optimal Health.*

Fueling Schedule: Phase I Using My Healthy Eating System

BREAKFAST	300–400 kcal
MID-MORNING FUELING	100 kcal
LUNCH FUELING	100–200 kcal
MID-AFTERNOON FUELING	100 kcal
DINNER	400 kcal
EVENING FUELING	100 kcal

Although it's best to treat lunch like any other 100-calorie fueling break, I've included an option for extra calories at lunchtime to accommodate business lunches or the demands of a high-energy job. If you opt to make lunch a 200-calorie meal rather than a fueling break, you can either choose two fueling-break options or remove the grain (starch) from your nine-inch plate meal selection.

In other words:

- Choice A: Two 100-calorie fuelings combined (for example, cottage cheese with olives and apple slices with walnuts).
- Choice B: The protein and vegetable/fruit components of your nine-inch plate meal (no grain/starch).

I've found that this plan works well for people with a wide variety of lifestyles and metabolisms. It will put you well on your way to learning two important Habits of Health—portion control and the proper proportion of the four major food groups. Both are essential habits that will help you reach and maintain an optimal sustainable weight.

If you're already at a healthy BMI, in Phase II you can graduate to my permanent healthy eating schedule, which is outlined in Part 2.8, *Healthy Eating for Life: Your Transition to Permanent Health.* You can then use the energy formula to calculate how many calories you should be consuming per day to fill out your eating schedule.

DR. A'S LOW-GLYCEMIC PORTION-CONTROL SYSTEM

The practical system you're about to use has three important benefits:

It's Automatic

Any system that teaches new habits needs to be simple, easy, and doable. My goal is to make your life so simple that when you go to a store or prepare a meal, your choices will naturally support optimal health. This needs to be as automatic as the drive to the window of any fast food joint.

It Supports Weight Loss

Weight loss is a critical first step to creating optimal health. What most people don't realize is that the USDA My Plate is designed to maintain a healthy weight, not to help you lose weight at the outset. Learning this system of healthy foods will support your goal of an optimal weight and help you remain that way. You can use the two-meals approach of my system to actually knock off a few pounds.

It Teaches You to Eat Healthy for Life

The principles, skills, and strategies you'll begin learning on day one of my system will become part of your permanent eating strategy. So, you can be reassured that every moment of your time is well spent!

This simple, effective strategy has its own basic guidelines. These are the most critical ones to understand at the beginning:

- You'll incorporate my two core principles of energy and insulin pump control.
- You'll eat breakfast within an hour of awakening (30 minutes is ideal).
- You'll eat something every three hours.
- You'll have a healthy dinner.
- You'll eat only lower-glycemic carbohydrates during Phase I (more information is available on this in Part 2.7, *The Science of Healthy Eating and Weight Loss)*.
- You'll gradually begin increasing your daily activity.
- You'll learn the key habits necessary to maintain a healthy weight, including support, monitoring, and reinforcement.
- You will be writing your new story in *Your LifeBook*.

If you're not already familiar with the basics of healthy eating, don't worry. The next few parts will explain in detail exactly how to choose and prepare foods that support optimal health. I'll show you how to shop for and plan great-tasting meals on your own, or you can simply follow my pre-planned menus found at HabitsofHealth.com. I'll even make it easy for you to prepare foods at work or while traveling.

Soon, with my guidance, you'll be able to:

- Shop for and prepare healthy low-glycemic meals that will turn off your insulin pump and use your excess fat as an energy source.
- Read food labels to distinguish healthy from unhealthy foods.
- Choose high-quality proteins and health-supporting fats.
- Understand portion size as a critical factor for energy consumption.
- Fill your plate the healthy way with my easy visual portion-control system.
- Master the logistics of eating healthy every three hours.
- Redesign your pantry, refrigerator, and freezer to support low-glycemic and healthy eating.
- Understand the importance of water.

> *Overwhelmed by the idea of shopping and cooking for yourself? If so, go back to Part 2.3 to learn more about using prepackaged low-calorie fuelings. They'll make it easier to learn the basics of healthy eating at your own pace.*

If you feel a craving coming on, take a big drink of water.

YOUR NEW FUELING PATTERN

Remember the chart on page 180, Modern Life's Disease Path? It showed you the dramatic spikes in blood sugar and insulin that result from the chaotic way most people eat. For most Americans, there's no pattern or rhythm to their meals. Throughout their busy days, eating becomes nothing more than a reaction to stress, hunger, boredom, and a million other problems. It brings instant relief, but leads to the overconsumption of high-calorie, nutritionally polluted foods that rob us of our health.

What many people don't understand is that it's not just the type of food they eat and the excess calories that cause weight gain, but the erratic nature of the fueling pattern itself. Learning how to fuel your body efficiently—through small meals every three hours—is one of the most basic and critical Habits of Health. In fact, it's what humans were designed to do. Just making this simple adjustment will have a dramatic effect on your body by:

- Turning on fat burning
- Increasing your metabolism
- Protecting muscle mass
- Naturally suppressing your appetite
- Improving your energy levels
- Lowering your cholesterol

And that's even before we start changing the quantity and quality of your fuel! Here's what your new healthy schedule might look like:

Your Optimal Eating Schedule: Glucose-Insulin Response Curve

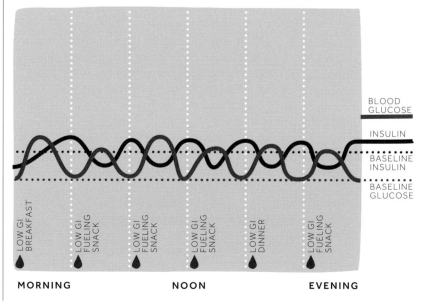

Your new healthy daily eating schedule starts with a solid breakfast and continues fueling you every three hours while you're awake with low-glycemic choices, including a healthy dinner. This plan helps keep blood sugar and insulin levels steady.

This steady fueling schedule starts with a solid breakfast and continues every three hours. My simple system, which we'll explore in the next few parts, will help you design a menu of low-glycemic choices.

As you can see in the illustration below, we have restored a normal insulin level by lowering your total calories, as well as changing to carbohydrates that don't flip those metabolic switches to fat burning. In the next part, we will give you a series of tools to help you always make choices that support long-term weight management and health.

"

A Habit of Health: Fueling your body every three hours.

"

2.4

Habits of Health Healthy Eating State: Healthy Waistline

BALANCED CALORIE HEATHY FUELING

FUEL FROM FOOD

NORMAL INSULIN STABLE WEIGHT

ANY EXCESS FUEL ENTERS FAT CELLS

FUEL FROM FAT CELLS BETWEEN MEALS

FAT CELLS NORMAL FUNCTION

As you build on your new healthy eating habits, you'll be able to eat whatever you want—in moderation—because you'll have integrated the Habits of Health, and your body will begin operating at peak efficiency. Once your body has gained back its full recuperative powers, even the occasional hot fudge sundae or slice of pizza will have no overall effect on your health, unless you have a high susceptibility to refined sugar and flour. To find out go to Element 16, *Dealing With Addictive Food,* in *Your LifeBook.*

In truth though, I doubt you'll even want these types of foods once you're fully aware of their negative effects. You'll begin to understand how processed food has robbed you of the almost spiritual experience of nature's flavors, and you'll be amazed how wonderful real food can taste and smell.

Speaking of great flavors, let's make this new healthy fueling pattern come alive.

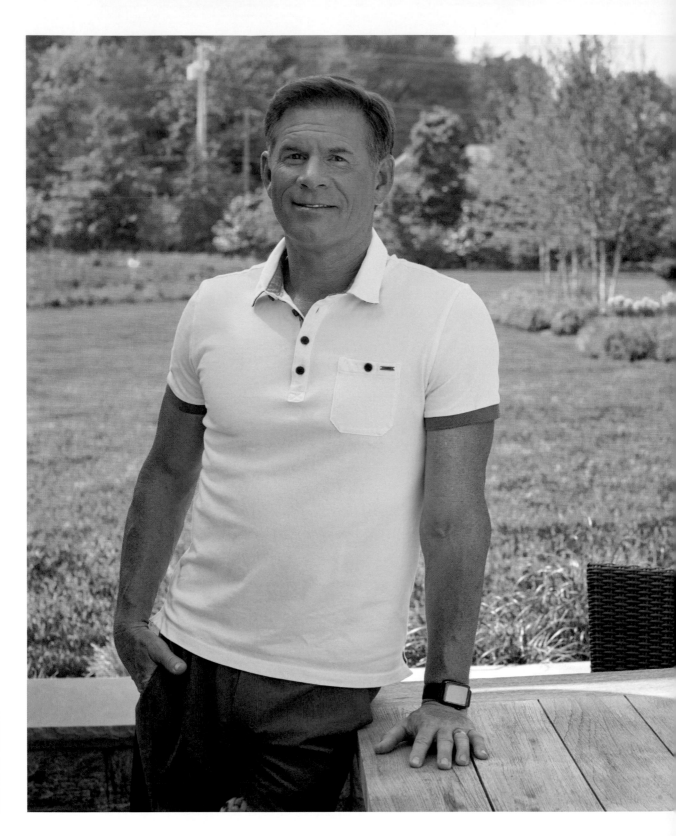

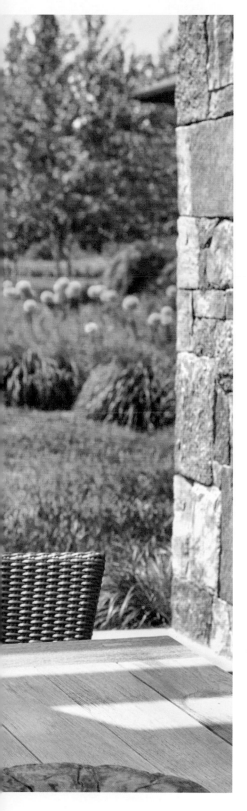

When I started with Dr. A, I had a background in fitness and managed my healthy weight through healthy exercise and movement. It really surprised me when I did my first health assessment that I was rated in the unhealthy category. Once I dug into the Habits of Health, I found the areas that I needed to work on.

I needed to get rid of my job because it was causing most of my unhealthy habits. I wasn't getting enough quality sleep, and I was able to correct that. I was a competitive cyclist and burned a lot of calories, but it allows you to eat some unhealthy things that don't really serve your health. I really struggled with sweets my whole life. I was getting sick a lot, and I knew that wasn't a natural thing to happen that somebody my age.

I have those habits under control now, and my health is fantastic. I rarely get sick. Before, I was taking antibiotics a lot, and that really manifests itself negatively. Everything was getting worse and worse (even though I still looked healthy) because I didn't have a lot of great healthy habits. Those are just a couple of the things that really made a major difference in my life.

I was a truck driver, and I was also a father. My real passion was my family, and I wanted to be there for them. I started working nights so I could split up my sleep to be at my son's games and support my children in their activities. But then I realized that the lack of sleep was really affecting me and how I showed up in the world.

One of the things I wanted was balance in life. The stress was actually a thing that manifested itself when I wanted to be somewhere and feeling guilty that I wasn't there. I even found that my mental health was worse than my physical health because I wasn't living a life fulfilled. I wasn't doing the things that were important to me, and I wanted to work my way back there. That's why I really wanted to become part of this optimal health community, because I could see an avenue of how I could get to where I wanted to be from where I was.

> " *I was getting sick a lot and I knew that wasn't a natural thing to happen to somebody my age.* "

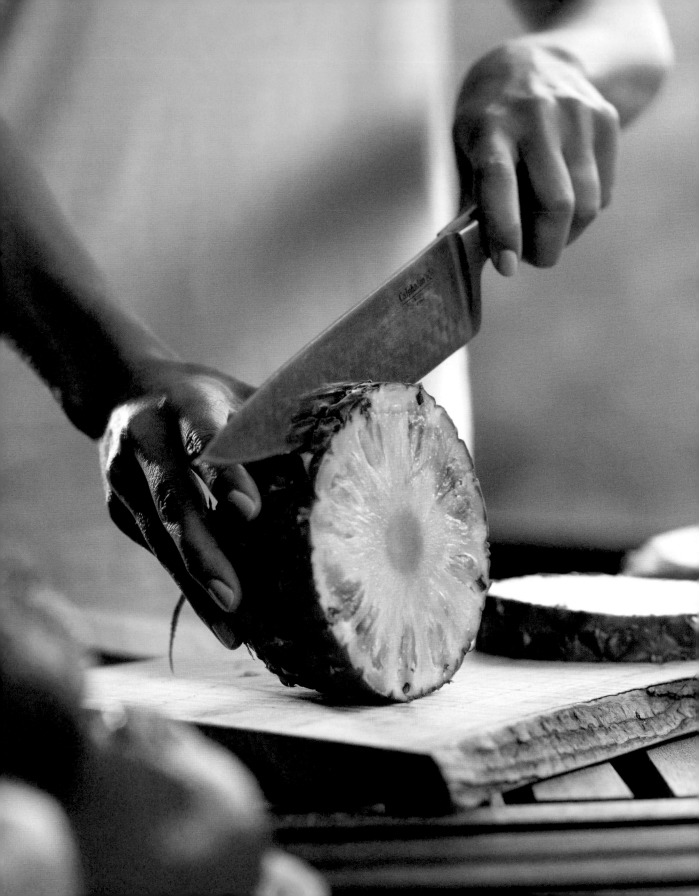

CHOOSING WISELY: DR. A'S COLOR-CODED SHOPPING SYSTEM

**HABITS OF
HEALTHY WEIGHT MANAGEMENT**

**THE HABITS OF
HEALTHY EATING AND HYDRATION**

The quality of the food you eat is actually more important than the quantity of calories we consume but both are critical to weight management and eating healthy for life. In Part 2.4, Dr. A's Healthy Eating System, we explained the first component of my simple eating system to manage the quantity of food you consume.

My innovative plate system was designed to overcome the confusing and complicated pyramid of the USDA approach. It has helped so many clients and patients take control of their energy intake, the USDA has followed my lead.

As I described in the last part, I have made two small adjustments so that My Plate and my system are interchangeable, thereby giving you access to multiple resources. I have taken the fruits and vegetable section which represents 50% of the nine-inch plate and separated it into two equal parts (25/25%) so you can follow their system. There will still be many times where you will want more of the 50% to come from vegetables, especially in the weight loss phase. I'll make those moments clear. I've also changed the starch category to grains to keep the categories consistent.

In this part, we will now shift our focus to the quality of the food you will be eating both for weight loss and also to eat healthier food for life.

We will introduce my color-coded system which will make shopping and eating out a breeze. It started as a simple way to distinguish healthy carbs because many experts in the medical establishment think that learning how to choose healthy, low-glycemic foods is just too difficult for most people to grasp, despite the proven health benefits. I disagreed! The color coded approach was so successful in helping people make healthy low-glycemic choices that I extended it to help with all of our food choices. Our simple color-coded charts now make it easy for people to master shopping for healthy proteins, grains, fruits, and vegetables. When combined with our easy visual portion-control system, this color-coded shopping system puts you well on the way to creating meals that help you lose weight and build optimal health.

And the color-coded system has been extended to give you easy ways to make healthy choices in all of the food groups—if you stay in the green you will stay lean (and healthy).

LOW-GLYCEMIC FOODS FOR OPTIMAL HEALTH

The message couldn't be simpler: staying away from refined sugar and flour and focusing instead on eating low-glycemic carbohydrates and healthy foods is the best way to lose weight and create health.

Many Western nations that, like the U.S., are experiencing obesity epidemics have embraced the glycemic index—a standard for measuring and communicating the glycemic content of food—as an important way to help people understand how to make healthy choices.

Sadly, the U.S. medical community has been slow to endorse this powerful tool, claiming that it's just too hard for most people to understand. Since the first edition of this book some leaders in nutritional research and obesity have started to come around. As I mentioned earlier, Dr. David Ludlow, a practicing endocrinologist and leading obesity researcher at Boston Children's Hospital and Professor of Nutrition at Harvard School of Public Health, has embraced glycemic index. His new book *Always Hungry* is based on glycemic

> " *Eat food.*
> *Not too much.*
> *Mostly plants.* "

MICHAEL POLLAN

Turn Down the Dial with These Easy Tips for Lowering the Glycemic Index!

Take low-glycemic eating even further. Here are some simple ways to help keep your blood sugar under control by lowering the glycemic influence in the foods you eat each day.

Note: We will address the science behind glycemic index in more detail in the Part 2.7, *The Science of Healthy Eating and Weight Loss.*

By changing your stomach and gut emptying times we can naturally reduce the entry of glucose into the bloodstream and lower the glycemic index which can be accomplished by the following:

- Use vinegar and lemon juice, pickle your vegetables, and select sourdough bread (not in Phase I) to slow down the rate of starch digestion and the rate at which your stomach empties.
- Undercook your spaghetti, oatmeal, and other pasta-like starches (in other words, cook them al dente) to slow digestion and prevent starch from gelatinizing.
- Use stone-ground rather than finely milled flours. Large particles (less refined) have a lower glycemic content.
- If you eat higher-glycemic foods (which should be avoided during weight loss), combine them with low-glycemic choices to lower the overall effect on blood sugar and the glycemic content of your meal.

index and load and supports what I have been teaching and the amazing results I have seen over the last 10 or more years.

If we move people away from the ultra-processed western diet and unhealthy carbs we can turn off insulin and the body stops behaving like a fat storage depot.

The system I have developed takes all of the confusion out of shopping and ordering at restaurants and makes choosing and preparing low-glycemic foods a breeze. At its core is a series of color-coded charts highlighting choices from each food group. You can use these charts when you're preparing meals at home, when you're shopping, or when you're ordering food in a restaurant.

Here's your rule of thumb for foods that contain carbohydrates:

Color Code for Glycemic Index

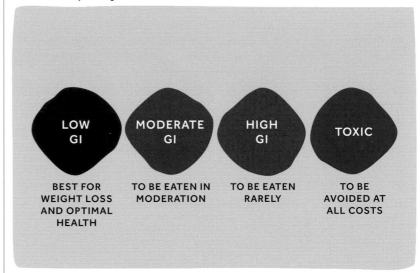

If you begin your journey in Phase I (weight loss), your healthy eating selections should come from the dark green charts. These foods are highly effective at turning off your insulin and fat storage and will facilitate reaching and maintaining an optimal weight. The light green charts list foods that are healthy but should be used sparingly in the first phase of our journey. Foods on the orange chart should be used with care, only after you've reached optimal health. And any food that is in the red is directly damaging to your health and should be eliminated completely from your diet, forever. However good they taste, they are just not worth it.

And, of course, the prepackaged low calorie fuelings are designed specifically to provide a high-quality, low-glycemic choice, and are always an excellent way to obtain a nutrient-dense, calorie-friendly fueling or meal. They are always designated dark green.

THE POWER OF FOOD

One criticism of current diet advice is that it really doesn't help people distinguish between healthy and unhealthy choices. One group is vilifying sugar and another is saying that high fat is the problem. The advice doesn't consistently discourage the consumption of red meats high in saturated fats, or encourage the use of health-enhancing oils. It gives equal classification to energy-giving whole-grain products and the health-robbing refined grains found in many processed foods.

My plan, however, teaches you to replace the processed foods with healthy foods that have a powerful healing effect on your body. By choosing healthy foods from the designated major food groups in this color-coded way, you will have a simple system to always be able to choose the healthiest options. This will allow you to tap into the natural ability of nutrient-dense foods to actually improve the health of your cells, thereby putting you in an ideal state to shed excess weight while moving you from non-sickness to optimal health.

In essence, as we eliminate the health robbing effects of unhealthy food we'll be using food to heal you instead of medicine to treat symptoms. Think of it as removing kryptonite so your body is no longer exposed to toxins and metabolic negative switches and is, instead, using health restoring quality meals that turn on healthy biological pathways and genes. It's all part of an exciting new discipline that lifestyle physicians like myself have defined as nutritional intervention—a much more powerful medicine than any pharmaceutical I've ever seen. And it's the very basis of creating optimal health and wellbeing.

So why would a critical care physician who spent over 20 years using pharmaceuticals now abandon a drug based approach for a healthy nutritional approach? Simple. In those 20 years I never saw one of my medications create radiant health but, over the last 17 years, we have seen that by providing nutritional intervention we can witness the almost miraculous reversal of multiple unhealthy conditions. Providing healthy food has the power not only to resolve pre-obesity, high insulin levels, and other unhealthy states without dangerous side effects. It also creates a platform for optimal health that traditional medicine cannot provide.

I like to call the healthy foods we'll be selecting "functional foods"—a term first used in Japan in the 1980s to describe foods that provide particular health benefits.

In my plan, I use the term to describe foods that add value to your body and move you up the path toward optimal health. It's one way of thinking of your nutritional intake as good medicine.

This new way of looking at food will unlock a whole new healthy world for you. Understanding how to select foods for optimal health is just as important as managing the total number of calories you consume—if not more so. In fact, the Habits of Health you're about to learn are among the most important daily decisions you can make.

The one thing we know for sure is when someone from anywhere

" *For your convenience, you can also download my color-coded shopping charts from HabitsofHealth.com or find them in the Habits of Health App.* "

2.5

A Habit of Health:
Choosing low-glycemic carbohydrates, lean proteins, and healthy fats.

DR. A'S COLOR-CODED SHOPPING SYSTEM

CHOOSING WISELY:

One reason people get confused about glycemic content and the glycemic index is that some foods that are low glycemic can be high carbohydrate. So how can you avoid picking the wrong foods? First, just choose foods from the dark green charts and, second, be sure that your portion size fits in the right compartment on your nine-inch plate. As long as you stick with these two basic rules, you'll keep your insulin level stable and your fat-storage machinery turned off. The charts are available for download on HabitsofHealth.com and they are also in Your LifeBook and the Habits of Health App.

in the world is exposed to the Modern American Diet (MAD) the result is the same: obesity, poor health and disease follows. I also know that we all have a body that we want to be healthier. I took an oath many years ago that stated I would first do no harm and help people improve in any way I could and the health benefits of an emphasis on eating healthy food far outweighs any benefit that comes from medicines that mostly just relieve symptoms.

Western Diet vs. Traditional Diets

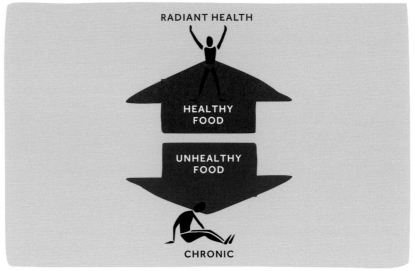

RADIANT HEALTH

HEALTHY FOOD

UNHEALTHY FOOD

CHRONIC

How do we make our choices all green to help us heal and improve our health and our wellbeing?

It's going to take a decision to make a nutritional intervention of your very own, along with some knowledge, some tools, some coaching, and some habit installations.

Let's start with some history and background of the evolution of eating and the birth of food technology in western countries.

What makes most of the MAD diet so bad for us and how do we stop the madness? The industrial revolution changed food forever. For over 10,000 years we ate a rather simple diet rich in fruits and vegetables, high in fiber and micronutrients, low in salt and sugar, and essentially free of trans fats and low in saturated fats. 100 years ago, food industrialization changed everything.

Starvation was a major international crisis and the food industry was asked to help eradicate this significant world issue. We asked for cheap, readily available, and easy to ship-and-store food to help feed the world. Unfortunately we forgot to ask for it to be healthy. Now, as amazing as this will seem, there are more people who are overweight and obese in the world than there are people starving.

What happened? It starts with refined flour. Grains are made up of three parts: the bran or hull, the germ, and the endosperm. Whole grains have all three while the principle component of refined grains is the least nutritious component. The advancements in technology created the ability to mill with a steel press and separate the starchy, white, endosperm away from the germ in a grain kernel. Overnight flour changed from being nutrient packed but with a short shelf-life, to a white powder that was highly digestible (high glycemic index), cheap, and long lasting but with almost no nutritional value.

Sugar follows a similar story. Originally, the coarse sugar found in beets and sugarcane was costly and difficult to purify. People chewed sugarcane raw to extract its sweetness. Over time, via advancing processing techniques, we now have refined sugar which, like flour, is a white powder that lacks any real nutritional value.

THE WHITE POWDER

Coca chewing and drinking coca tea is carried out daily by millions of people in the Andes. It is considered sacred within indigenous cultures and does not cause any harm: in fact, it is beneficial to human health. But as you will know, the coca leaf can be refined and turned from a healthy natural food into a dangerously addictive substance.

That is exactly what has a happened with sugarcane and flour. They have been turned from a healthy food with great nutritional value into cheap readily available calories that have little or no nutritional value and create metabolic and inflammatory havoc. They're also highly addictive.

When subjects are placed in fMRI machines that are designed to show areas of the brain activated after consuming sugar or foods made with refined flour, the subject's pleasure and reward center lights up like a firework display. The hyperactive area, known as the nucleus accumbens, releases large amounts of dopamine, which creates a pleasurable feeling and leads to the desire for more.

Brain on Sugar (left), Brain on Cocaine (right)

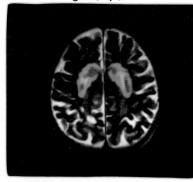 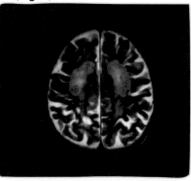

"Nutritional intervention is a more powerful medicine than any pharmaceutical and it's the very basis of health."

2.5

Excess sugar has been shown to accelerate aging and inflammation and is like candy for cancer cells.[1] It also leads to a smaller brain! Studies show that as your blood sugar increase to the higher end of normal your brain begins to shrink.[2] There is no reason to add sugar to your diet beyond what you get from fruits and vegetables!

Some of us are more susceptible than others. We will have you take a survey in *Your LifeBook* to determine how susceptible you are. It will make a difference to your long-term success!

DR. A'S COLOR-CODED SHOPPING SYSTEM

CHOOSING WISELY:

One of the biggest changes in modern wheat is that it contains a modified form of gliadin—a protein found in wheat gluten. Gliadin unleashes a feel-good effect in the brain by morphing into a substance that crosses the blood-brain barrier and binds onto the brain's opiate receptors. Gliadin is a very mind-active compound that increases people's appetites. People on average eat more calories a day when eating wheat, thanks to the appetite-stimulating effects of gliadin.[1]

It is the identical response that occurs when subjects are given cocaine.

This addiction creates a pathologic feedback loop that makes the desire for more and more sugary and flour products almost unavoidable. Your body needs more and more sugar to mimic the pleasurable sensation in an addiction-habit loop that becomes hard to break.[2]

Isn't it ironic that in their raw state coca, sugarcane, and wheat are all healthy, and yet when we process them into a white refined powder they all become deadly. Then there's gliadin in new strains of refined wheat! See the sidebar for more information on this.

And those powders form the basis of not just breads and buns, but also for a huge variety of processed foods, from cereals, crackers and pizza dough to cookies, cakes, and ice cream cones. As a result, the average American now eats 10 servings of refined grains each day. And, as we showed you in Part 1.1, *It's Not Your Fault That Your Struggling*, refined sugar is in everything; in fact, we are consuming an average of over 150 lbs of refined sugar and flour products a year.[3]

GETTING READY TO SHOP

Today's supermarkets can be confusing places, with far too many choices. Before you head out to the store, here are a couple of guidelines to steer you toward foods that promote health and away from those that lead to disease.

- Fresh is better than frozen, canned, or in a jar.
- Natural is better than processed.

That's all well and good, but what do these terms really mean, and how can you know you're getting what you think you are?

SO WHAT DO WE MEAN BY FRESH?

It's a tricky question. Too often what's advertised as fresh really isn't, as in the following examples:

Problem: Those greens may have been fresh at one time, but since then they've sat in a warehouse for weeks losing vitamins and nutrients. By the time you buy them at the store, the freshness is depleted.

Solution: When possible, buy locally grown produce. It will be picked closer to the sale date and have spent less time traveling.

How Do I Know If It's Organic?

The term organic can mean different things on food labels, depending on how it's used. Here's a quick guide to some common labeling terms:

- 100% certified organic: all the ingredients are certified organic
- Organic: contains at least 95% organic ingredients
- Made with organic ingredients: at least 75% of the ingredients are organic. Some packages may not state organic on the label, but still list some ingredients that may be organic.

Problem: Many commercially grown foods are "protected" with chemicals designed to preserve freshness. But do they? The veggies maintain their color and texture but lose their flavor and much of their nutritional value.

Solution: A local green grocer may carry fruits and vegetables that haven't been treated. You will get healthier, better-tasting food that's higher in nutritional value than the supermarket variety.

NATURAL, PROCESSED, ORGANIC: IS THERE REALLY A DIFFERENCE?

The short answer is yes. Take peanut butter, for example. Natural peanut butter consists of peanuts and a bit of salt. That's it! Processed peanut butters, including most of the familiar national brands, contain peanuts and salt as well as sugar or high-fructose corn syrup, along with other ingredients that are completely unnecessary and which can have a negative effect on your health. And—just as an aside—once you've become used to the real thing, the processed stuff tastes like plastic.

Today's farm raised beef, lamb, pork, and poultry are fed the same unhealthy Western diet that we are. They eat much higher levels of saturated fats and their levels of inflammatory omega-6 are high. And since producers try to decrease time to market, animals are fed growth hormones and become sick; this means that they need antibiotics. So most of them test positive for antibiotics and even growth hormones—a practice that increases production for the food industry, but brings its own set of problems, including increasing bacterial resistance to antibiotics. If you can, try to buy meats that aren't processed—those labeled natural—to indicate that the animal hasn't been given antibiotics or growth hormones.

A wide assortment of these foods, as well as grass-fed meats, can usually be found at stores like Whole Foods Market.

And what about organic? Organic products are becoming more accessible, even in the large supermarket chains. For products to be labeled certified organic by the USDA, the producer needs to uphold a rigorous set of standards that go beyond natural. As demand for organic grows, so does the organic food industry. In time, this could prove a tremendous counterforce to "big food", which all too often is more concerned with high production and profit than with quality. Yes, organic products usually cost 10–20% more, but the difference is worth it. You're better off eating less meat and dairy products and going organic, than eating more processed stuff.

What is Organic Food?

Organic foods are produced according to certain production standards, meaning they're grown without the use of conventional pesticides, artificial fertilizers, human waste, or sewage sludge, and processed without ionizing radiation or food additives. Livestock are reared without the routine use of antibiotics and without the use of growth hormones. In most countries, organic produce cannot be genetically modified.
Going Organic? Look for the 9s!
Discover whether the produce you're buying is organic or conventionally produced by checking the PLU (price look-up) code—the four or five-digit number usually located on a small sticker affixed to fruits and vegetables. If the code has four digits, it's conventional. If it has five digits and begins with the number nine, it's organic.

2.5

mHoH

Before you try a new food, read the nutrition label. The contents and calorie count may surprise you.

> *Functional foods have particular health benefits that enhance your meals and move you toward optimal health. They're nutrient dense, calorie friendly, and contain healthy fiber. Dysfunctional foods rob you of your health and promote disease. They're energy dense, nutrient poor, and usually over-processed.*

THE ECONOMICS OF HEALTHY FOOD

When your body's working well, it needs less food. Let's do the numbers. Say you spend $100 a week for food right now. Once your body wants less to eat, you can spend the same amount, but you'll be able to buy higher-quality food.

Better food costs more, but you need less of it. When you eat bad processed food, your body is never really satisfied and so you eat more and more, even if you're stuffed to the gills. So much of our food is energy dense but nutrient poor, leaving the body deficient in the nutrients it so desperately needs. With higher-quality food, your eating habits change because you are eating nutrient-dense food that fulfills the body's requirements. And when your sense of taste is satisfied, your body is satisfied, and as a result you're able to stop eating before you're too stuffed. You'll find yourself leaving the table before you've eaten everything in sight, and you won't even want to make that midnight raid on the refrigerator!

READY? LET'S GO SHOPPING!

The charts that follow are designed to steer you toward foods that rev up your health. Think of them as the octane-disclosure sheets at the gas pumps. Watch your engine's performance improve as you switch from regular gas (the low-octane, nutrient-poor foods you're eating now) to premium (functional foods that are nutrient-dense, highly efficient fuels that turn down your insulin pump and turn on fat burning).

As you shop, remember to visualize your nine-inch plate, with its divisions based on the proper proportion of foods for optimal health and weight loss. You'll need to have plenty of vegetables and fruits on hand, as well as fewer quantities of healthy complex grains and lean proteins to create healthy, delicious meals.

Healthy Eating and Weight Management: MacroHabit Principles to Keep in Mind:

Here are the main points and Habits of Health from your healthy eating system. Keep them in mind as you plan your daily meals.

- Choose all your carbohydrates (vegetable, fruit, and grain components) from the green lists, with the majority from the dark green sections.
- Remember to serve your new, healthy food choices on a nine- inch plate.
- Maintain the proper proportions for healthy eating and weight loss: 50% vegetable/fruit (mostly vegetables during the weight-loss phase), 25% grain (starch), and 25% protein.
- Select healthy fueling-break foods from the choices provided, choosing those that you enjoy and fit your lifestyle. Remember to choose from the healthy periphery of the store, not the interior aisles that are full of unhealthy processed foods!
- If you are using my eating system to lose weight maintain your Phase I meal schedule: two meals (400 calories each) and four fueling breaks (100 calories each).

Before You Shop

- Be sure you've created the microenvironment of health we discussed in Part 2.2, *Your Blueprint: Safe Weight Loss and Health Gain*. That means clearing your house of all junk food. Have fun doing it! Imagine that you're getting rid of your bad food demons, and renewing your kitchen as a source of health, life, and energy.
- Arm yourself with a shopping list before you enter any sort of food shop to avoid impulse buying. Stay along the outer aisles of the store, where the produce, meat, fish, and other fresh, healthy items are found. Avoid the tempting processed foods on the inner aisles.
- Never go shopping when you're hungry!

Remember: You buy your willpower at the store! If you don't bring it home you will be much less likely to eat it!

> *Fresh foods are critical for optimal health. If you're not sure which foods are fresh, ask your grocer.*

2.5

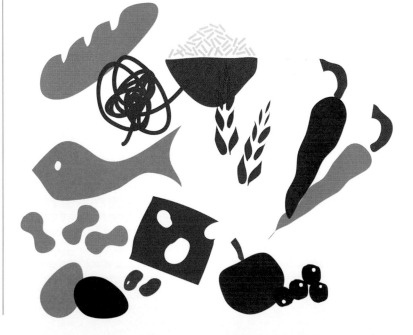

Specific Receptors for Specific Fruits & Vegetables

Recent research is showing that there are specific receptors for different fruits and vegetables. That is why it is so important to have diversity in our consumption of fruits and vegetables. Each plant family has a unique combination of phytonutrients that may bind to specific proteins within our body.[4]

Half of fruit servings are taken up by just six foods: OJ, bananas, apple juice, apples, grapes, and watermelons. And half of vegetables are made up of iceberg lettuce, frozen potatoes, fresh potatoes, potato chips, and canned tomatoes.[5]

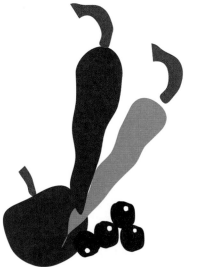

To estimate the correct portion size, visualize a healthy portion of vegetables and fruits together as being about the size of a small paperback book or 50% of your plate.

VEGETABLES AND FRUITS:
25%+25%: 50% OF YOUR PLATE

Functional:
Rich in vitamins, minerals, phytochemicals, and fiber, vegetables and fruit are at the core of your long-term plan to reach and maintain optimal health. And because they're low in calories and provide plenty of bulk to fill you up, they're a great tool to help you take charge of energy intake.

Dr. A's Health Eating Plate System for Life

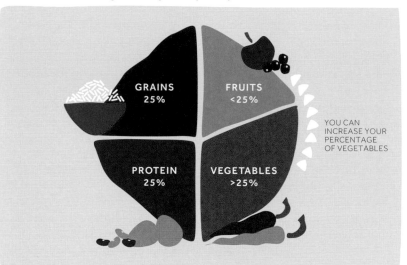

GRAINS 25%

FRUITS <25%

YOU CAN INCREASE YOUR PERCENTAGE OF VEGETABLES

PROTEIN 25%

VEGETABLES >25%

When you're shopping, think about the meals you're planning. A meal on your nine-inch plate should be made up of 50% vegetables and fruits, 25% protein, and 25% grain from my healthy food choices. Remember you can always add more vegetables and less fruit to the percentage. You could even skip the fruit and use all vegetables every now and then.

Note: If you are using the Optimal Weight 5&1 Plan as your Phase I weight-loss program, you are not allowed fruit during this phase.

Dysfunctional:
The fried vegetables typical of fast food chains and other restaurants, as well as many common packaged fruit juices have both been stripped of their nutrients and are loaded with fat and sugar.

Vegetables and fruits represent half of your meal in our eating system. These essential foods provide nutrient-dense functional support to help you lose weight, as well as a wealth of antioxidants and anti-inflammatories for building optimal health. And you'll never tire of their abundant variety of flavors and textures: sweet to sour, crunchy to smooth, from mild lettuces to power-packed blueberries.

Healthy vegetable and fruit choices:
A wide variety of vibrant foods including salads, crunchy raw vegetables, and nutrient-packed berries.

Proportion of your meal:
50% of your nine-inch plate between the two. However, you have to limit your fruit intake to 25% but you can increase the percentage from vegetables.

Portion size:
About the size of a small paperback book with about 100 pages, but green low-glycemic vegetables are so beneficial, you could probably even use a great big Tom Clancy book as your point of reference and still not overdo it!

Note: If you are using my healthy eating system as your Phase I weight-loss program I would limit your intake to a small amount of low-glycemic fruit on occasion or avoid totally; this is because fruit is higher glycemic and more calorie dense, and so they should be the minor contributor to your vegetable/fruit group in this phase. Once you've reached a healthy weight and transition to Phase II, you'll be able to increase the amount of fruit in your diet.

Vegetable Choices

	15 OR LESS				
VERY LOW GI	• Zucchini		• Arugula		• Broccoli
	• Spinach		• Asparagus		• Chives
	• Peppers		• Fennel		• Leeks
	• Onions		• Cucumber		• Celery
	• Mushrooms		• Cabbage		• Cauliflower
	• Lettuce		• Squash		• Chili peppers
	• Alfalfa sprouts		• Brussels sprouts		
	• Artichokes		• Bell peppers		
	20 OR MORE				
	• Eggplant	20	• Green beens	20	• Carrots (raw)	30
HIGH GI	**50 OR MORE**				
	• Peas	50	• Corn	65	• Carrots (cooked)	80
	• Taro	54	• Red beets (canned)	64	

Vegetables and fruits make up a whopping 50% of your meals, so it's especially important to select the lowest-glycemic varieties. Although a small amount of low-glycemic fruit is permitted while you're optimizing your weight (not on the *Optimal Weight 5&1 Plan*), it's best to focus on vegetables for your vegetable/fruit component. The charts are arranged from lowest glycemic (dark green) to moderate glycemic (light green) to high glycemic (orange). If you see a red chart avoid at all cost! Red can make you dead! Okay, so it won't kill you instantly but it will, predictably, over time.

> " *Fruit juices may seem like a healthy choice, but they're usually loaded with sweeteners and empty calories that don't fill you up but rather lead to weight gain.* "

2.5

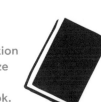

One fruit and vegetable portion is about the size of a small paperback book.

Vegetables from the dark green charts have very little effect on blood sugar and insulin and should be used freely. In fact, if you find that you absolutely need a little something extra as you're settling into your new eating strategy, you can always select from this component. Celery is a great crunchy choice!

Unhealthy Vegetables and Fruits: A Habit of Disease

It's truly criminal what the processed and fast food industries do to once-healthy fruits and vegetables. Think of such "delights" as the Bloomin' Onion™, tempura vegetables and, sadly, the number-one selling vegetable in our country: French fries. A potato is already a very high-glycemic, high-carbohydrate tuber vegetable to be avoided completely in the weight loss phase but it can be made so much worse by the manner in which it's prepared and eaten.

A recent study found that most Americans eat fewer than two servings of vegetables and fruits a day—far below the recommended five to seven daily servings.[8] Even more troubling, half of those respondents named French fries as one of their daily choices![9]

Fruit choices

	30 OR LESS					
VERY LOW GI	• Olives	15	• Lemons	20	• Grapefruit	25
	• Avocado	10	• Raspberries	25	• Cherries	25
	• Limes	20	• Blackberries	25	• Tomatoes	30
	50 OR LESS					
LOW GI	• Apples	30	• Pears	35	• Apricots (dried)	35
	• Nectarines	30	• Strawberries	35	• Plums	35
	• Peaches	30	• Oranges	35	• Figs	40
	50 OR MORE					
HIGH GI	• Apricots	57	• Kiwi	50	• Pineapple	59
	• Bananas	60	• Grapes	53	• Watermelon	76
	• Blueberries	53	• Mango	51		
	• Cantaloupe	50	• Melon	60		

But what about fruit juices? Surely that's a healthy choice? The sad reality is that most packaged juices contain nothing more than high-fructose corn syrup with a little fruit "waved" over them. As such, they contain a high level of non-nutritive calories in a form that's so hard for the body to detect that it doesn't even sense it's being overloaded with calories. The result is excess weight and a whole host of diseases, including an epidemic increase in childhood obesity.

Unhealthy fruit and vegetables

UNHEALTHY: HABITS OF DISEASE		
• French fries	• Onion rings	• Fruit juices

Total intake of vegetables and fruits is a powerful predictor of overall wellbeing. Your wellbeing goes up with each additional serving of fruit or vegetable.[6]

A study of almost 5,000 breast cancer survivors found a 62% reduction in mortality for women whose consumption of vegetables was in the top fourth![7]

PROTEIN: 25% OF YOUR PLATE

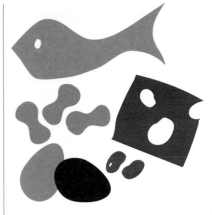

Functional:
Lean proteins form the building blocks of your vital tissues and organs. They contain amino acids that protect your muscles during weight loss and are the best macronutrient to help you feel full.

Dysfunctional:
Many common forms of protein are high in unhealthy saturated fat.

Healthy protein choices:
Very lean meats, eggs, fish, seafood, white-meat poultry, low-fat yogurt, low fat milk and cheeses, legumes, nuts, seeds.

Proportion of your meal:
25% of your nine-inch plate.

Portion size:
About the size of a deck of cards (after cooking).

Proteins are a critical component of weight loss. Most protein sources, including fresh meats, poultry, and fish, contain no carbohydrates at all, so their glycemic level is negligible. And to top it off, calorie-for-calorie they're better than any other food at giving you a sense of fullness and satisfaction. Research suggests that protein stimulates cells that keep us thin and alert. To support weight loss and optimal health, choose lean proteins that are low in saturated animal fats. Great sources include eggs, fish, and white-meat poultry, as well as vegetable sources such as soy and other legumes, which I'll discuss later. While dairy products are included in the protein category, bear in mind that they can contain considerable amounts of carbohydrates as well.

The following charts don't list glycemic levels for meat, fish, or poultry because the glycemic content for these foods is negligible. However, the charts do include total fat and saturated fat levels for meats. To guide your choices for optimal health, just choose any fish from the charts, or any meats that fall in the green area.

Fish and Seafood
When you eat fish, you're not only choosing a great protein source, you're also significantly reducing your risk of disease.[10-19] Eating fish one to three times a week is an important Habit of Health and can have a profound impact on your wellbeing over time. In fact, one serving of fish a week may reduce your risk of fatal heart attack by 40%!

Note: Pregnant women and young children should limit their intake of fish to once a week due to the potential for high mercury content in some fish.[10-19]

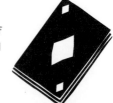

One serving of protein should be about the size of a deck of cards.

"

With their power to eliminate hunger and renew muscle for optimal health, healthy protein selections are highly supportive of weight loss.

"

Healthy Fish and Seafood

FRESH FISH	CANNED FISH
• Atlantic and pacific salmon • Smoked salmon • Atlantic and Pacific mackerel • Bluefin tuna • Oysters • Squid (calimari)	• Salmon • Sardines • Mackerel • Tuna (in water, canola, olive oil, tomato sauce, or brine)

Meat

It's an important Habit of Health to lower your consumption of meat. But if you're like me and once in a while need that savory taste of meat, just minimize the amount of saturated fat so you can enjoy this great protein source and still stay healthy.

Did you know that wild meat—the kind our ancestors ate 10,000 years ago—contains much less saturated fat than farm-raised meat? Our cattle are fed on high-glycemic foods and, as a result, contain an unhealthy amount of fat. By eating them, we concentrate our ingestion of fat and calories. Farm fed cattle have high levels of omega-6 which we already have too much of in our diet. If you do eat beef then make sure it is grass fed.

Wild meats, such as buffalo and elk, contain very little fat and have a much higher level of omega-3 which is what you want. I've found both of these very enjoyable, as well as venison (deer) which, although a bit powerful in flavor, can be quite good if prepared properly. Many of these wild meats are available in grocery stores such as Whole Foods Market. Traditional American beef is fine if you select cuts such as filets and sirloins rather than those that contain excess marbling from fat.

Fat Content of Meat

	TOTAL FAT	SATURATED FAT
Buffalo, elk, venison	17%	7%
Pork loin	26%	9%
Round steak	27%	10%
Veal chop	39%	17%
Canadian bacon	41%	14%
Filet mignon	42%	16%
Sirloin steak	44%	16%
Flank steak	44%	19%
Lamb ribs	48%	22%
Spare ribs	52%	22%
Ground beef (very lean)	58%	23%
Sausage (beef)	80%	33%

Unhealthy Proteins: A Habit of Disease

With our processed lunch-meats, hot dogs, and hamburgers, most of us eat far too much protein that's high in saturated fat. Foods like these stimulate inflammation and have a profoundly negative effect on your heart, your blood vessels, and your brain. They create oxygen free radicals that attack the lining of the vessels in all your organs and contribute to heart disease, high blood pressure, strokes, and cancers and accelerate aging.

One of the largest studies of its kind found that those who ate just one daily serving of processed red meat, a hot dog or two slices of bacon had a 20% greater chance of dying during the 28 years of the study.[20]

To make matters worse, we stick these fatty meats on the "barbie" to char them. This creates extremely dangerous substances called advanced glycation end products (AGES), which can make these foods up to 200 times more immuno-reactive, and which also attack your body with a vengeance. The challenge is that AGES are very deceptive and the char that forms when grilling smells and tastes great is the least healthy part to eat![21] (For more information on the dangers of inflammation, see Part 2.14, *Inflamation: Dousing the Flame*). As you can imagine, eliminating these foods can have a dramatic effect on your health!

Unhealthy Protein Choices

UNHEALTHY: HABITS OF DISEASE		
• Fatty meats	• Hot dogs	• Hamburgers

Poultry

Chicken, turkey, and other forms of poultry are healthier choices than red meat. But be careful! The health value and calorie content of poultry can vary significantly depending on the type of bird, which part you eat, and how it's prepared and cooked. For example, while a skinless turkey breast is 18% fat, the fat content of a skinless chicken breast is 24%. And manufactured products such as sausages, hot dogs, and burgers made from turkey and chicken aren't really much healthier than their meat counterparts.

Fat Content of Poultry

	SKIN?	TOTAL FAT	SATURATED FAT
Turkey breast		18%	6%
Chicken breast		24%	7%
Chicken breast	yes	36%	10%
Turkey breast	yes	38%	5%
Chicken dark meat		43%	12%
Turkey dark meat	yes	47%	14%
Turkey sausage		50%	15%
Duck	yes	50%	19%
Chicken dark meat	yes	56%	16%
Cornish game hen	yes	63%	28%
Turkey hot dog		70%	19%

As a general rule, avoid eating; however, it is a dark meat (legs and thighs) and always remove the skin before eating—though it is a good idea to keep the skin on while you bake, grill, or broil your

"

Learning to eat healthy for life is about much more than numbers on the scale. Don't forget to measure your other successes, like creating a new healthy recipe, walking farther than you thought you could, or enjoying an evening out while making good food choices.

"

2.5

poultry to help lock in flavor and maintain moistness without adding significantly to the fat content of the finished dish. As far as portion size is concerned, you should ideally end up with a piece that fits in the 25% protein portion of your plate (about the size of a deck of cards)—around 3.5 oz of cooked poultry.

A final piece of advice: free-range or organic poultry can help you avoid the antibiotics and growth hormones that are given to many commercially raised birds.

Eggs

Eggs are an incredible source of protein that deliver all the amino acids, B2, B12, folate, and vitamins D and E. The whites are a wonderful digestible source of iron as well. While eggs are low in saturated fat, they're a major source of cholesterol and, even though we now know that saturated fat actually has more impact than dietary cholesterol on blood cholesterol levels, you should still limit your daily intake of dietary cholesterol to 200 mg—the amount in one small egg. There's no limit to the amount of egg whites you can eat, as long as they fit the 25% of your plate devoted to protein.

Legumes

Legumes, a group that includes beans, peas, and lentils, are one of my favorite functional foods and probably my top pick for an all-around health food. They're a good protein source and almost always low glycemic, making them a wonderful alternative for vegetarians or for anyone looking to meet their protein needs while lowering their intake of meats and saturated fats.

What else is great about legumes? They're full of riboflavin, niacin, folate, calcium, potassium, iron, and phosphorus. They're high in soluble fiber, which naturally lowers cholesterol. They're less expensive than meat and dairy products, and can be made into a wide variety of creative, flavorful dishes. In fact, when it comes to legumes, there's just no downside!

A cup of legumes gives you 110 to 150 calories of the best fuel you can buy. Choose from any of the varieties in the chart for the protein portion of your meal—all are low glycemic and do an excellent job of turning off your insulin pump.

Legumes GI Chart

VERY LOW GI	30 OR LESS					
	• Soy beans	18	• Chickpeas		• Lentils	25
	• Edamame	20	(Garbanzo beans)	20	• Black beans	25
LOW GI	50 OR LESS					
	• Lima beans	32	• Chickpeas	35	• Black-eyed peas	42
	• Kidney beans	35	• White beans	35		

A Habit of Health: Legumes!

Make daily consumption of legumes—beans, peas, or lentils—a part of your healthy eating strategy.

A Word about Soy

One particularly amazing legume stands out—soy. Soybeans have twice as much protein as other legumes and provide nearly as many essential amino acids as animal protein, without all the saturated fat. They're a good source of calcium as well, making them a great alternative to dairy products. In addition, soy is full of naturally occurring isoflavones—phytonutrients that protect against cardiovascular disease, especially in the Asian population.[22]

In fact, I think so highly of soy that it's my top choice for the protein component of our portion-controlled packaged meals and fuelings are a great way to make **using this healthy** legume as your protein component a breeze![23]

Dairy Products and Cheese

Dairy products are not a necessary food group once we are grown and because they can wallop a lot of calories, so I suggest you avoid them at least during weight loss. If you enjoy them, they can be a good source of calcium, protein, and other nutrients. They are the one protein source that can be quite high glycemic. Despite what the dairy industry would have you believe, dairy products can contribute to poor health if you are overweight and taking in too many calories, if not selected appropriately. Whole milk dairy products are not only high glycemic but also high in saturated animal fats—a double unhealthy wallop that pumps up insulin while creating ready stores of fat.

However, if consumed in portion-controlled amounts there is growing evidence that they may lower your cardiovascular risk and the risk of diabetes. There may be some benefits from the fatty acids in whole milk that potentially could help hormone regulation, cause you to store less fat, and rev up your metabolism. Skim milk is stripped of these fatty acids but one thing we know is that the sugar load is similar. Skim milk simply removes the fat but the sugar content remains the same.

Also dairy products are an excellent source of calcium—which has been shown to aid weight loss—but so are many of the fruits, green vegetables, and whole-grains you'll be eating.

In fact, dairy products should be used sparingly and confined to low-fat, low-sugar servings during Phase I until you reach your optimal weight and not at all if you're using the prepackaged fuelings. Once you've reached your healthy weight, you may opt to include two to three servings of dairy a day. You can choose low or high fat, unless you have high cholesterol or you are eating saturated fats from some other source. Then you should steer clear of whole-fat products and focus on skim (non-fat) or low fat. Good choices include non-fat yogurt (six ounces), non-fat milk (one cup), and cheese (one ounce), especially low-fat cheeses such as ricotta or cottage cheese. Remember, though, a one-ounce serving of cheese is a very small amount—about the size of two AA batteries.

> " *A one-ounce serving of cheese is about the size of two AA batteries.* "

2.5

Recent research indicates that the walnuts may be even more important than olive oil in creating the health-boosting effects of the popular Mediterranean diet.

Cheese with Calories per Ounce

Cheese	Calories	Cheese	Calories
Cottage	20	Soy	43
Ricotta	50	Feta	75
Mozzarella	90	American	94
Brie	95	Blue	100
Provolone	100	Gouda	101
Monterey Jack	106	Swiss	108
Havarti	106	Jarlsberg	110
Parmesan	110	Colby	112
Cheddar	114		

Seeds and Nuts: Your High-Octane Fuel Source

These health-giving, low-glycemic, protein-rich foods are also just chock full of healthy fats. But nuts and seeds are also extremely energy dense, meaning that they pack a lot of calories into a small amount. Those calories can add up in a hurry—in fact, a serving size is no more than a handful.

Nuts and seeds are about 15–30% proteins, with the remainder primarily made up of mono- and polyunsaturated fats—the healthy fats. They're also rich in thiamine, riboflavin, vitamin E, calcium, phosphorus, potassium, and iron. And, as an added bonus, they're full of an amino acid that contributes to your body's ability to relax blood vessels, decrease blood pressure, and inhibit clot formation. The steady, powerful fuel they provide makes nuts and seeds great snacks for fueling breaks, with enough protein to give you a pleasant, long-lasting feeling of fullness. Just limit yourself to a small handful to avoid excess calories.

Seeds and Nuts: Your High-Octane Fuel Source

VERY LOW GI	30 OR LESS					
	• Peanuts	15	• Sunflower seeds	15	• Hazlenuts	15
	• Brazil nuts	15	• Pecans	15	• Walnuts	15
	• Pumpkin seeds	15	• Almonds	15		

GRAINS: 25% OF YOUR PLATE

Functionally
Whole grains are a great slow-burning fuel, rich in fiber and loaded with B vitamins, calcium, potassium, and phosphorus. In their natural, low-glycemic state, they're critical for optimal health.

In their intact form, grains are made up of three parts: the bran or hull, the germ, and the endosperm. Whole grains have all three while the principle component of refined grains is the least nutritious component, or endosperm. Whole grains are not associated with BMI changes, and actually create lower fasting insulin levels, higher folate levels, and decrease chronic diseases.[24]

Refined Grains
The advancement in technology changed flour from a grey nutrient packed flour that needed to be eaten quickly before it spoiled, to a white powder which is principally made from the endosperm which has little nutritional value and is highly digestible (high glycemic index). It's also cheap and can be stored for longer, but it's lost all its nutrients. It has been implicated in weight gain, obesity, inflammation, and cancer.[25]

Dysfunctional
When refined and processed, grains are really unhealthy starches or are perhaps better described as an energy-dense, high-glycemic poison that turns on your insulin pump and puts you in fat-storage mode.

It may seem melodramatic, but it's true: your grain selections set the stage for success or failure. Starches come in a vast array of options. Sadly, most of the options developed and promoted by the fast-food and processed-food industries are bad for you. Healthy starches, however, are a nutrient-rich source of slow-burning fuel and long-lasting energy.

When looking at starches, it's essential to consider their position on the glycemic index. Most processed and prepackaged starches score high on the index, meaning that they deliver large amounts of carbohydrates and must be avoided. Instead, shop for healthy, low-glycemic starches using my color-coded system—your reliable guide in this vast and sometimes confusing food group.

Healthy Starch Choices:
Bread, pasta, noodles, and breakfast cereals made from whole grains such as rice, oats, wheat, barley, and rye. Potatoes, though a vegetable, act more like a refined starch due to their high glycemic and high carbohydrate content. Starchy foods include peas, corn, potatoes, beans, pasta, rice, and grains. Starches are a more concentrated source of carbohydrates and calories than fruits, nonstarchy vegetables and dairy, but many of them are excellent sources of fiber, vitamins, minerals, and phytonutrients.

> *Eating unhealthy carbohydrates like soda, french fries, candy, and doughnuts brings your fat-burning machinery to a halt.*

2.5

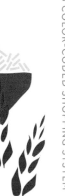

Your grain (starch) choices can set you up for success or failure—low-glycemic, whole-grain starches are critical for optimal health, while refined and processed high-glycemic starches put you in a fat storage mode. Remember, we are using grain and starch interchangeably to be able to use the tools presented in the My Plate System to guide you on healthy and unhealthy choices.

Proportion of Your Meal:
25% of your nine-inch plate.

Portion Size:
About the size of a tennis ball.

Grain Choices:
There's a wide variety of grains out there, many of which fall into the unhealthy, high-glycemic category. Just stay in the green and you'll be fine! (I've included potatoes, actually a vegetable, in the unhealthy starch section because their high-glycemic, high-carbohydrate content means they function more as a starch in most meals.)

Cereals, Breads, and Pastas GI chart

LOW GI	50 OR LESS			
	• Quinoa	35	• Buckwheat	45
	• Muesli (natural)	30	• Pasta (whole-grain)	45
	• Rye bread	30	• Whole wheat bread (with bran)	45
	• Unrefined flour:		• All-bran cereal	48
	bread	40	• Sourdough bread	35
	pasta	40		

HIGH GI	50 OR MORE			
	• Oatmeal (from steel-cut oats)	58	• Corn flakes	70
	• Semolina (cream of oats)	60	• White bread (enriched)	71
	• Hamburger roll	61	• Bagel (white)	72
	• Couscous	65	• Dinner roll (white)	73
	• Cereals (refined)	70	• Kaiser roll (white)	73
			• Crackers	80

Commercial Breakfast Products

LOW GI	50 OR LESS	
	• All-bran®	34

HIGH GI	50 OR MORE					
	• Frosted Flakes®	55	• Kellog's Raisin Bran®	73	• Rice Krispies®	82
	• Special K®	56	• Bran Flakes	74	• Crispix®	87
	• Nutri-grain®	66	• Coco Pops Snax®	77	• Shredded Wheat	75
	• Fruit Loops®	69	• Kellog's Corn Flakes®	77	• Wonder® Bread	80
	• Honey Smacks®	71	• Corn Pops®	80	• Oatmeal (instant)	82

A healthy portion of grain (starch) is about the size of a tennis ball.

Pastas, Potatoes, Rice GI Chart

LOW GI	50 OR LESS					
	• Wild rice	35	• Spaghetti		• Sweet potatoes	46
	• Yams	37	(durum)	40	• Brown rice	50
	• Spaghetti		• Basmati rice	50		
	(whole wheat)	40				

HIGH GI	MORE THAN 50					
	• White pasta	55	• Potatoes (mashed)	80	• Risotto	70
	• Potatoes		• Potatoes		• Rice cakes	85
	(with skin, baked		(instant mashed)	88	• Rice (precooked)	90
	or boiled)	65	• French fries	95		
	• Potatoes					
	(peeled and boiled)	70				

Note: Gluten Intolerance (Celiac disease and reported gluten sensitivities). There appears to be a rising prevalence of gluten sensitivities in the U.S. In those individuals the elimination of grains is helpful. For the main population there is no health benefit of eliminating gluten any more than there would be to eliminate peanuts to improve the health of people that are not allergic to them.

Unhealthy Grains (Starches): A Habit of Disease

What about the choice so many of us make—the starches that poison our body? Unhealthy starches like the ones in the following illustration are convenient, inexpensive, readily available, and tempting, thanks to the food industry's heavy use of advertising. They fulfill a need for comfort and satisfy cravings and hunger for a short time. But they also rev up your insulin pump, turn on your fat-storage system, stimulate inflammation, and can lead to the myriad health problems that make up metabolic syndrome—the path to disease. In the end, they leave you with nothing but fatigue, excess weight, more cravings, and poor health.

What's more, consuming unhealthy starches like these during Phase I of your weight loss will bring your fat-burning machinery to an abrupt halt for several days. Once you've reached a healthy weight, your body should be able to tolerate some of these foods on occasion but I recommend that you eliminate them permanently. You'll soon find that the meals I teach you to prepare using healthy starches will be just as convenient, taste much better, and bring you to a state of energy, vibrancy, and health.

Starches and Sugars (Carbohydrates)

UNHEALTHY: HABITS OF DISEASE		
• Doughnuts	• Cookies	• French fries
• Sodas	• Candy	

" *Eliminating all ultra-processed unhealthy food filled with refined sugar and flours can have a dramatically positive effect on your health!* "

2.5

Top sources for healthy fat:

- Fatty cold-water fish, especially salmon
- Soybeans
- Olive oil
- Nuts, especially almonds
- Avocados, guacamole
- Flaxseed products

FATS

Eating the right type of fats in the right amount can have a dramatic impact on your health and is an important component of our healthy eating strategy. The typical Western diet takes about 34% of its calories from fat—the vast majority from saturated, animal-based fat. According to the USDA, fat should make up between 25–35% of your daily caloric intake, with no more than seven percent coming from saturated fat. It's no wonder that Western societies, which eat too much of the wrong fat, lead the world in heart disease, diabetes, obesity, and several types of cancer.[26]

Take a look at the chart above, and notice how fat intake in the U.S. compares to that of other countries that have a lower incidence of these diseases.[27]

Fat as a Percentage of Calories in Daily Diets

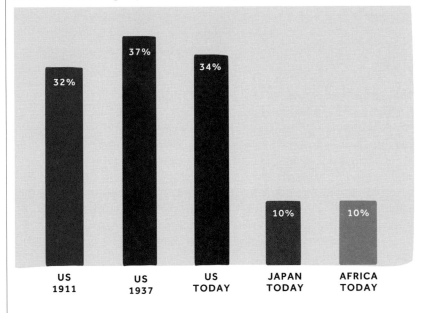

US 1911	US 1937	US TODAY	JAPAN TODAY	AFRICA TODAY
32%	37%	34%	10%	10%

Unhealthy Fats

The type of fat you consume has far-reaching effects on your health. In general, the fats to avoid are saturated, hydrogenated, and partially hydrogenated fats.

Saturated fats derived from animals and occur in high levels in foods such as hot dogs, hamburgers, bacon, and fatty meats leading to a 20% increase in death.

Hydrogenated fats, also known as trans-fats, are found in most processed foods, where they're used to extend shelf life. Directly linked to heart attack and stroke, they've also been found to oxidize the brain, accelerating the loss of memory and cognitive function.

In fact, they represent such a health hazard that progress has been made to ban hydrogenated fats entirely.

Partially hydrogenated vegetable oils were first developed with the launch of the low-fat, low-cholesterol craze in the 1980s, when saturated fats were found to contribute to heart disease and stroke. Polyunsaturated fats were known to be healthier than saturated fats, but they spoiled more easily, so food scientists devised ways to increase their stability by heating them and altering their molecular shape. This was the invention of partially hydrogenated vegetable oils, derived from corn, soybean, and cottonseed oils. These so-called "trans-fats", which were unsaturated and had no cholesterol, were thought to be a healthier choice than butter. In the end, however, they were determined to be even more dangerous, causing oxidative stress, radical formation, and an inflammatory state.

Back in the 1990's, most types of margarine were full of unhealthy trans-fats. The margarines were reformulated and today contain less than one percent trans-fats. However, butter has no trans-fats but it's loaded with cholesterol and saturated fat. So how does it all stack up?

Butter
- No trans-fats
- Seven grams of saturated fat per tablespoon (63 calories)
- 33 mg of cholesterol per tablespoon

Margarine
- Cheap solid and cooking margarine could potentially have small amounts of trans-fat see the label (the nutritional panel on the bottom of the tub) for more information. It should list the trans-fat content as less than 0.1 g per 100 g or <0.1%*
- Low in saturated fat
- No cholesterol

Remember that as a general rule—and as a Habit of Health—you should limit yourself to no more than 10–15 g of saturated fat and 200 mg of cholesterol per day (assuming your cholesterol level is in the normal range).

Healthy Fats
My plan makes it easy to stay within the USDA guidelines for fat intake by building in strategies for healthy fat consumption. You'll get about 20–25% of your daily calories from fat, mostly through mono- and polyunsaturated fats like those found in olive, canola, and flaxseed oils. You'll also consume small amounts of fat through fish, skinless white poultry, and healthy lean and wild meats.

So what exactly are these healthy fats, and how do they serve as functional foods to support weight loss and put you on the path to

*Semi-solid (tubs) and liquid margarines contain much less trans-fats than solid (stick) margarine.

"

Are all margarines bad for you? No. Several types of semi-solid margarine are free of trans-fats, including brands such as Smart Balance and Benecol (though the latter cannot be used for cooking).

"

2.5

optimal health? Healthy fats—what scientists call essential fatty acids—may also be known to you by the popular name of omega fats. They're wonderful foods that have very specific and helpful roles in weight loss. Among other benefits, they turn off insulin, unload unhealthy triglycerides from your fat cells, increase your metabolism, and protect your muscle membranes and your brain against memory loss.

It's worth noting, however, that all fats and oils, while rich in health benefits, are a calorie-dense food with 120 calories in just one tablespoon. Therefore, they should be used sparingly, particularly during Phase I, when it's important to maintain a lower energy intake.

Healthy Fats and Cholesterol

How exactly does eating "good fat" alter your cholesterol level and improve your health? A diet high in monounsaturated fat decreases your level of unhealthy triglycerides and LDL (the so-called "bad cholesterol") without decreasing HDL (the "good cholesterol").

Think of LDL as the trucks that deliver unhealthy fats and cholesterol to your blood vessels, and HDL as the trucks that cart them away. By increasing the amount of monounsaturated fat in your diet, you'll keep removing just as much of the bad stuff, while letting less of it in. As you progress, I'll show you natural ways to continue bringing in those good HDL trucks and rid your body of even more unhealthy fats and cholesterol.

Cooking and Salad Oils

One benefit of oils high in monounsaturated fats is that when they're heated they develop fewer free radicals than polyunsaturated oils. That means they're great for cooking. Note, however, that olive oil—my favorite healthy oil for just about everything else—cannot be used for high-temperature cooking because its low smoking point will cause it to smoke, impair flavor, and become degraded. So if you're really cooking, canola oil may be a better choice.

Cooking and Salad Oils GI chart

	OMEGA TYPE	MONO-UNSATURATED	POLY-UNSATURATED	SATURATED
Olive	0-9	75%	8%	17%
Canola	0-6, 9	55%	38%	7%
Sesame	0-6, 9	39%	43%	18%
Coconut	0-6	34%	45%	21%
Corn	0-6	20%	66%	14%
Soy	0-6	19%	65%	16%
Safflower	0-6	13%	79%	8%
Sunflower	0-6	11%	80%	9%
Peanut	0-6	5%	2%	93%

The Omega Fats: Omega-3, Omega-6, Omega-9

Think all omegas are alike? Think again. There are different types of omegas, some healthy and some not so healthy.

Omega-3 is the flagship of healthy fats. It can have a profound effect on your waistline, muscles, and brain, and can help you move quickly toward optimal health. The effect on brain health is significant. A daily consumption of omega-3 fatty acids can decrease anxiety levels by 20% and promote a significant reduction in inflammation.[28] As you can imagine, we'll want to make sure to provide you with the right amount. Fish is a great source of omega-3, especially salmon, which you'll learn more about in the next part's discussion on buying healthy protein. Liquid flaxseed oil is another prime source. It can't be used as cooking oil, but it's great to use on salads or breads or added to soups. And, of course, it's also contained in walnuts!

Omega-6 is a healthy fat if it's consumed in a 1:1 ratio with omega-3s. Unfortunately, for the most part, our consumption of omega-6 far outweighs our intake of omega-3. The ability to make seed and vegetable oils was another result of the industrialization of the food industry. They are easy to produce, cheap, and most vegetable oils, including soybean, corn, sunflower, and safflower oil, contain heavy concentrations of omega-6. Increasing your use of olive and canola oil, and adding flaxseed oil to your diet, will help restore a healthier ratio and provide a better balance to support health.

Omega-9, another very healthy omega, is found in olives, avocados, and nuts. Olive oil, particularly extra virgin olive oil, is an ideal way to get enough omega-9. Use it for sautéing or to add a marvelous flavor to cooked foods and salads—just make sure you don't cook at very high temperatures, and, as with all oils, keep track of the amount so you don't consume too much!

DR. A SAYS…

" *Fats and oils are extremely calorie dense, and should be used sparingly.* "

2.5

FIBER

You've probably heard that fiber is an important part of a healthy diet. But the different types of fiber can be a little confusing. Here's a guide so you can be sure to include both types in your daily food choices. There are about three grams of fiber per cup or piece of the foods listed here.

Soluble fiber dissolves in water. Its benefit to your body includes slowing the breakdown of complex carbohydrates and helping to reduce blood sugar. When you eat it in a large enough quantity, it can help lower cholesterol as well. Good sources of soluble fiber are grains such as rye, barley, and oats; vegetables and fruits; legumes.

Processed food is loaded with salt. Lowering your **salt intake** has important health benefits, including helping to lower your blood pressure. Here are some tips for eliminating excess salt from your diet:

- Follow the Habits of Health, including my Healthy Eating for Life system.
- Lower or eliminate your intake of processed foods.
- Don't add salt to your food.
- Fill your salt shaker with half salt, half pepper.
- Use salt-free seasonings.

Insoluble fiber doesn't dissolve in water and is not absorbed or digested by your body. But it does reduce hunger (it's filling!), helps keep your gastrointestinal tract clean, and aids in regular bowel movements by pulling water into the colon. Good sources of insoluble fiber are brown rice; whole-wheat breads and cereals; seeds; fruit and vegetable skins; legumes.

PREBIOTICS, PROBIOTICS, AND POLYPHENOLIC COMPOUNDS

Our digestive tract is extremely important for our overall health. The gut microbiome is made up of over a trillion microorganisms and is responsible for maintaining the integrity and health of our intestinal lining. With the consumption of a highly processed diet the gut flora suffers, leading to the potential for more weight gain, inflammation, and poor digestion of vital nutrients. This can lead to leaky gut which has been linked to Alzheimer's, multiple sclerosis, asthma, eczema, arthritis, psoriasis, irritable bowel syndrome, chronic fatigue syndrome, depression, and more unhealthy states. With a proper diet the bacteria produce more fermentation that nourishes the gut flora.

So what can we do to improve gut health? It starts with adding probiotics, which are live healthy bacteria found in certain foods and supplements (more on that later). The second part is to consume more prebiotics which come from the rich fiber sources we mentioned above. The third part is to provide the polyphenolic compounds that come from fruits and vegetables which slow the growth of the toxic microbes so that the healthy bacteria can flourish.

Polyphenols, like curcumin found in the spice turmeric, can be found in curry-based foods. This can actually enter the bloodstream to have an anti-inflammatory effect on the whole body. Eating whole plant foods and live fermented products can really improve gut health. Great sources of probiotics come from several sources that most people do not eat that often. Fermented pickles (not those made with vinegar), sauerkraut, kimchi, and kefir are all great sources along with live yogurt cultures.

TOPPING IT OFF WITH HERBS AND SPICES

Herbs and spices are a great way to enhance flavor without adding calories, fat, or other unhealthy substances. And many do much more than that—they actually help you lose weight while providing particular health benefits as well. Try these great choices:

- Toss foods with a simple mixture of sea salt, black pepper, olive oil, and vinegar.
- Add red pepper to an egg-white omelette to decrease hunger and increase metabolism.
- Add a pinch of turmeric, source of the substance curcumin, to add a hint of mustard flavor and reduce inflammation.
- Don't forget garlic, cilantro, parsley, and basil, which add so many flavors and have numerous health benefits.

WATER

What's water doing in a discussion of our major food groups? It, along with your Habits of Healthy Eating, allows us to make sure we always stay hydrated.

Water is a critical component of your body, making up between 55–60% of your weight. Your body can't store water—unlike fat—so you need to replenish it often. That's why drinking at least eight glasses (eight ounces each) a day is a core Habit of Health.

Water plays a key role in supporting health, particularly during weight loss when it helps remove toxins and other unhealthy substances stored in your fat cells. Being well-hydrated helps all your organs and systems function properly. In fact, every function in your body takes place in water. It's the solvent that moves nutrients, hormones, antibodies, and oxygen through your bloodstream and lymphatic system. It also removes waste. And, of course, it's essential to your kidneys' ability to filter and eliminate metabolic byproducts and toxins. If you don't drink enough, your body is forced to recycle dirty water, diminishing the efficiency of every metabolic function.

What you may not realize is that we actually lose nearly twelve cups of water every day: two cups through perspiration, six cups through urine, two to four through breathing, and nearly one cup through the soles of our feet! Also, in high altitudes or dry environments, you lose even more, so you can get dehydrated in a hurry.

During Phase I of your weight-loss plan, there are even more good reasons to make a conscious effort to drink your eight glasses a day. Here are a few:

- It's calorie free, but helps you feel full and satisfied.
- It keeps you from overeating. Studies have shown that when we feel hungry, some of the time our bodies are actually signaling for water.[29]
- It facilitates the removal of toxins, such as pesticides and preservatives, from your cells.
- It prevents dehydration as your body eliminates excess salt and water from a diet of too many processed foods.
- It minimizes or eliminates fatigue, lack of energy, headaches, and unclear thinking.

> *Liven up your water by adding a squirt of lemon or some fresh mint leaves and try to start your day with a couple of glasses before you hit the coffee pot.*

2.5

- It speeds up metabolism. A recent study showed that drinking two eight-ounce glasses of cold water increased metabolic rate by 30% for 90 minutes.[30]
- It helps your liver convert fat to energy.
- It compensates for the loss of glycogen stores as you lose weight.

Water FAQs

What's the best source for my eight glasses a day? *Plain water is the best beverage for quenching thirst. It's cheap, calorie free, and contains no sugar, caffeine, or other additives. However, tap water should be filtered first to remove chlorine and other contaminants.*

What about bottled water? *Bottled water is fine, as are sparkling waters flavored with lemon or lime. Just make sure they haven't been enhanced with sugary substances and calories!*

What about distilled water? *Distillation takes out both impurities and minerals, including calcium, magnesium, and sodium, which may provide clinically important portions of your recommended dietary intake. I encourage you to check the mineral content of your drinking water, whether tap or bottled, and choose the water most appropriate for your needs. If you do use distilled water, you should supplement your mineral intake through your diet in order to maintain proper health.*

What about reverse osmosis? *Reverse osmosis produces distilled water, so the above cautions apply. And because it removes all of the impurities, minerals, and toxins, its filter requires considerable maintenance and cost.*

I'm just not thirsty. *Do I still need to drink water? Don't use thirst to guide your water intake! Thirst is a late warning symptom of dehydration. Waiting until you're thirsty to drink means that your body must function at less than optimal efficiency for several hours.*

How do I know if I'm not drinking enough? *If you start feeling tired, have trouble thinking, develop a headache, or notice that your urine is darker than usual, these are late-stage signs that you need to drink more water! Your urine should be almost colorless, unless you've just taken vitamins.*

How much water should I drink? *It is recommended that you drink eight glasses (eight ounces) of water each and every day. This should be your guide unless you have a specific medical condition that requires you to restrict your fluid intake, such as renal failure or severe congestive heart failure, or if you've recently performed intense physical activity in a hot environment, in which case you should consume an electrolyte-enriched drink.*

A Habit of Health:
Drinking plenty of water

Drink a glass of water as soon as you wake up, before every meal, and any time you feel the urge to put something in your mouth, because in addition to water's other wonderful benefits, it helps suppress appetite.

HEALTHY HYDRATION	UNHEALTHY HYDRATION
• Purified water • Bottled water • Reverse Osmosis water • Tea • Coffee • Infused water (calorie free)	• Fruit juices • Sodas • Almond, coconut milks • Diet soda • Energy drinks • Sports drinks • Alcohol

Coffee is a diuretic—it makes you go to the bathroom more often, so it must dehydrate you, right? Well, not so. Turns out that this idea dates back to a 1928 study, and it wasn't exactly rigorous research. Nonetheless, the results spread like wildfire and, ever since, caffeine has been considered a diuretic. Now, a recent study finds that coffee—and caffeine in other drinks—won't in fact cause dehydration.[38]

Above is a list of healthy choices of how to keep yourself hydrated. Teas, both hot and iced, have all kind of health benefits but make sure you do not add milk which inactivates the healthy phenolic compounds and—naturally—don't add sugar.[31] Green tea, in particular, is full of health benefits from decreasing inflammation and preventing cancers to improving your learning and memory.[32]

Coffee studies are showing many benefits because of the high levels of antioxidants. Studies show it decreases depression, reduces the risk of some cancers, and may help you live longer, and slow down cognitive decline, boost mood, increase stamina, and may even protect against adult onset diabetes.[33] And, by the way, coffee and tea are not diuretics!

Infusers that are designed to provide additional vitamins, minerals, or other healthy supplementation are a great way to make sure your body is adequately hydrated throughout the day and evening.[34] It's important that any infusers you use have minimal calories. We have a Purposeful Hydration™ system that supplements as well as makes it easier to fulfill your habit of drinking eight glasses of water a day.

One of the Habits of Disease is consuming sugary sodas, fruit drinks, and the many sweet beverages out there with added sugar, syrups, and concentrates. Half of the U.S. population consumes at least one sugary drink a day even when excluding fruit juice, diet soda, sweetened milks and sweet tea! [35] These sugary drinks can lead to diabetes and some forms of cancer.[36] Each sugary drink you consume increases your risk of heart disease by almost 20%. It is estimated that 180,000 people a year lose their lives by consuming these sickening sweet elixirs![37]

The unhealthy drinks on the list above not only stimulate insulin and drive glucose into the fat cells, thereby worsening your weight issues, but will actually make it harder to stay hydrated!

So that's it—my easy shopping system for long-term healthy eating and reaching an optimal weight. When combined with the prepackaged system you learned about in Part 2.3, *The Catalyst to Reaching a Healthy Weight,* you now have a comprehensive strategy for reaching and maintaining optimal health.

When you think of the hours we spend shopping for clothes, electronics, even pet supplies, it really makes sense to take the time to learn and use this simple system. Once you do, you can be sure that you're giving your body the best-quality fuel available, through foods that boost your ability to function and put you on the path to optimal health.

2.5

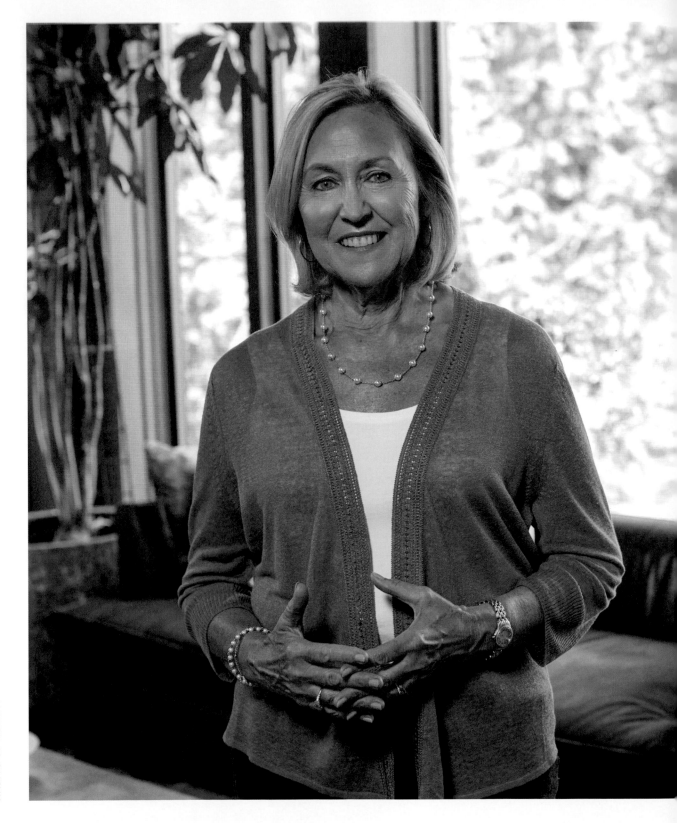

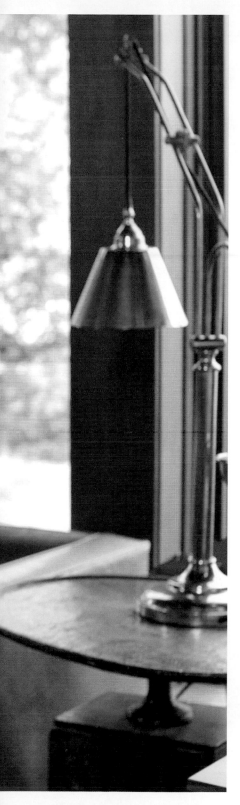

TRANSFORMATION: MARY BELL

I had been on yo-yo diets ever since I was a teenager. I had been up and down with my weight and that last 10 or 15 lbs was always a challenge. But when I read Dr. A's book, I saw a way that I could incorporate his daily habits into my life to make permanent changes towards optimal health.

I had to tweak my habits quite a bit because I had been cooking kind of the wrong foods, but now I know what to cook: healthy lean and green meals. When I go to the grocery store, I make sure I go down the produce aisle, and I try to get organic produce. I also go for lean meats and fresh fish. I also make sure I have my proper hydration each day—for me, that means at least eight glasses of water a day.

Dr. A's book on healthy habits helped me realize that even small amounts of sugar was not very good. I pretty much cut out the sweet tea—which I used to drink a lot of—and desserts. I really did change my cooking habits, and it has shown up in our family health pattern. I cook for our grandkids too; I do not let them have the candy that they beg for.

I have four grandchildren and one on the way, and my goals in life are to try to be as healthy as I can as I age. I do a lot of very active things with my grandkids. They're young, and they always want me to either give a piggyback ride or do active games with them—running up and down the hall or the yard. I really do have it as a goal in my life to stay as active, fit, and healthy as possible so that I can enjoy a lot of years with my grandkids as they get older and get into sports.

For me, the Habits of Health were a day-to-day journey, not just a diet that you go on, lose some weight, and then go back to your old eating habits. It was very important to remember that I had to change my life on a day-to-day basis, one habit at a time, and that's what I try to do.

2.5

" I had been up and down with my weight and that last 10 or 15 lbs was always a challenge. **"**

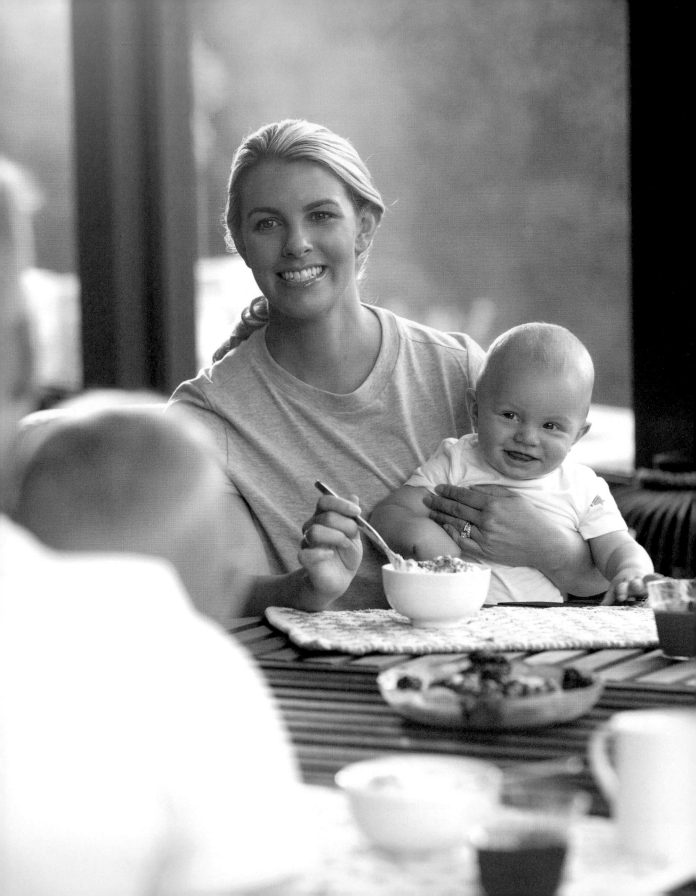

BUILDING HEALTHY MEAL PLANS FOR OPTIMAL HEALTH: HOW TO MAKE HEALTHY EATING AUTOMATIC

You've learned about portion control using my divided plate system, how to make the healthiest choices from the major food groups, and the ins and outs of shopping for healthy foods using my color-coded shopping charts. Now it's time to put it all together in the third piece of the system. We're about to look at how to plan meals that are quick, convenient, affordable, portable and, most of all, healthy. This will help you reach and maintain your first goal: a healthy weight!

HABITS OF HEALTHY PREPARATION

A new body of research is uncovering that how you prepare food may be more important than the type of food you eat. I am going to give you some easy and quick ways to cook up juicy and flavorful food without adding tons of unnecessary extras. Most of us know that we should not fry our food, but when cooking up healthy meals, we may not think about how our cooking method affects the nutritional makeup of our meals.

Heat can break down and destroy 15–20% of some vitamins in vegetables, especially vitamin C, folate, and potassium. Some people have stopped cooking their food altogether, claiming that uncooked food maintains all of its nutritional value and supports optimal health. Studies suggest certain foods actually benefit from cooking. When cooking carrots, spinach, tomatoes, sweet potatoes, and peppers, the heat helps to release a greater amount of antioxidants.[1]

THE TECHNIQUES

Microwaving

The cooking method that best retains nutrients is one that is quick, heats food for the shortest amount of time, and uses as little liquid as possible. Microwaving meets these criteria. Using the microwave with a small amount of water essentially steams food from the inside out. This keeps in more vitamins and minerals than almost any other cooking method and shows microwaved food can indeed be healthy.

While microwave cooking can sometimes cause food to dry out, you can keep things moist by splashing the item with a bit of water before heating or placing a wet paper towel over the top of your dish. Regardless, the way that microwaves cook food eliminates the need to add extra oils. You can microwave just about anything to preserve nutrients in veggies.

Boiling

Boiling is quick, easy, and requires nothing but water and a touch of salt. But in addition to the high temperatures, the large volume of water dissolves and washes away water-soluble vitamins and 60–70% of foods' minerals.

While this method can dissolve vitamins and minerals in some foods (especially vegetables), it's not the worst way to cook food. Some antioxidants become more available when cooked in this way, such as lycopene in tomatoes. The level of beta-carotene also increases after carrots are cooked.

Steaming

Steaming anything from fresh veggies to fish fillets allows them to cook in their own juices and retain all that natural goodness. It's always good to add a little seasoning first, whether that's a sprinkle of salt or a squeeze of lemon juice. If the carcinogen-fighting components in broccoli are important to you, some research suggests steaming is the best to release isothiocyanates, which can inhibit the growth of cancer cells.[2] The main drawback is you don't get a lot of flavor from steaming, which can lead to reaching for excess butter or salt.

Poaching

Poaching means cooking food in a small amount of hot water just below boiling point. It takes slightly longer, but it's ideal to gently cook delicate foods like fish or fruit. It's also the best way to cook eggs.

Broiling

Broiling means cooking food under high, direct heat for a short period of time. Broiling is a great way to cook tender meat, but may not be ideal for cooking vegetables. The high temperature can easily dry out the veggies and decrease the enzyme potency in the produce, causing more nutrient loss.

Grilling

In terms of getting maximum nutrition without sacrificing flavor, grilling is a great cooking method. It requires minimal added fats and imparts a smoky flavor but still keeps meats and veggies juicy and tender. While these are definitely healthy benefits, as we mentioned in the previous part, Advanced Glycation End Products (AGES) can result from charred fat, making grilled food potentially inflammatory and cancer-causing. They are chemicals that have been linked to oxidation (free radical production), inflammation, diabetes, cancer, and other chronic diseases. Stated simply, AGES age us! You can still grill but just limit it to lean cuts of meat that require less cooking time and rare to medium preparation.

Sautéing

While this method does require oil in the pan, it's effective for meat, rice and quinoa, and thin-cut veggies like bell peppers, julienned carrots, and snow peas. A small amount of olive oil may increase the antioxidant capacity like the heart-healthy Mediterranean diet.

Raw

Many studies suggest there are benefits to incorporating more raw (mostly plant-based) foods into the diet because they provide more vitamins, minerals, and fiber, as long as they are consumed with no added sugars or fats from cooking. The problem is that without cooking, you do not destroy potentially dangerous microbes. And while some raw items might be super healthy, studies have found that cooking tomatoes, carrots, spinach, sweet potatoes, and peppers enhances the availability of antioxidants to you.

A Habit of Health: Selecting and preparing healthy foods.

QUICK AND EASY TOOLS FOR "AUTOMATIC EATING"

For most of us, eating processed, microwaved, or fast food is an easy alternative to preparing meals that seem too hard, too time-consuming, and messy. Cooking just doesn't seem worth it! One of my goals is to make preparing healthy foods as easy as stopping into a fast food restaurant. First, let me introduce you to some of my own favorite tools that will make your new healthy eating strategy a breeze.

Microwave
This appliance is an easy way to cook just about anything and, despite some lingering doubts, it's considered safe for all foods and is best at preserving nutrients in veggies. You do, however, want to make sure you use microwave-safe containers to prevent burns and reduce the potential for plastic elements to leach into foods. And please don't stand in front of your microwave watching your food go around as there is a potential of developing cataracts if you do.[3]

Portable Cooker
These portable, self-contained countertop appliances make preparing portion-controlled meals a breeze! Portable cookers actually provide a miniature range that cook your meals quickly (in about three to 10 minutes) without any dishes. Both the two-portion and four-portion models allow you to cook on a non-stick surface, eliminating the need for extra fat or oil, and the cooking process doesn't even require turning, so there's no hassle! And what's really great is that you can take this portable device to your workplace. I use a portable cooker all the time to make great-tasting meals.

Portable Blender
This compact tool lets you mix up great-tasting fruit smoothies, healthy frozen shakes, and other tasty meals and snacks without the mess.

Shaker Cup or Jar
This is a great way to quickly prepare the portion-controlled meals that we introduced in Part 2.3, *The Catalyst to Reaching a Healthy Weight*. These meals fit very nicely into my system and can be a useful part of your fueling strategy in the healthy eating plan as well.

Wok
The indispensable ancient Chinese implement for fast, healthy cooking. A wok's main advantage is that cooks can create healthy meals in a relatively short amount of time. Little oil is used in preparing vegetables, meats, or seafood. Vegetables retain a crisp, crunchy texture, while the meats and seafood do not absorb large amounts of oil, which makes them heart healthy. Woks also eliminate the need to cook with a number of pots and pans. One wok can hold a variety of ingredients. Woks also are useful for sauteing, stir frying, or steaming.

What are you waiting for?

Before you start your journey, I suggest you schedule a visit to see your healthcare provider. No doubt your healthcare provider will be excited that you've decided to lose weight and create health in your life. After all, it makes their job easier! In the appendix, you'll find a sheet of information to give your physician that explains this "health makeover" you're doing. It's also available for download at my website at www.HabitsofHealth.com.

A Special Note for Those With Type 2 Diabetes

Checking in with your healthcare provider before you change your diet is particularly important if you have type 2 diabetes. As you switch to my low-calorie, low-glycemic eating plan, your blood sugar may lower immediately, and your level of medication may need to be reduced accordingly. The great news is that this is a signal of your body's initial step toward health. Your disease progression is being arrested! But do remember to watch your blood sugar closely in the beginning to make sure your medications are properly adjusted.

Bamboo Steamer
Make delicious steamed foods inside your wok. The steamer is convenient and allows the placement of multiple steaming baskets on top of each other and the base is where the water boils. You can place meat, veggies, or rice in the baskets. Make sure that you keep the fastest steaming agent at the top and follow this hierarchy downwards. This reduces the cooking time, while ensuring that food bacteria is destroyed. It is also inexpensive to buy and look after.

Zipper-Style Plastic Bags
Pop extra meals and snacks into these to keep one jump ahead when you need to fuel at home and on the go.

Portable Cooler
An insulated, lightweight cooler keeps prepared meals fresh and is easy to transport.

Why all this emphasis on quick and easy? It's because humans react to hunger and stress, often in ways that don't promote health. We need to create an automatic eating system—my healthy version of fast food—to fuel your body before you cave in to cravings. Planning meals in advance, having them ready to go and, perhaps most importantly, sticking to my every-three-hour healthy eating schedule helps you to stay in control.

What happens when you're in control?
- You'll reach a healthy weight over time.
- You'll develop permanent Habits of Health.
- You'll improve your health and possibly reduce your reliance on medications for certain weight-related health conditions.
- Your work performance will improve.
- Your quality of life will improve.
- You'll eliminate cravings.
- Your mental focus and energy will improve.
- You'll save money.

YOUR CUSTOMIZED DAILY MEAL PLAN USING MY HEALTHY EATING SYSTEM

So what does a day on your new meal plan look like? Remember the basic principles of reaching an optimal weight:
- Eat breakfast.
- Eat a small amount of food every three hours.
- Eat a healthy meal at dinner time.

To create your daily menu, you're going to design a healthy breakfast and dinner using your nine-inch plate, supplemented by four fueling breaks. Each of your two meals provides about 300 – 400 calories through:

Dr. A's Healthy Eating System for Life

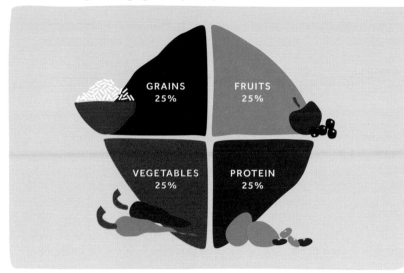

- A combination of vegetables and fruits* (50% of your plate; 25% vegetables and 25% fruits) which is about the same size of a small paperback novel of about 100 pages.
- A healthy, low-glycemic grain (25% of your plate—a tennis ball).
- A healthy protein (25% of your plate—a deck of cards).

Dr. A's Healthy Eating for Weight Loss Phase I

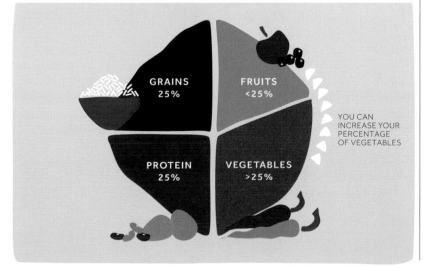

YOU CAN INCREASE YOUR PERCENTAGE OF VEGETABLES

"
Reduce your exposure to pesticides by washing and scrubbing fresh produce, discarding the outer layers of leafy greens, and trimming the fat and skin from meat and poultry.
"

*Remember to use fruit sparingly during the weight-loss phase and choose only those with a glycemic index below 30 for both fruit and the vegetables (from the dark green section of the charts). If you are using the 5&1 do not eat any fruit and go back go Part 2.3: *The Catalyst to Reaching a Healthy Weight*, for instructions.

Your fueling breaks provide about 100 calories each. If you wish, you may add a second fueling break item at lunchtime (for a total of two 100-calorie items), or opt for a light lunch (a regular nine-inch-plate meal without the starch component). The prepackaged portion control meals function as the perfect fueling, and you'll find a list with plenty of ideas and options for foods you can use for fueling breaks later in this section.

This eating strategy gives you a steady, balanced stream of energy throughout your waking hours for a total of 1,200 calories per day. Let's go through a day's sample menu to see exactly what we're looking at:

7:00 a.m.	**Breakfast**	**300–400 calories**
Vegetable/fruit	*Strawberries/peaches*	*Small paperback*
Starch	*¾ cup rolled oats*	*Tennis ball*
Protein	*½ cup low-fat milk*	*Deck of cards*
10:00 a.m.	**Fueling break**	**100 calories**
	Handful of almonds (12) or fueling	
1:00 p.m. option 1:	**Fueling break plus another fueling serving if needed**	**100 calories**
	1 cup vegetable soup and 4 Wheat Thins crackers	
Option 2:	**Light lunch**	**200 calories**
Vegetable/fruit	*½ tomato and 1 cup lettuce with oil and vinegar*	*Small paperback* *No starch*
Protein	*5 oz cooked turkey breast*	*Deck of cards*
4:00 p.m.	**Fueling break**	**100 calories**
	Yoplait non-fat French vanilla yogurt or fueling	
7:00 p.m.	**Dinner**	**400 calories**
Vegetable/fruit	*Fresh asparagus*	*Small paperback*
Starch	*Whole-grain pasta*	*Tennis ball*
Protein	*Grilled salmon*	*Deck of cards*
10:00 p.m.	**Fueling break**	**100 calories**
	Frozen non-fat yogurt (3 oz) or fueling	

WHAT TO EXPECT ON DAY ONE AND ONWARD

So what can you expect after your first day on the meal plan? For one thing, you probably won't have any hunger pangs or cravings, and your energy level should be consistent, balanced, and high.

Your first experience is just a starting point. Over the next few weeks, it's going to get better and better. Your internal clock is being changed, along with your body's expectations. You're feeding your body healthy food (it likes that!) and giving it regular nourishment through small meals throughout the day, which is just what your ancient, 10,000-year-old programming wants. By feeding it smaller meals, you're giving your body the ability to process food without being overwhelmed and having to work too hard. And, as a bonus, you'll rediscover your flavor palate as you move further and further from processed foods with excess sugar and salt.

PLANNING YOUR FUELING BREAKS

Your fueling breaks are an extremely important part of your day and a critical component of my healthy eating plan. To make sure you always have healthy fuel on hand, it's a good idea to prepare these small meals ahead of time and bring them with you to work or wherever your day takes you. You can use the prepackaged low calorie meals, or you can prepare and transport whole foods. That's where the zipper-style plastic bags and portable cooler come in: just fix up your days' worth of fueling breaks, pop them into the plastic bags, and take them with you in the cooler with an ice pack or two.

The following fueling break ideas are healthy, easy to prepare, and perfect for transporting. Each contains around 100 calories, making them ideal for the fat-burning state you want to encourage if you're working on reaching or maintaining your optimal weight. Remember, you can add one extra fueling break item at lunchtime if you wish, or opt to have a light lunch instead by preparing a regular nine-inch-plate meal without the starch component.

SAMPLE FUELING BREAKS

- Prepackaged low calorie fuelings. These make excellent fueling breaks and assure that you're getting a 100-calorie, low-glycemic, nutrient-dense healthy food source.
- One portion (size of two AA batteries) of natural cheese, such as cheddar or Monterey Jack, with one sliced tomato.
- Endive and tuna salad. One endive leaf with one tablespoon tuna salad, prepared with hummus in place of mayonnaise.

If you haven't reached your optimal weight yet, be sure to check the glycemic index of any snack before you choose it. It's important to eat only lower-glycemic snacks during weight loss—that is, foods that fall in the green zone (preferably dark green), with a glycemic index of less than 30.

Mediterranean Delights makes delicious, organic, low-fat hummus flavors like tomato basil, and low-glycemic endive makes a handy container for the tuna salad.

- 3 oz mixed nuts (a small handful)
- 10 almonds and a celery stick
- 29 pistachios
- 12 cashews
- 20 peanuts
- 2 tbsp sesame seeds
- 4 Brazil nuts. Great for boosting your selenium levels!
- ½ sliced apple with 3 walnuts
- ½ apple with 2 tsp natural peanut butter. Make sure it's all-natural peanut butter: just peanuts and salt.
- ½ cup fresh strawberries with 2 tbsp light whipped topping
- 1 cup fresh cherries
- 1 medium apple
- ½ cup blueberries (high glycemic) or strawberries (lower glycemic) with a dollop of yogurt
- 1 orange
- 1 pear
- ½ peach with 2 tbsp yogurt
- 2 cups raspberries
- 30 raisins
- Fresh veggie mix. 1 cup broccoli, red pepper, cauliflower with 1 tbsp low-fat ranch dressing.
- 6 pieces basil, sliced tomato, and hummus. My wife Lori's creation: put a dab of hummus and tomato on top of a basil leaf—delightful!
- Herbal lentils and one tomato
- Celery sticks with 1 tbsp natural peanut butter
- 1 cup fresh spinach salad with olives
- ¼ cup egg salad with lettuce or endive
- Half small avocado
- Cauliflower (size of paperback)
- 1 cup tomato and cucumber soup
- ¼ cup guacamole. Combine avocado, tomato, lime juice, and hot pepper to taste.
- Basil, tomato, and hummus (1 tomato)
- Grilled Portobello mushroom sprinkled with cheese
- 5 cherry tomatoes with one portion cheddar cheese (size of two AA batteries)
- ½ cup endive and cottage cheese spread. In a food processor or blender, mix cottage cheese, red pepper, fresh parsley, chives, and chopped jalapeño and then spread it on an endive leaf.
- Eggplant pizza slice. Sprinkle a slice of eggplant with oregano and roast. Melt cheese on top.
- 1 cup vegetarian chili
- ½ cup edamame (soybeans)
- Half red bell pepper dipped in 3 tbsp hummus
- ½ cup cucumber slices

- 1 large dill pickle
- 1 Carrabolla (starfruit)
- 2 cups baby carrots
- 3 celery sticks with 1 tsp natural peanut butter
- ¼ cup hummus and avocado dip with 3 celery stalks
- 1 cup mashed lentils and tomatoes
- Vegetables and dip. Choose either ½ cup cucumber slices, 6 celery sticks, 6 slices red pepper, or ½ cup raw broccoli florets and dip into 2 oz fat-free, sugar-free ranch dressing.
- 1 cup bean and chickpea salad. Toss diced celery, green pepper, cooked red beans, cooked chickpeas, and fresh parsley together with low-calorie balsamic vinaigrette.
- ⅓ cup low-fat cottage cheese with 4 olives
- Yogurt with ¼ cup berries. Yoplait Light plain yogurt is a great choice.
- ½ cup cottage cheese and ½ medium tomato
- 1 Yoplait Light Smoothie
- ½ cup low-fat cottage cheese with 5 strawberries
- 1 serving of string cheese
- 3 oz frozen non-fat yogurt
- 1 square 70% cacao or higher dark chocolate with 5 almonds
- 1 whole deviled egg. Cut a hard-boiled egg in half, mix the yolk with hummus, and fill the egg.
- 1 cup of soup (cream of tomato, cream of chicken, chicken noodle, or vegetable)
- 1 slice Wasa crispbread with 1 oz smoked salmon
  1 slice whole-grain bread (such as Fiber for Life) with 2 oz fat-free turkey breast
- ½ cup couscous with celery sticks
- 4 slices Melba toast
- 1 slice Wasa crispbread and ½ sliced tomato

Once you've reached a healthy weight, you can add these to the list as well:

Cottage Cheese and Cantaloupe
Top ½ cup of low-fat cottage cheese with ½ cup of diced cantaloupe. That ½ cup of cantaloupe delivers 50% of the daily recommended values of vitamins A and C—two vitamins that may help promote clear skin.

Red Pepper and Goat's Cheese
Slice up one medium red pepper and enjoy with two tablespoons of soft goat cheese. Goat's cheese is tangy and flavorful and has about one-third fewer calories and one-third the fat per ounce compared to cow's milk cheese.

Pumpkin Yogurt
Combine ½ cup nonfat plain Greek Yogurt with ¼ cup pumpkin

mHoH

Have a back-up healthy meal that is quick and easy to make if you ever find yourself short on time or creativity.

If you're short on time or just don't feel like preparing these 100-calorie meals, remember that prepackaged portion-controlled meals are an easy and great option for fueling breaks!

purée. Sweeten with stevia, ¼ teaspoon vanilla extract, and pumpkin pie spice blend (or cinnamon). Pumpkin is a low fat way to increase this snack's fiber and flavor profile.

Broccoli and Tzatziki Sauce

Whip up a quick tzatziki-like sauce by combining two tablespoons plain non-fat Greek yogurt, one teaspoon lemon juice, and one tablespoon minced cucumber. Dip six florets into the sauce. The healthy bonus here is that eating broccoli raw may help maintain the green veggies cancer-fighting nutrients.

Apples and Cheese

Pair a Laughing Cow Mini Babybel Light cheese wheel with half a baseball-sized apple, sliced. The cheese has six grams of protein and 20% of the daily recommended value of calcium.

Kiwi and Coconut

Slice one large kiwi and top with 1 tablespoon unsweetened shredded coconut. One kiwi has all the vitamin C to meet the daily recommended value.

Dark Chocolate

Let's be honest, this snack doesn't need any friends. Enjoy three squares. A bit of the dark stuff can help regulate levels of the stress hormone cortisol.

Protein Shake

Shake up one scoop vanilla whey protein with one cup of unsweetened almond milk. This one's perfect for post-workout snacking too because whey protein has been shown to help rebuild muscles after exercise.

Frozen Grapes

Grapes make a great snack fresh or frozen, but if you opt for the chilly state, they last way longer. Nosh on one cup (about 28 grapes). Feeling fancy? Use them as fruity ice cubes in a tall glass of water to stay hydrated while snacking.

Baked Apple

A simple low-calorie version: core a tennis-ball sized apple, dust it with cinnamon, and bake at 350 degrees for 20 minutes or until tender, but not mushy.

Once you are maintaining a healthy weight these fruits can be used judiciously as well:
- 1 cup fresh mango
- 1 cup cantaloupe
- 1 medium banana
- 1 small bunch of grapes (28)

This list should help you get started on ideas for your own small meals. Remember, each one should be low-glycemic and no higher than 100 calories.

PLANNING YOUR MEALS

When it comes to healthy eating, planning ahead is the key to success. You can go to HabitsofHealth.com and download two weeks' worth of healthy breakfasts, dinners, and fueling breaks, which should give you a good start. Feel free to mix and match meals or substitute fueling break ideas from the list above. Or make it easier on yourself by sticking to the sample menus for the first two weeks, and if you've enjoyed them, start the cycle again at week three.

Using these sample menus is a great way to learn how to prepare healthy meals—an important Habit of Health. And to top it off, you'll find recipes for all the evening meals in the appendix. Together, the meals I've planned for you are easy to prepare, give you lots of great flavors, and support your ability to stay at your optimal weight.

Note: Selecting a healthy, scientifically formulated meal can provide an excellent, nutritious, 100-calorie exchange for as many of the four fueling ideas as you desire.

SAMPLE MEALS

Learning to shop and prepare meals differently can feel intimidating, and I know from my work with thousands of people like you that this step in the journey can be one of the most challenging. To simplify your life, I have created a two-week meal plan complete with recipes and tips to give you a clear, easy-to-follow prescription for making your own healthy fuelings. Visit HabitsofHealth.com to download the guide and to explore dozens of other delicious healthy recipe options.

As you become more comfortable and confident in your shopping and cooking habits, don't be afraid to experiment and become adventurous. You can make all kinds of healthy entrees, as long as you:

- Keep the proper proportions of 50% vegetable and fruit with at least 25% of it coming from vegetables, 25% from protein, and the final 25% from healthy grains or starch.
- Use my shopping menus.
- Stay in the green zones.
- Choose from the food charts that contain "very low" and "low" glycemic selections.

Don't skip breakfast! It's one of the keys to successful weight maintenance. In fact, according to studies, 80% of people who've maintained a 35 lbs or greater weight loss make breakfast a part of their day, every day.

Remember, you can mix and match you fueling breaks too, as long as you stay within the guidelines. WIth this approach, you will discover a world of foods that are both healthy and delicious.

CHECKLISTS FOR CHANGE

So there you have it—a very simple method to help you reach and maintain your optimal weight while learning crucial dietary habits, including:

- Eating every three hours
- Eating breakfast
- Making healthy food choices
- Eating low-glycemic foods
- Planning your meals

Once you have a handle on these habits, you'll have the framework for success—not only for weight loss, but for a lifetime of maintaining your healthy weight and optimal health. Before you begin your weight-loss plan, make sure you've taken these important first steps:

- You've created a microenvironment of health.
- You've gone shopping and stocked your pantry and refrigerator with groceries selected using the color-coded shopping system.
- You've taken the wellbeing evaluation and are starting to write and progress in *Your LifeBook* by tracking your daily and monthly progress sheets.
- You've created a structural tension chart for your first goal of reaching a healthy weight. (For more information, see Parts 1.4 – 1.6 in this book).
- You've bought a journal and are regularly recording your daily eating habits, tracking your daily and monthly progress sheets, and/or using *Your LifeBook* and tracking choices that support optimal weight and health.

Once you're on the move, here are some tips:

- Get through your first few days of new healthy eating successfully.
- If you need some extra motivation, review Parts 1.3 – 1.4 on motivation for change, fundamental choice, and the discipline of daily choices.
- By day four you should feel great, with lots of energy as your body starts to respond to healthy fueling. After a week, if you're ready and feel good enough, start slowly increasing your daily activity.
- Drink at least eight (eight-ounce) glasses of water every day.
- Eat slowly.
- Use your support system. Tie into your surrounding support,

community and, if you have a coach, call her or him or consider requesting one.
- Make sure you're writing and progressing in *Your LifeBook*. This is a great way to monitor your progress and help you focus.

If you're using the healthy eating system to knock off those couple extra pounds and have reached your healthy weight (with a body mass index below 25), you're ready to transition to your permanent schedule.

In Phase I, we've laid the foundation for a more efficient energy management system by teaching you how to control the types of foods you choose, your portions, and the timing of your meals.

You're now eating healthy, you're at a healthy weight, and you're ready to take the next step of your journey. As you transition to Phase II, we'll boost both your energy intake and expenditure. The thread that connects each phase is the relationship between energy in and energy out. Let's take another look at the energy diagram. Notice that the colored boxes in Phase II highlight our three key focal areas: a healthy body mass index, or BMI (green); increased activity and exercise (tan); and increased caloric intake (blue).

Not Losing Fast Enough?
Low on Energy?

If your weight loss is slower than you expect or your energy level is low, eliminate the grain (starch) component and double up on vegetables until you notice an improvement. Avoiding fruit for a couple of days until your weight loss picks up is often helpful.

2.6

Energy Management in Phase I Graph

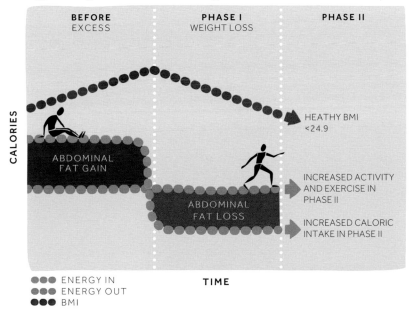

Energy Management in Phase I: Moving into transition. Before you transition to Phase II, you'll have decreased your daily energy intake (blue) as well as your body mass index, or BMI (green). Once you've reached your healthy weight and BMI and have begun to develop the fundamental Habits of Health, you're ready to begin transitioning into Phase II.

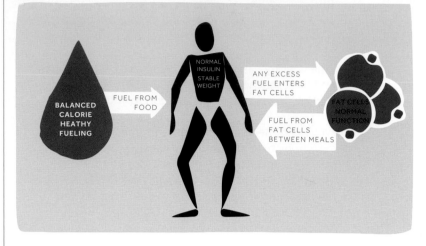

Your fat cells are now reaching equilibrium and ready to make the adjustment to utilizing energy in a balanced way that will maintain long-term weight management and metabolic stability.

In the next part, we'll review the science of weight loss and maintenance and teach you more great ways to control your energy intake and your insulin pump. There's a lot of great material there, but if you're at a healthy weight and eager to increase your calories, feel free to move right ahead to Part 2.8, *Healthy Eating For Life: Your Transition to Permanent Heath.*

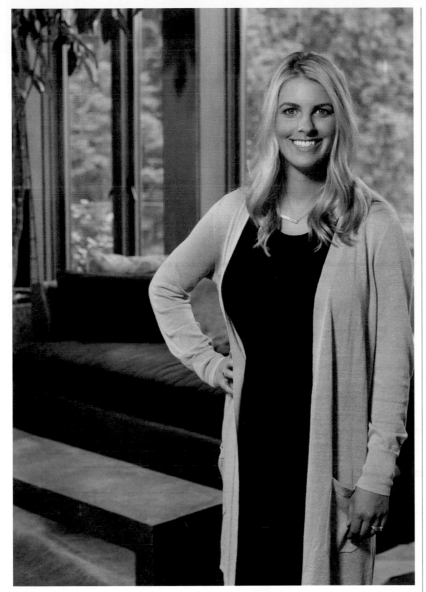

TRANSFORMATION: ASHLEY MILLER

When I began my journey with Dr. A, I was working 60 hours a week, six days a week, commuting at least an hour and half each way. Sleep was on the back burner.

I went on to use the Habits of Health Transformational System and philosophies to lose 55 lbs* after my first son. Now I have a seven-month-old, and I've lost another 30 or 35* just using the Habits of Health and living the lifestyle that Dr. A teaches us.

I think what Dr. A teaches about how to create the rituals to wind down and then also to wake back up really affected me. I learned how much better I can be when I am awake if I value my sleep in the ways that he teaches.

At 21, you don't have a lot of experience learning sustainability with your mindset, and you don't know a lot about sleep, at least in my experience. Those were parts of the Habits of Health that really impacted me as I got older. It gave me the ability to have more sustainable energy and the energy to be a coach and do what I love, be the mom I want to be, the wife I want to be, and the friend I want to be.

> "
> *I learned how much better I can be when I am awake if I value my sleep in the ways that Dr. A teaches.*
> "

2.6

*Average weight loss on the Optimal Weight 5 & 1 Plan® is 12 lbs.

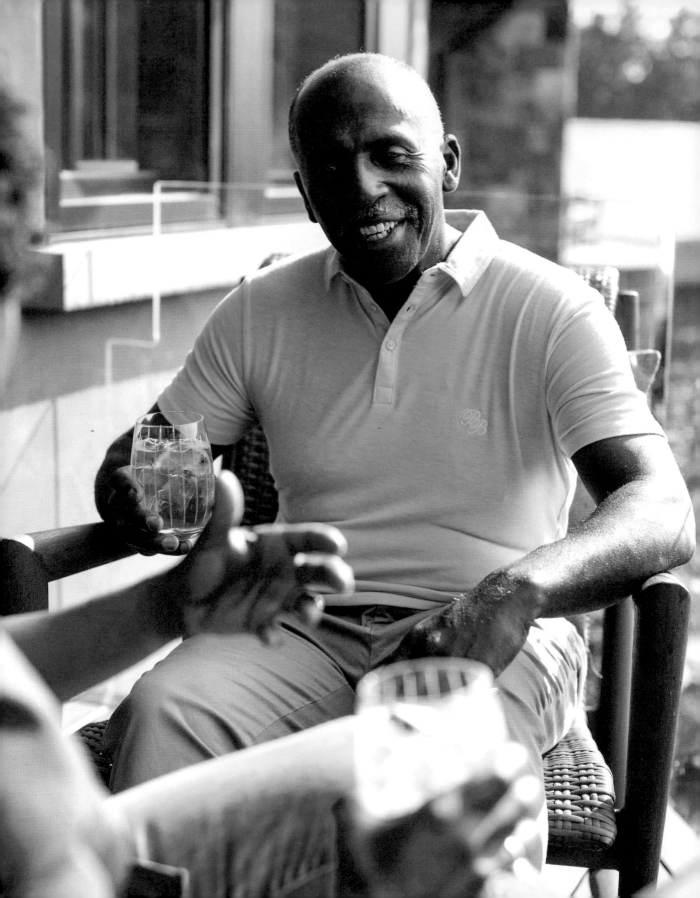

THE SCIENCE OF HEALTHY EATING AND WEIGHT LOSS

The ability to create optimal health and wellbeing is based on the progressive mastery of six MacroHabits of Health.

Although they are all important and all interdependent, the ability to eat at an optimal level—because of its critical role in our physical and mental health—sets the cornerstone in creating a foundation for radiant wellbeing. We live in a time when it seems difficult to discover what is best for us when the dietary guidelines appear to change constantly, influenced by fad diets, the latest book, or a celebrity success story. The daily messages of dieting wisdom, controversial theories, conflicting opinions, and research have left the public paralyzed.

In this part, we will present the science that supports the lifelong transformations in weight management that so many are already experiencing using the Habits of Health.

THREE CORE PRINCIPLES

You can rest assured that my eating system is based on irrefutable science and predictable components of success. It produces a comprehensive healthy eating system aligned to the cutting edge of medical science. Plus it is founded on three core principles that are essential for reaching and maintaining a healthy weight with a practical and simple way to create health in this chaotic world.

We have seen tens of thousands of people who have transformed their lives and their health over the last decade based on the science and techniques that I wrote over 10 years ago. In fact, many of my strategies are now being incorporated as the conventional guideline, like my plate system and the NEAT system for daily movement, which we will discuss shortly in order to help you with health and energy balance.

This material is to expand your understanding of why this system was so successful over this last decade and why it will continue to be over the decades to come, especially compared to all of the fads and quick fixes that come and go and do not work long term!

We will focus on the three unchanging core principles that will make my healthy eating system foundational and effective for the rest of your life.

- Fuel control—Mastering calories and insulin
- Hunger control—Satiety: the science of fullness
- Waist control—Removing excess visceral adiposity (fat)

Let's look at each of these core principles.

CORE PRINCIPLE 1:
FUEL CONTROL—MASTERING CALORIES AND INSULIN

The healthy eating system you're learning is built around the Habits of Health that give you the ability to control the quantity and quality of your energy intake. Most people aren't able to master this fundamental principle even after a lifetime of struggle. They're relying on their internal programming to select their food choices. But, as we've discussed, that programming—which was optimal for a different time, when we needed to grab onto and hoard every calorie we consumed—is no longer helping us.

Today, unlike 10,000 years ago, we have no system for disposing of all that excess energy. So, if we consume more than we need to run our body, the extra calories get stored away as fat. That fat around your middle is a symptom of an imbalance between your energy intake and energy output, with your intake set higher than it should be. The type of food you eat flips certain metabolic switches. We will help you gain mastery so food will serve your health, not hurt it.

> *Three out of four people surveyed find that ever-changing dietary guidelines have made it harder to eat healthy. Half said that it is easier to figure out their income taxes than to know how to eat right!*

2.7

THE SCIENCE OF HEALTHY EATING AND WEIGHT LOSS

Here are the methods built into our system.

1. Portion Control

We have two important tools at our disposal to help us cut down the total amount of food we eat. The first, scientifically formulated portion-controlled meals, such as the ones we discussed in Part 2.3, *The Catalyst to Reaching a Healthy Weight: Healthy Fuelings*, are backed by a wealth of scientific research that documents their effectiveness. For many people, particularly those with busy lifestyles who need instant access to healthy, nutritious fuel, this high-quality "fast food" has become a permanent tool for weight maintenance, not just weight loss. Hopefully you have already added them to your eating system.

The second, my nine-inch-plate system, is a simple visual technique that keeps you mindful of portion size for all four categories in our user-friendly system: protein, grains (starchy carbohydrates), fruit, and vegetables. Together, they offer the ability to create long-term success because they allow a balanced eating system that provides a balanced amount of the right energy. The correct amount keeps excessive energy being deposited in the fat cells and leaves available energy able to run the power-hungry organs (like the muscles, brain, and kidneys), and keep insulin levels under control. The right energy makes sure we are keeping the metabolic switches, specifically insulin and leptin, at a level to facilitate proper glucose and energy balance.

Our system works both for weight loss and sustaining an optimal weight long-term because we can simply dial up and down the portions to match whether we are in the weight loss or long-term weight management regulation.

2. Three-Hour Fuelings

Eating every three hours fits right into our nature as hunters and gatherers. Paired with low-glycemic eating, it turns off our insulin pump, keeps us at an even energy level, and helps us avoid wide swings in glucose (blood sugar) and other key nutrients. It also decreases the body's workload, which has been shown to reduce dangerous oxygen radicals that lead to inflammation and disease. And, of course, it reduces the chances that you'll overeat due to cravings! We have discussed above the importance of having the right fuel, and in the right amounts. Let's look at how our system uses the right timing.

We, as humans, alternate between a fed and a fasting state. Let's look at where the fuel comes from when we go through the cycles of the fed and the fasting state.

Three Stages of Energy Availability

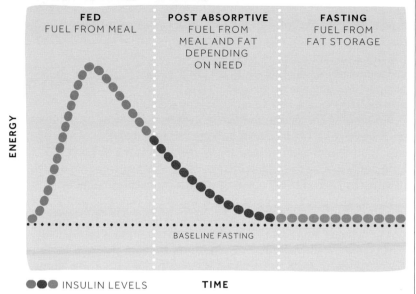

FED
FUEL FROM MEAL

POST ABSORPTIVE
FUEL FROM MEAL AND FAT DEPENDING ON NEED

FASTING
FUEL FROM FAT STORAGE

ENERGY

BASELINE FASTING

●●● INSULIN LEVELS   TIME

Your body is in the fed state when it is digesting and absorbing food. Typically, the fed state starts when you begin eating and lasts for three to five hours as your body digests and absorbs the food you just ate. When you are in the fed state, it's very hard for your body to burn fat because your insulin levels are high.

After that timespan, your body goes into what is known as the post-absorptive state, which is just a fancy way of saying that your body isn't processing a meal. The post-absorptive state lasts six to eight hours after your last meal, which is when you enter the fasted state. It is much easier for your body to burn fat in the fasted state because your insulin levels are low. When you're in the fasted state, your body can burn fat that has been inaccessible during the fed state.

Stages of Energy Availability

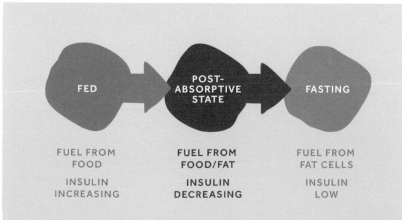

FED

POST-ABSORPTIVE STATE

FASTING

FUEL FROM FOOD

FUEL FROM FOOD/FAT

FUEL FROM FAT CELLS

INSULIN INCREASING

INSULIN DECREASING

INSULIN LOW

" *The current fad of fasting with long periods of not eating at all, tries to do what our system does naturally, putting the body into fat burning state. Unfortunately like most diets, it creates a non-sustainable restrictive period that violates the way we live our lives.* **"**

The three-hour system with portion control works so well because we don't overfeed. The fed state is then shorter because the energy load is much less than that of traditional meals. We also don't over stimulate insulin, so we have adequate insulin to ensure that energy entering the muscles, brain, and kidneys doesn't stimulate fat storage.

In the post-absorptive state, the body will start using fat to complement any energy needed by the body. At night the body goes into a fasting phase that helps burn any extra fat.

By keeping the three-hour schedule, you will not be hungry, you will have a constant source of energy, and your blood fuel and sugar will not undergo wide fluctuations. The current fad of fasting with long periods of not eating at all tries to do what our system does by getting the body into fat burning state, but once again creates a non-sustainable restrictive period that violates the way we live our lives.

So far, the research studies evaluating intermittent fasting have been relatively short and have enrolled only a limited number of participants. In one, published July 1, 2017, in JAMA Internal Medicine, 100 overweight people were assigned to one of three eating plans: restricting daily calorie intake by the same amount every day (similar to a traditional diet plan); fasting on alternate days; and continuing with normal eating habits. At the end of the 12-month study, both diet groups had lost weight compared with the normal eaters. However, the fasters didn't fare any better than the conventional calorie cutters.

3. Fueling Percentages

Your body runs on three different types of fuels, or macronutrients: carbohydrate, fat, and protein. A fourth type of fuel, alcohol, contains a significant number of calories but has no nutritive value. Using these fuels in just the right proportions is a critical part of weight loss and optimal health. Let's look at each group, one by one.

Macronutrients as Fuel

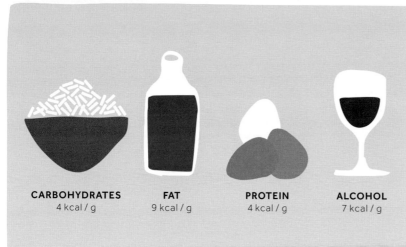

CARBOHYDRATES	FAT	PROTEIN	ALCOHOL
4 kcal / g	9 kcal / g	4 kcal / g	7 kcal / g

Macronutrients— carbohydrates, fats, proteins, and alcohol—are the body's main fuel sources. The number of calories per gram differs, with fat containing the most calories, alcohol the second most, and carbohydrates and protein the least.

CARBOHYDRATES: 50% OF YOUR DAILY CALORIES (RANGE 40 – 50%)

One of the primary drivers of my healthy eating system is the relationship between the carbohydrates you eat and your body's production of insulin—the key hormone in energy management. When you eat carbohydrates, your blood sugar or glucose levels rise, causing your pancreas to secrete insulin. This flood of insulin unlocks the gates that allow your body's tissues (especially muscle: your greatest energy consumer) to use glucose as an energy source.

As a result, your blood sugar returns to normal. In a healthy individual, glucose level peaks about 30 minutes after a meal. Insulin levels rise accordingly, just behind the rising glucose level. It's a fine-tuned cycle that keeps blood sugar precisely controlled, as you can see in the following chart.

"When our insulin levels are too high for too long— a result of eating unhealthy, high-glycemic foods— we move quickly from a state of health to non-sickness and disease."

2.7

THE SCIENCE OF HEALTHY EATING AND WEIGHT LOSS

> *Right now, over eight million Americans have diabetes and don't even know it!*[1]

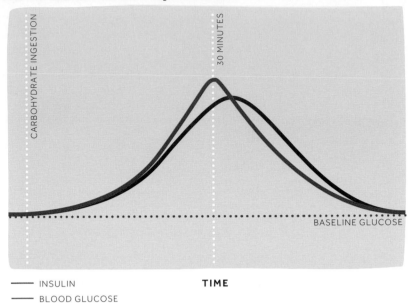

Normal Glucose-Insulin Response Curve

CARBOHYDRATE INGESTION

30 MINUTES

BASELINE GLUCOSE

TIME

—— INSULIN
—— BLOOD GLUCOSE

In a healthy individual, blood sugar (glucose) levels rise and peak about 30 minutes after a meal. Insulin is secreted in response, at a precisely controlled level that lags just behind that of blood sugar.

One of insulin's key roles is to determine whether the body takes more of its energy from carbohydrate or from fat. When insulin levels are low, as they are just after you get up in the morning, your body burns mainly fat.

Having a healthy low-glycemic breakfast can keep you in this fat-burning state, as can a little early morning activity. When you follow this pattern, your body uses those healthy breakfast carbohydrates right away for energy instead of storing them away as fat. Conversely, when insulin levels are high—for example, after you eat a high carbohydrate meal—your body burns mainly carbohydrates and stores fat.

Habits of Health Healthy Eating State: Healthy Waistline

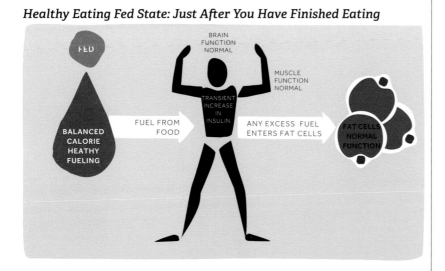

In fact, of the major food groups, carbohydrates (starches and sugars) are by far the greatest stimulators of insulin. That's why it's so important to eat low-glycemic carbohydrates, which don't raise blood sugar as much as high-glycemic carbohydrates do, which puts less demand on the pancreas to produce insulin.

As you look at the healthy eating state, let's summarize why it is important to have the right fuel, in the right amounts, and at the right times.

Healthy Eating Fed State: Just After You Have Finished Eating

As you finish one of your healthy meals, the body starts absorbing the food. In response to the portion-controlled, low-glycemic meal your blood sugar and (to a lesser extent) your blood fat and protein levels increase. However, the carbohydrate causes the release of insulin to help the glucose enter the muscles' cells and important organs, and the meal provides the energy. Once the meal has been fully digested, we enter the post-absorptive state.

Healthy Eating Post-Absorptive State: Once You Are Done Digesting Your Food

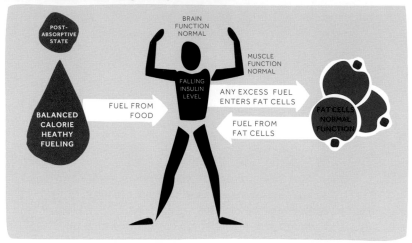

In the post-absorptive state, the body will continue to use the glucose from the meal. But since we have not overstimulated insulin, fat can start leaving the fat cells in order to provide any additional calories the body needs. Additionally, the lack of excessive calories, high insulin, and glucose peak prevents the blood glucose level from dropping below the baseline. This helps the fat calories maintain normal brain energy levels, which decreases cravings and mood swings.

Healthy Eating State: You Are in a Fasting State

Now that we're in the fasting state, we then use the fat from our fat cells as the energy source until we have our next fueling. This is an extremely gentle, sustainable way to fuel and keep our weight and health optimal.

This is all done without the difficult task of not eating carbohydrates—which are what give our food its variety—or the other option of fasting where you simply don't eat for many hours or a day at a time. We are all about making it easy, simple, and sustainable.

The benefits are immediate! Our system avoids the prolonged high levels of insulin that can lead to diabetes in susceptible individuals. When that happens, the pancreas can no longer produce the right amount of insulin to control blood sugar (which can cause type 2 diabetes) and may eventually be unable to make insulin at all (which can cause type 1 diabetes).

Unfortunately, as we go about consuming our supersized meals in bliss, the damage begins without us noticing. Deep inside, high insulin levels are creating a state of inflammation, decreasing the flexibility of our blood vessels and causing the premature aging of our cells. The warning signs are poor sleep, low energy, headaches, thirst, cravings, and hunger.

For many of us, these signs seem like nothing more than one more reason to stop at the fast food drive-thru or local drugstore to grab a soda or some painkillers. In fact, over seven million Americans right now have diabetes and don't even know it![2] The good news is that once you get your fueling mixture correct through my healthy eating program, you're going to feel unbelievably better. It will be like switching to high-performance fuel! And what's more, it has the power to prevent diabetes or even stop it in its tracks.

Note: The CDC just released in July 2017 that more than 100 million U.S. adults are now living with diabetes or prediabetes![3]

THE POWER OF LOW-GLYCEMIC EATING

Remember, food can be used in one of two ways—as an energy source or stored away in fat cells. When you eat a high-glycemic meal, those cells respond by turning on insulin and stimulating an enzyme that ramps up for your fat-storage system. Low-glycemic eating, however, shuts down your fat factory. Let's see how that's going to work in Phase I. Right now, you're probably eating too many calories, mostly from unhealthy carbohydrates like soda, bread, cookies, pizza, corn flakes, instant rice, or any number of cheap, plentiful (and tasty!) high-glycemic foods. To find out just what happens to our bodies when we eat foods like these day in and day out, let's first take a look at the glycemic index—a great tool that makes it easy for you to choose carbohydrates that support health.

mHoH

If you have to eat out, reference the glycemic index charts at HabitsofHealth.com or your Habits of Health App before you order. Remember, stay in the green to stay lean!

The glycemic index (GI) was created in 1981 by Dr. David J. A. Jenkins and it provides a standard for determining which foods raise blood sugar the most, thereby stimulating insulin production and weight gain. Using pure glucose, or sugar, as a reference point, Dr. Jenkins fed a variety of foods to his subjects and studied what happened to their glucose and insulin levels. Take a look at the following chart to see the results from eating pure glucose, which has a GI score of 100 on the 0–100 scale.

Note: The glycemic index of food is the percentage area under the curve compared to glucose.

Glucose Reference Curve: Glycemic Index

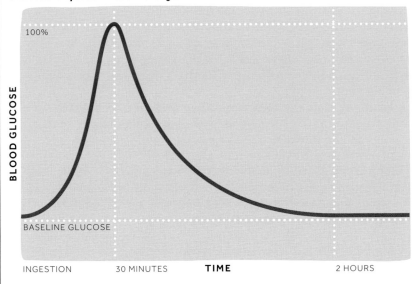

When you eat pure glucose (sugar) your blood glucose (blood sugar) level rises steeply and then falls. Glucose has a score of 100 on the glycemic index, a standard measure of glycemic content in foods. The glycemic index uses a scale of 0–100.

Now let's see what happens when you eat a low-glycemic food like lentils. (FYI these small green legumes make a great-tasting soup).

Lentils: Glycemic Index 28

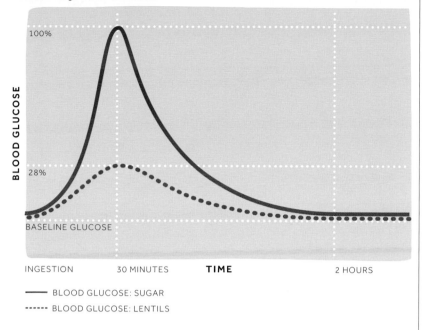

Compare the rise in your blood glucose level when you eat lentils (green
line) as opposed to pure sugar (yellow line). The curve is much less steep
when you eat lentils, which have lower glycemic content.

As you can see, lentils raise blood sugar only 28% as much as glucose
does, thereby creating far less demand on the pancreas to secrete
insulin. The release of sugar is much slower because the body has to
breakdown the lentils to obtain the energy whereas in the pure sugar
its absorption is almost instantaneous.

Your body can handle high-glycemic food some of the time.
But when you eat such foods daily, you create a chronic state of
hyperinsulinemia—the first step on the downward path to non-
sickness and diabetes. Not to mention that this constant high level
of glucose and insulin turns on fat storage and converts all that extra
energy to—yep, you guessed it—fat. And what do you think happens
after your blood sugar level peaks? It drops, of course, to below
normal. The result is hunger pangs and cravings that soon enough
have us running for the next vending machine.

Here's a closer look at what happens when we eat high-glycemic
versus low-glycemic foods.

Half of an eight-ounce bag of potato chips weighs about 100 g and contains 534 calories. You can easily eat that in one sitting and probably follow it up with a couple of beers. Even though this is a lot of calories, high-fat, high-energy, high-carb processed foods like these may even trigger us to eat more food.

Compare this to a 1,000g (2.2 lbs serving) of broccoli, which has 340 calories. The weight is 10 times greater and imagine how many days it would take to eat that amount. Energy density and volumetrics are powerful allies in helping us curb our hunger and create healthy eating habits.

Insulin Response to High vs. Low GI

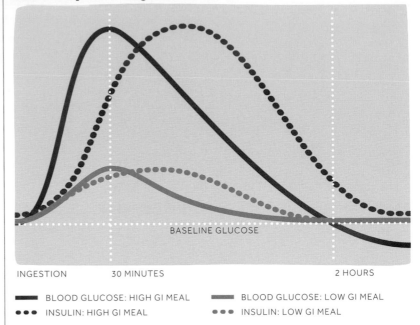

BASELINE GLUCOSE

INGESTION   30 MINUTES   2 HOURS

— BLOOD GLUCOSE: HIGH GI MEAL   — BLOOD GLUCOSE: LOW GI MEAL
●●● INSULIN: HIGH GI MEAL   ●●● INSULIN: LOW GI MEAL

When you eat low-glycemic foods (solid blue), your blood sugar and insulin levels don't rise as dramatically as they do when you eat high-glycemic foods (gradient). As a result, you don't get a rebound effect that can cause your blood sugar to dip below normal between meals and lead to cravings and hunger pangs.

Now look what happens when we eat high-glycemic foods all day.

Modern Life's Disease Path: Glucose—Insulin Response Curve

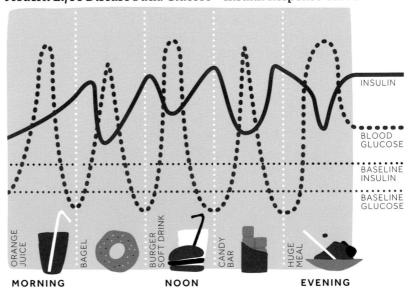

INSULIN

BLOOD GLUCOSE

BASELINE INSULIN

BASELINE GLUCOSE

ORANGE JUICE   BAGEL   BURGER SOFT DRINK   CANDY BAR   HUGE MEAL

MORNING   **NOON**   **EVENING**

If you eat unhealthy high-glycemic foods all day, such as in the typical Western diet, you will experience enormous swings in blood sugar levels—peaks that then dip down to lows between meals. Your insulin levels stay high, causing you to store energy as fat, putting an enormous burden on your pancreas, and paving the way to metabolic syndrome and insidious diseases such as diabetes.

As you can see, constant spikes in blood sugar are interspersed with dips between meals that bring about cravings for yet more quick carbohydrates, and the insulin level remains elevated continuously.

Today, over 45 million people in the U.S. alone suffer from hyperinsulinemia as a result of Habits of Disease like these.[4] In Phase I, we're going to turn off your insulin pump by limiting your intake to low glycemic carbohydrates—foods that are 30 and under on the glycemic index (your dark green charts). Then we'll add nutrient-dense but lower-calorie fuel sources to help you feel full and gain control over your intake. It all adds up to a fat-busting, inflammation-soothing combo that would make Mother Nature herself proud!

Now let's turn to our second major food group: fat.

2.7

DR. A SAYS…

" *Try this tip: Fill up faster by starting with a broth-based (not cream-based) soup or a big, low-density salad as a first course.* "

Satiety:
The state of being full.

Leptogenic: Likely to cause someone to become thin.

THE SCIENCE OF HEALTHY EATING AND WEIGHT LOSS

Heart disease in France is 60% lower than in the U.S.[5] Could it be the red wine? Once you reach Phase II, read my guide to red wine and longevity at HabitsofHealth. com.

"

FAT: LESS THAN 25% OF YOUR DAILY CALORIES (LESS THAN 7% FROM SATURATED FAT) ESPECIALLY IN PHASE I (RANGE 20–35%)

How big a role does fat ingestion have on blood sugar and insulin response? Let's take a look.

Pure Fat Load: Glucose-Insulin Response

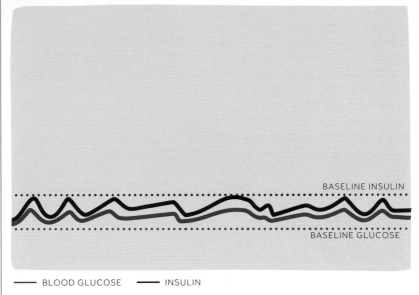

BASELINE INSULIN

BASELINE GLUCOSE

—— BLOOD GLUCOSE   —— INSULIN

Fat, unlike carbohydrates, has little effect on blood sugar and insulin levels. However, fat is extremely energy dense, meaning that even a small amount contains lots of calories.

The effect is pretty negligible, as you can see. Fat's role in weight gain and weight loss is related to its energy density rather than its effect on glucose and insulin. In fact, with nine calories per gram, it provides over twice the energy per gram as carbohydrates! That caloric density helps explain why it's so easy to overdo our calorie intake by eating too much fat, and why doing so leads quickly to obesity—it's easy for our bodies to store it in virtually unlimited amounts. To help you keep fat in control, my healthy eating system encourages you to eat only healthy fats and to carefully monitor your overall fat consumption.

The Mediterranean diet provides a general guideline for healthy fats.

Your fats should come from avocado, nuts (especially walnuts, almonds, pistachios), olives, and olive oil, coconut oil, fatty fishes like salmon and tuna, eggs, dark chocolate, ground flaxseed, and occasional grass-fed beef or pork. It is important to stay on the lower percentage of your diet during the weight loss Phase I.

PROTEIN: 20–25% OF YOUR DAILY CALORIES

While protein provides energy, it's also our body's building block for cellular structure, immune function, and a myriad of health-giving processes. Under my eating plan, where every meal includes a highly digestible protein source, you benefit from a consistent supply of this important nutrient. This keeps your body from using muscle as a fuel source—a common problem on many other weight-loss plans. And regular protein means that your body has adequate building material for the repair and growth of critical support structures. Additionally, studies have shown protein to be highly effective in spurring weight loss and maintenance—first, by helping you feel full and, second, by requiring more energy to digest than carbohydrates and fats do. You'll find out more about protein as a weight-loss tool in the next section, when we discuss satiety (the science of fullness).

Animal products have always been part of human consumption, but the quality of animal protein is very dependent on whether it is from grass fed range animals that live natural lives versus factory raised animals. Industrial animal production also raises major environmental and ethical issues of animal treatment. And the saturated fats, hormones, and antibiotics are good reasons to avoid eating factory raised animal products, including meat, poultry and fish.

You can get all of the necessary protein from plant-based sources, whether through a vegetarian diet with eggs and dairy or vegan diet that contains no animal products at all. The Nurses' Health study showed a 30% reduction in heart disease for those that ate their protein from vegetable sources.[6] There are some thoughts that the higher levels of amino acids in animal protein may stimulate a higher release of insulin versus plant protein.

THE ROLE OF ALCOHOL

Alcohol isn't really a nutrient since it doesn't provide nutrition per se, but it does play a role in managing—or not managing—your weight. Not only is alcohol high in calories, it lowers inhibitions, making you more likely to overeat or to eat unhealthy foods. In fact, it can halt the fat-burning state in its tracks and diminish your ability to control your energy intake, and it should be avoided entirely during Phase I. If you do drink, you can resume doing so in Phase II—though you may want to change your drink of choice to red wine once you learn in Phase III and IV about the healthy, longevity-producing properties of some of its ingredients!

Red wine is a part of the Mediterranean lifestyle, although it should be avoided in the weight loss Phase I.

Now that you've gained a better understanding of how your body uses the energy you feed it, let's take a look at some important

A Habit of Health:

Asking yourself if you're really hungry before you eat.

Could You Be Thirsty?

Sometimes when we think we're hungry, it's really a sign that our body's craving water. Here's a tip: next time you feel hungry, grab a big glass of water and drink the whole thing. Wait 15 minutes or so and ask yourself if you're still hungry. About 30% of the time, what we think is hunger is something else entirely.

THE SCIENCE OF HEALTHY EATING AND WEIGHT LOSS

A Habit of Health:
Avoiding foods with too
many ingredients

When you're shopping, be sure to check the food labels and avoid any grocery items with lots of ingredients. Studies show that if a product contains fewer than three ingredients, you're less likely to overeat.

techniques that can help you use that energy more effectively and fight hunger as you burn fat.

CORE PRINCIPLE 2:
HUNGER CONTROL—SATIETY: THE SCIENCE OF FULLNESS

The emerging science of appetite control has given us a number of important ideas that can make your new leptogenic world—the world of thinness—that much stronger. Most of these principles are already built into your healthy eating strategies, so they should be pretty easy to grasp. We'll focus on five principal areas that can help you fight hunger:

- Volumetrics
- Energy density
- Sensory-specific satiety
- Protein enhancement
- Fiber

VOLUME: THE KEY TO SATIETY

Research shows that we eat about the same volume or weight of food every day. So, if you want to feel fuller quicker, it makes sense to eat foods that are low density (that is, contain a lot of water) and high volume (meaning there's a large amount of food per calorie). Vegetables and fruits are good examples.

In addition to being high in water content, they contain lots of nutrients, so they create a sense of fullness. That's why making foods from this group a large part of your meals—as you do when you use my healthy eating system—is so effective for weight loss and maintenance. With its color-coded listings and high percentage of vegetables and fruits, my system is designed to help you increase your intake of filling, low-density foods in the proper proportions.

CONTROLLING YOUR INTAKE THROUGH
ENERGY DENSITY (ED)

Knowing the energy density (ED) of foods can help you choose ones that promote weight loss and maintenance. This is a particularly useful tool when you're choosing foods that aren't part of the glycemic index, such as meats. In fact, the ED number is already an important part of food labels on products in Europe and Canada.

But since we don't yet have this information on our food packaging, we need to calculate the ED ourselves. To do so, divide the number of calories in one serving by the weight of that serving in grams. For example, if one serving of peanut butter contains 190 calories and weighs 32 g, divide 190 by 32 for an ED of 5.9. Once you have the ED, you can use this simple guide to determine which foods are good choices:

- Best: ED less than one. Includes vegetables and fruits. Eat mostly foods from this group, which makes up 50% of our plate system.
- Good: ED between one and two. Includes whole-wheat pasta and skinless meats.
- Limit: ED above two. Choose these foods sparingly, but if you really want some, go ahead and enjoy them as a special treat.

When you use our healthy eating system, you'll automatically choose the right proportion of foods that help you feel full and minimize energy density. But, for additional guidance, here's a diagram that categorizes some common foods based on their ED:

Food Groupings by Energy Density (ED) Level

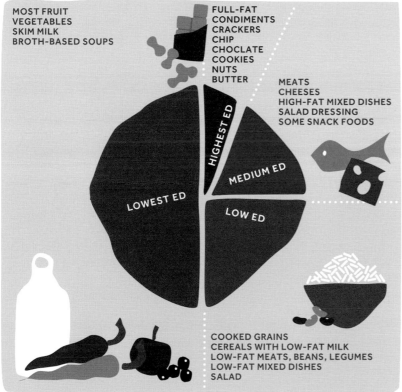

MOST FRUIT
VEGETABLES
SKIM MILK
BROTH-BASED SOUPS

FULL-FAT
CONDIMENTS
CRACKERS
CHIP
CHOCLATE
COOKIES
NUTS
BUTTER

MEATS
CHEESES
HIGH-FAT MIXED DISHES
SALAD DRESSING
SOME SNACK FOODS

HIGHEST ED

MEDIUM ED

LOWEST ED

LOW ED

COOKED GRAINS
CEREALS WITH LOW-FAT MILK
LOW-FAT MEATS, BEANS, LEGUMES
LOW-FAT MIXED DISHES
SALAD

To feel satisfied while keeping calories in check, choose mostly foods from the lowest-ED section (dark green), followed by those from the low-ED section (light green). Eat foods from the highest-ED section (dark red) sparingly, and never when you're hungry.

FLAVOR ENHANCEMENT: THE FOOD INDUSTRY'S DIRTY LITTLE SECRET

Did you know that flavor can either stimulate or suppress the brain's appetite control? While science is just beginning to understand how it all works, the food industry has been using this trick for decades, overloading our senses with processed foods filled with salt, sweet, and sour flavors to encourage us to overeat.

One classic way the food industry overstimulates our appetite centers is by masking ingredients. It may surprise you to know that some cereals actually contain more salt than potato chips! As a result, we keep eating in order to satisfy our salt appetite center, even once our sugar senses are full. Flavors can work the other way as well. Experts at Yale's Prevention Research Center found that people tend to feel fuller and stop eating sooner when a meal contains fewer flavors.[7] So, limiting the varieties of flavors that you eat may actually help you lose weight!

What's the best way to do that? Limit your intake of processed foods and beat the food industry at its own game! Instead, let your color-coded shopping charts be your guide to buying healthy whole foods with flavors that are naturally satisfying and true.

BATTLE HUNGER WITH PROTEIN

Don't skimp on protein. Studies have shown that protein makes us feel fuller than other macronutrients, such as carbohydrates and fats. A recent Washington School of Medicine study showed that participants on a controlled higher-protein diet (up to 30% of their daily intake from protein) felt less hungry than those on a lower-protein diet (as little as 15% protein). And when given as much to eat as they wanted, the higher-protein group lost considerably more weight than the lower-protein group.[8]

Another benefit of protein is that your body uses more energy to break it down, and that means you're burning more calories just to digest it. So the total number of calories you need to maintain your weight might be a little higher if you eat the right amount of protein.

Macronutrients Ranked by Level of Satiety

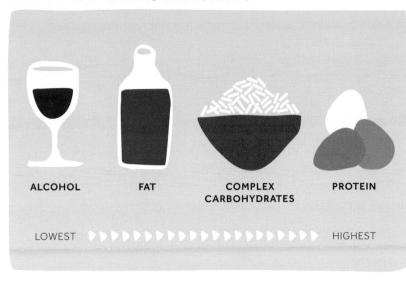

| ALCOHOL | FAT | COMPLEX CARBOHYDRATES | PROTEIN |

LOWEST ▶▶▶▶▶▶▶▶▶▶▶▶▶▶▶▶▶▶▶▶ HIGHEST

Which types of foods make us feel the fullest? Protein is the most filling, followed by complex carbohydrates, then fat. Alcohol is at the bottom, making it a poor choice when you're trying to maintain your weight.

That's one reason we've been careful to include the proper proportion of healthy low-fat proteins in our healthy eating system (25% of your plate), as well as ample portions of low-density complex carbohydrates (50% of your plate). That way you know you're choosing the most satisfying and filling foods available.

Remember, though, that some high-protein foods can be extremely energy dense because of their fat content. Grabbing a handful of nuts may stave off hunger, but it comes at the price of high calories. Just be sure to keep your intake moderate.

FILL UP WITH FIBER!

Not only does fiber provide critical health benefits, it also fills you up so you're less tempted to overeat. As we discussed in Part 2.5, *Choosing Wisely: Dr. A's Color-Coded Shopping System*, both soluble and insoluble fiber are important. Soluble fiber slows the breakdown of complex carbohydrates, thereby helping to reduce blood sugar. In the right quantity, it can even help lower blood cholesterol. It is found in rye, barley, oats, vegetables, legumes, and fruits. Insoluble fiber can't be absorbed or digested by the body, but it still provides a number of benefits, including reducing hunger and cleaning your digestive tract by pulling water into the colon, which stimulates regular bowel movements. Insoluble fiber is found in brown rice, whole-wheat breads, cereals, seeds, vegetables, fruit skin, and legumes.

" *Suffering from back pain? Maintaining a healthy weight is the number one way to strengthen and protect your back, according to the American Council on Exercise.* "

2.7

THE SCIENCE OF HEALTHY EATING AND WEIGHT LOSS

ARE YOU SURE YOU'RE HUNGRY?

Stress, socializing, watching TV, and eating out with friends can all contribute to mindless eating. Our three-hour fueling strategy should fulfill your body's energy needs most of the time. So, if you find yourself wanting to eat outside of your planned meals and fueling breaks, you may well be responding to something other than hunger.

If this is the case, remember the tools that keep you on your path. Eat slowly and pay attention to all the sensory input you experience through your food. You'll feel full and satisfied sooner. In time, eating mindfully will become second nature. Becoming more aware of your eating habits and experiences will help you stay focused and encourage you to make the best secondary choices to support your primary goals.

You now have a comprehensive understanding of your healthy eating strategy and know how to use tools, such as portion-controlled meals, a nine-inch plate, the four major food components, and the color-coded system, to stay on top of your energy intake and hunger for life. A recent study showed that simply by decreasing portion size and energy density by 25%, people were able to maintain their healthy weight.[9]

And now, so can you. Combine your new understanding of portion control and energy density with your knowledge of healthy protein, grains (starch), vegetables and fruits, and you have the Habits of Health to support a lifetime of healthy eating!

CORE PRINCIPLE 3: WAIST CONTROL— REMOVING EXCESS VISCERAL ADIPOSITY

You now know a bit more about how the extra energy you take in leads to extra fat storage. But how exactly do you go about unloading this dangerous substance? Many people think the answer is exercise. Well, that's true if you're close to your healthy weight and just want to maintain the status quo. But intense exercise simply isn't the best way to lose weight. And, for someone who is overweight and out of shape, it's a downright terrible way! For starters, I've seen far too many overweight people strain their knees, develop tendonitis and lower-back pain or worse from pounding the pavement in a desperate attempt to lose weight. Plus, it's not even effective!

People join gyms in droves in January, but by April—when those very same gyms are a ghost town—those super-enthusiastic New Year members have resigned themselves yet again to being overweight. In fact, holding off or at least cutting back on exercise for the first few weeks of Phase I is critical to reaching a fat burning state and experiencing safe, effective weight loss. So, why is it the difference between success and failure? At this beginning stage, exercise can actually slow weight loss down by stimulating stress hormones.

In addition, as your body uses up its glycogen stores and adjusts to a lower insulin level and salt intake during the first week, it will eliminate any excess water it was holding onto.

The resulting decrease in blood pressure can make you fatigued, lightheaded, or dizzy if you exercise prematurely. Besides, steering clear of exercise for now gives you time to learn and slowly begin applying important Habits of Health, such as stretching, progressive movement, and eventually weight resistance training. It's all about sequencing for success, and it's one of the elements that sets this program apart from many others. We will use your early success to generate more success.

It is the Halo Effect of habit installation we talked about back in Parts 1.5 and 1.6. As we generate momentum, you will find it easier and easier to do more and more. And because we are sequencing, each microHabit will build on the next.

So, our Habits of Health weight management and healthy eating system is the most effective way to first unload and then maintain a healthy fat distribution. It just makes sense. Keeping you in a fat-burning state is the most efficient way I know to unload excess fat. Let's look at a couple of examples to help you understand just how this smart approach to weight loss works. In order to increase our understanding of what sources within your body are available for use as energy sources, we are going to create a visual model. Remember, there are only three macronutrients that we can use because alcohol has no nutritional value and we cannot store it anyway.

Our first example is a healthy male who weighs 167 lbs and has a BMI (body mass index) of 24. The chart shows you his energy storage percentage for each major energy source.

Energy Storage System: Healthy Male

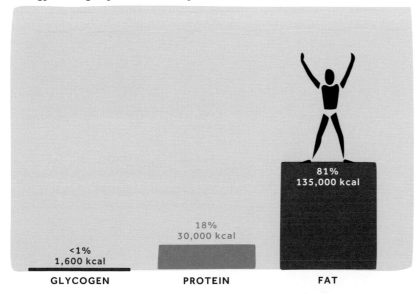

Energy Storage: This man has a healthy proportion and amount of fat, protein, and glycogen (carbohydrates) stored away.

Protein represents 18% of this man's energy stores and is designed to be used for energy only in emergencies, such as starvation. Our program, unlike many diets, is designed to protect against a dangerously low protein level, which can lead to cyclical yo-yoing. Glycogen, the body's store of carbohydrates, is less than one percent in this man. However, fat is plentiful and provides a rich reservoir of energy—over 135,000 calories in this example.

Now look at the following chart to compare this healthy individual to someone who through poor daily choices—perhaps as little as one soda a day. This person has reached a BMI of 30 and is medically obese. At 209 lbs, he's accumulated 42 lbs of unhealthy fat, each of which contains the energy equivalent of 3,500 calories. His fat-storage facility has sequestered an excess 147,000 calories.

This obese male has doubled his fat stores to a whopping 282,000 calories! He needs to offload all this extra energy before it precipitates a heart attack, stroke, or other health crisis.

Energy Storage System: Unhealthy Male

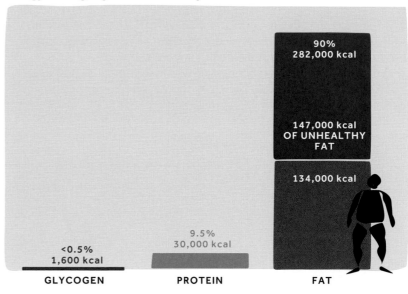

At 209 lbs, this obese individual has accumulated 42 extra pounds of dangerous visceral fat around his organs.

Now, what if he were to try to do this through exercise alone, while maintaining his normal eating pattern? Let's see: so running a marathon race consumes on average about 2,600 calories and so if we assume that our obese friend here could even manage this level of activity (which I definitely wouldn't recommend!), he'd have to run more than 56 marathons to burn off his excess weight. If he were to run one marathon a week, it would take him over a year to offload those calories and that's using one of the most intense forms of exercise there is! It's not a very effective strategy, but countless obese people are out in the summer heat jogging along the side of the road. *The Biggest Loser* TV show used a version of that tactic, which failed miserably.

Let's contrast that scenario with our healthy eating strategy. We could help this same unhealthy man reach his healthy weight and offload those 147,000 calories of fat in a relatively short period of time —safely, without significant loss of muscle, and without exercise. How? We induce a natural fat-burning state while protecting, and even enhancing, the body's protein stores. First, you limit your energy intake through our portion-control system, lowering your total daily calories to below your current energy expenditure. This discrepancy causes your body to burn through its limited supply of stored carbohydrates (glycogen) in the first few days, while your low-glycemic, decreased-carbohydrate diet helps turn down your insulin pump. As a result, your body sends out signals that it needs energy.

The ensuing hormonal changes convert your fat cells from storage centers to little fuel tanks full of triglycerides, which is a substance that the liver converts into useful energy through a process called ketosis—in other words, fat burning (not to be confused with ketoacidosis, an unrelated condition that occurs in diabetes). Once you enter this controlled fat-burning state, you can offload your fat in a progressive fashion until a normal BMI, waist circumference, and percentage body fat is your new state of health as you move into Phase II, which we will address shortly.

You can see why it just doesn't make sense to try to reach your healthy weight through exercise alone. A much easier, safer, and more effective method is to tap into this excess fat reserve and use it as an energy source. There will be plenty of time to add activity and exercise once you're feeling better and, in fact, when the time's right, I'll guide you through a progressive series of easy-to-learn steps to help you develop habits that support greater flexibility, cardiovascular health, and muscle strength.

2.7

THE SCIENCE OF HEALTHY EATING AND WEIGHT LOSS

Your New Weight-Loss and Health Path: Glucose-Insulin Response Curve

Once you begin to control your energy intake by eating frequent low-glycemic meals and snacks, your body's internal response will quickly level out, reducing the blood sugar spikes and dips that lead to cravings and the high-insulin output that leads to dangerous inflammation and disease.

In the meantime, our healthy eating system is designed to bring order to your day and restore function to your body. Just take a look at the illustration above to see the difference in your blood sugar and insulin level once you begin to unload excess calories, turn off your insulin pump, and turn on fat burning by mastering your energy intake!

   Best of all, once you've reached your healthy weight, you can use this very same system (with expanded variety and calories) to maintain it. Soon, with the addition of my healthy movement program, you'll be burning enough extra calories to stay at your ideal weight indefinitely! It's all part of my balanced plan to move beyond weight loss to a state that supports you for life—optimal health.

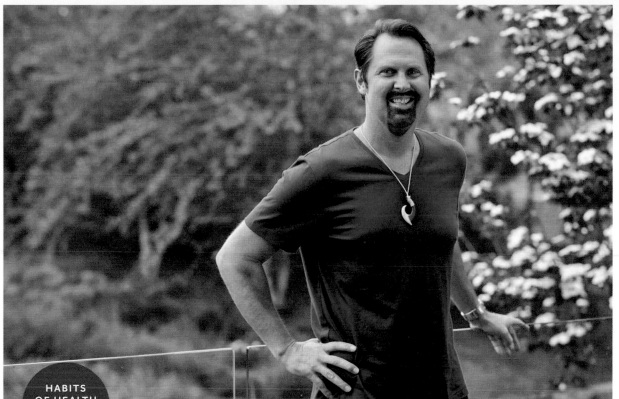

TRANSFORMATION: GREG REX

> *I had one big meal a day and no matter how much exercise I did, I couldn't lose any weight.*

At age 53, I feel like I'm in the best shape of my life, but before I had the habits, I was completely out of balance: fifty pounds overweight, out of balance emotionally. I had a lot of stress in my life and I was eating like a sumo wrestler. I had one big meal a day and no matter how much exercise I did, I couldn't lose any weight.

I got to the point of giving up until I met Dr. Andersen. I learned about these habits and I made a couple of shifts and I lost 50 pounds in less than a couple of months. But more importantly, I made these habits part of my lifestyle. I have a healthy mind, I surround myself with healthy people, and that's one of the reasons I've kept it off for sixteen years.

What I love about the Habits of Health system is that it's comprehensive. It doesn't just focus on exercise or diet. Within the first week or two, I knew I could do this for the rest of my life. It was a total transformation, and I'm so glad I embraced it.

*Average weight loss on the Optimal Weight 5 & 1 Plan® is 12 lbs.

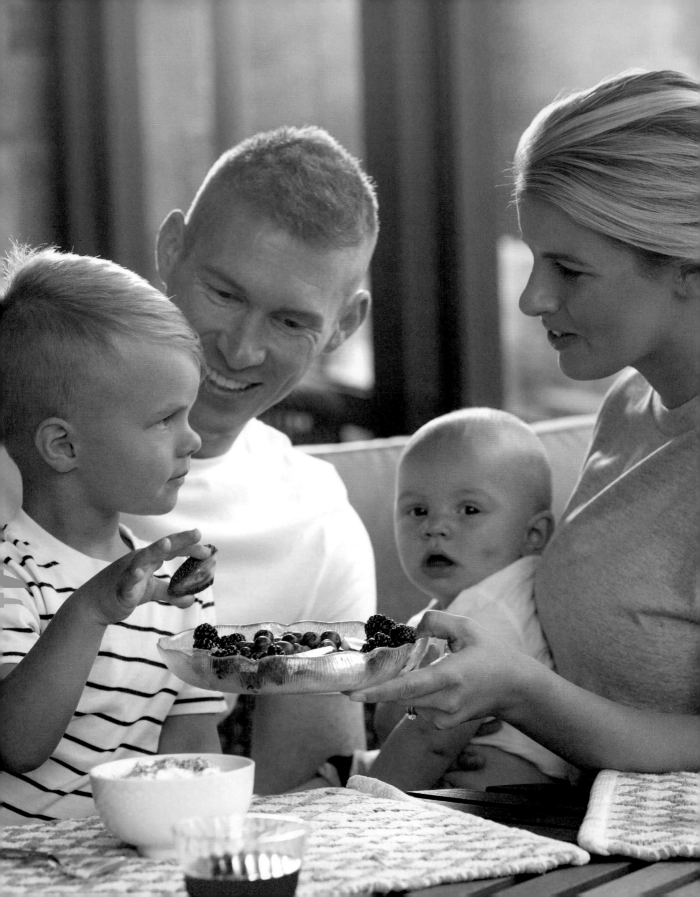

PART 2.8

HEALTHY EATING FOR LIFE: YOUR TRANSITION TO PERMANENT HEALTH

HABITS OF
HEALTHY WEIGHT MANAGEMENT

THE HABITS OF
HEALTHY EATING AND HYDRATION

Your discipline throughout Phase I has paid off. You've reached a healthy weight, which is the first important milestone on the path to creating optimal health. And that means you're ready to transition to Part Two. In Part Two, we'll start by expanding and developing the eating plan you used during Part One to create a strategy you can use for life.

Part Two is also the time to learn how to make many of the daily choices that will assist you on your journey to optimal health. First, let's review the Habits of Health you've learned so far, which form the foundations for the success to come.

BE SLIM

Six of the Habits of Health you're learning while you're losing weight spell out the acronym "BeSlim". It's a tool I created to help you begin to focus and understand some of the key behaviors essential to maintaining a healthy weight. Now we're going to take these beginning steps and start developing them into your comprehensive long-term optimal health plan.

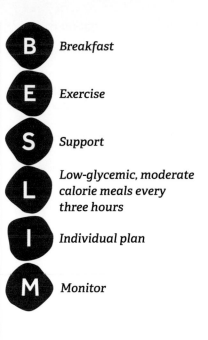

B Breakfast

E Exercise

S Support

L Low-glycemic, moderate calorie meals every three hours

I Individual plan

M Monitor

Breakfast

By now, you're in the habit of beginning each day with a healthy breakfast (which may be in the form of a portion-controlled meal). It's an important routine that's critical for long-term weight loss, according to the National Weight Control Registry.

Exercise

As your weight has decreased, and I am sure you are feeling much better. Perhaps, you've started adding more activity, using the stairs instead of the elevator, for example, or taking the dog for a walk. If you've been in Part One for a while, you may have started learning my progressive movement systems for sustainable exercise, as outlined in Parts 2.9 to 2.12. Whatever your current level of physical ability, my plan is designed to give you an easy entry into the world of fitness. You've been hearing me talk about the relatively minor role exercise plays in weight loss. Well, that was true in the beginning of Part One. But increasing your activity level becomes very important as you move from Part One into Part Two and beyond. After the first three weeks of Part One, your body is ready for increased motion. You're lighter, you have more confidence, you're physically healthier, you have the right motivation, and you're in the process of installing the *Habits of Health Transformational System*. My NEAT and EAT plans for physical movement are doable and are designed to fit your current level of health and fitness. Over time, these systems will put you on track for long-term success!

Support

I'm a big believer in seeking help on your journey to optimal health and wellbeing. While I can serve as your immediate mentor through this book and *Your LifeBook*, connecting with a coach—like a healthcare professional or a trained coach—can add tremendous value. We discussed this in detail in Part 1.7, *Optimizing Your Surroundings: Creating Your Microenvironment of Health*. Additionally, your family, friends, weight-loss buddy, or group can be helpful for encouragement and moral support. This is all a part of developing your Habits of Healthy Surroundings MacroHabits that are embedded throughout the rest of the book!

Low-glycemic meals every three hours

You're now in the habit of eating smaller meals every three hours,

Monitor Your Weight and Measurements Regularly

Monitoring your weight, waist measurements, and (if possible) your percentage of body fat are important surveillance tools that provide an accurate picture of your current reality. Remember, the scale and tape measure are your friends!

Here are some tips:
- **Set up a regular schedule for weighing and measuring. I believe that once a week is the most reliable schedule for tracking a trend, but daily is fine, especially during transition!**
- **Weigh and measure yourself in as little clothing as possible.**
- **Weigh and measure yourself on the same scale and at the same time of day. Most people are at their lowest weight in the early morning.**
- **Use my favorite technique to check inches and weight: monitor yourself regularly by trying on a favorite pair of jeans or pants whose proper fit you know well. If you have to get on the bed and hold your stomach in, you'll know you're putting on weight and need to adjust your calories accordingly!**

which is a very powerful Habit of Health. And low-glycemic, lower-unhealthy- fat, moderate-calorie eating has been shown to be a key factor in long-term weight management. This is a great time to review the lessons of healthy eating. In fact, there will never be a better time. You're feeling better, you're tuned into the proper motivation and healthy choices, and you're learning how to choose and prepare foods that support your health.

Your permanent eating strategy now includes meals that:

- Are low-glycemic
- Satisfy your hunger
- Control your caloric intake
- Contain healthy fats in moderate amounts
- Keep to a three-hour eating schedule

These basic behaviors form the key Habits of Health that you'll need to keep in mind as you head into Part Two.

Now, as you begin your transition, we're going to expand the food choices available to you (while keeping within our healthy guidelines) and add calories to your three-hour meals until you reach equilibrium between your energy in and energy out. That's how we'll make our healthy eating system into a complete plan that teaches you how to eat for a lifetime of health.

Individual plan

Now that you're past the initial weight-loss stage, you're ready to build a permanent plan that gives you control over your energy intake and long-term strategies for life. Each of us is a little different, and it is this curiosity and openness to learn and grow that will put you in control of those 200 food choices you make every day for the rest of your life!

Monitor

You've become used to checking your weight weekly. Keeping an eye on your energy balance helps you make sure you're not loading fat. Now that you've solidified your understanding of these key Habits of Health, let's look ahead to what's next—learning how to use these important new behaviors to maintain your weight loss and build optimal health for life!

THE TWO KEYS TO MAINTAINING YOUR HEALTHY WEIGHT

There are two main reasons why most diets fail: a lack of understanding of energy balance and a lack of understanding of proper motivation.

1. Energy Balance: The First Key to Maintaining Your Healthy Weight

The fat cells in your body use energy. When you lose weight, you decrease your metabolic demands because your fat cells empty and you have less energy needed to run them. As a result, you experience a lower level of daily energy expenditure. If you simply go back to your old, pre-diet eating habits (as dieters so often do), your energy needs will be out of balance, and your new, lighter body will be taking in more energy than it can use. And, as a result, your weight can balloon. It's the classic yo-yo pattern, which is caused by an ever-widening gap between energy in and energy out.

Even worse are unbalanced diets that lower calories so severely that your body is forced to cannibalize its own muscle, or diets designed to fabricate weight loss by manipulating macronutrients such as fats and carbohydrates, thereby producing an imbalance in the amount of energy you take in from each group. Diets like these are hard to sustain. The body isn't shy about letting you know it has a macronutrient deficit, and soon enough the cravings will begin. Even if you do manage to stay with one of these diets long enough to lose some weight, once the diet is over, it's off to the races to replenish that deficit. That's why a low-carbohydrate diet has no chance of long-term success. Nature knows best!

We have talked a lot about how we can control our overall weight by paying attention to the quantity and quality of food we eat. In the next sections, we will begin looking at how we can increase your energy expenditure as this is essential for long-term weight control, optimal health, and longevity.

Let's spend a moment talking a little more about how our body regulates our weight from a central command control.

There is a very complex system that helps us keep our weight within a fairly close range or set point. It's easiest to explain by thinking of the thermostat that determines your room temperature in your heating and air conditioning system. It's known as the Body Set Weight (in medical literature it's called the appestat or obesistat).

We have many different feedback loops that work extremely well when we are not overwhelming the body with huge meals of sugar, flour, saturated fats, and other ultra-processed foods. From stretch receptors and satiety hormones, leptin is released when the fat cells are full to signal us to stop eating. When the stomach is empty, ghrelin is released, which stimulates hunger. When the stomach is stretched, secretion stops.

These satiety mechanisms make a lot of sense from a survival point of view. Our body is designed to stay within certain body fat parameters. If you are too skinny, you will die during the hard times of famine or winter, and if you are too fat, you will not be able to catch food, and you might just get eaten yourself because you cannot avoid capture. The following illustration shows how the body would adjust. The right side shows when somebody is getting too heavy and leptin levels increase to decrease appetite and raise energy expenditure.

> " *A Habit of Health: Monitoring your weight and measurements regularly.* "

On the left, it shows how when we are too thin, we turn off leptin to increase appetite and slow down movement to conserve energy.

So why is this important to know? In the world we live in, the problem is almost always being too heavy because of the obesigenic conditions. Let's look closer at these metabolic switches.

The two key players in determining your set point are leptin and our old friend insulin. Just like the heat and cool elements of your HVAC system, these two hormones help regulate your set point. When we have eaten a meal and the body has adequate energy, the fat cells release leptin to tell the body it's full and to stop eating. In addition, it tells the body to be more active. This mechanism is represented on the right side of the illustration.

Body Set Weight Thermostat in Weight Control: Balanced System

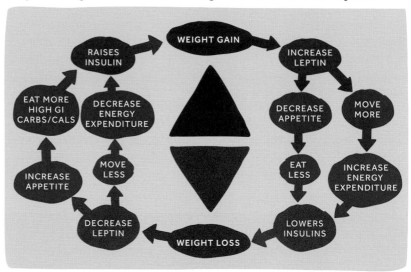

However, if you are eating food that stimulates high insulin, it tells the fat cells to overstuff and store more and more energy as fat. These two hormones that control body fat percentage have directly opposite effects on our energy management system. As you can see if you increase the set point or push the red arrow it shifts to the left and we create a new higher set point. This would be helpful if we moved to a colder climate. If we need to naturally lower our set point or push the green arrow we shift to the right side and leptin wins. If leptin wins, then we are able to reduce appetite and increase basal metabolic rates sufficiently to burn off the excess calories being eaten. Look at the following illustration.

Body Set Weight Thermostat: Habits of Healthy Eating Keeps You in the Green

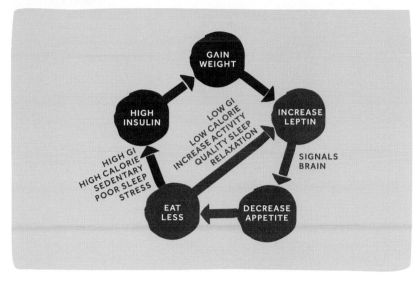

As we eat the wrong foods and we stimulate insulin, the size of the fat cells increase and this stimultates an increase in the release of leptin. This signals the brain to decrease the appetite, which then causes our body to eat less.

If you start eating the right foods, as outlined in the Habits of Healthy Eating strategy, your set point will lower itself naturally. You'll stay healthy and in the green zone, which will help you to maintain a consistent energy balance, and the natural balance between your insulin and leptin will stay in a healthy range without you having to think too much about it.

But when you continue to eat unhealthy food, your set point will increase, and you'll reach hyperinsulinemia, which prevents leptin from doing its job. Hyperinsulinemia tells us to eat more and sit on the couch. Your leptin levels will continue to rise because of the increased level of fats, it won't be effective. You'll eventually develop leptin resistance as well as your insulin resistance, and your weight will cascade out of control. See the following illustration.

Increasing Body Set Weight Thermostat: Weight Gain and Leptin Resistance

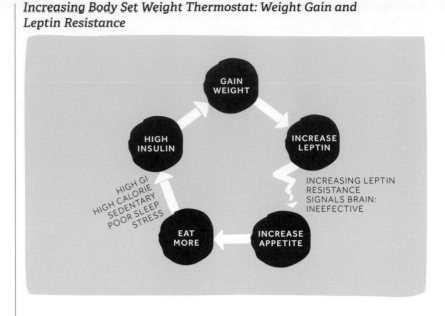

The scientifically formulated low-calorie meals and my Healthy Eating for Life System deliver a proper balance of macronutrients in the form of healthy, great-tasting, low-glycemic foods that will keep you satisfied for a lifetime and protect your muscles from attack. It will gradually lower your set point to make it easier and easier to maintain your healthy weight.

Keeping insulin low is the key to long-term health and weight management. Here are the basic factors in keeping insulin levels under control:

1. *Eat less sugar*
2. *Eat less refined grains*
3. *Eat moderate protein and natural fats*
4. *Eat more whole foods*
5. *Eat food, not too much, mostly plants (Michael Pollan)*
6. *Balance macronutrients (see Optimal Daily Intake of Macronutrients below)*
7. *30 minutes of active exercise a day*

Optimal Daily Intake of Macronutrients (According to the 2015–2020 Dietary Guidelines for Macronutrients Optimal Range)[1]

	ENERGY PER GRAM	PERCENTAGE OF TOTAL DAILY CALORIE INTAKE
CARBOHYDRATES	4 kcal/g	45 – 65%
PROTEIN	4 kcal/g	10 – 35%
FAT	9 kcal/g	20 – 35%
		<10% SATURATED

Your body needs a balance of macronutrients—carbohydrates, proteins, and fats—in order to run at its best. Some diets manipulate macronutrients, producing an imbalance of energy from each group. But these diets are hard to sustain.

2. Proper Motivation:
The Second Key to Maintaining Your Healthy Weight

Many people go on a diet with the sole purpose of losing pounds and so when their weight-loss goal is reached, they think they're done. And they're glad, because their diet has been a period of great deprivation, and they can't wait to get back to their old way of life. But with our plan, reaching a healthy weight is just the first step on your path. Your underlying motivation is inspired by your fundamental choice—the choice of optimal health that you adopted during your preparation for this journey.

Hopefully by now, you're writing your new story in your companion, *Your LifeBook*. You're progressing through the Elements adding the principles that will lay a solid foundation for a series of new habits, choices, and ways of thinking that will assist you in your lifelong transformation. Make sure you're doing all the exercises focusing on motivation and choice. This is a good time to take a look, especially those in the first five Elements, if you haven't done so already. Make sure you have a firm grasp on how to support the motivation behind your decision to lose weight and attain optimal health. These new habits are integral to your success as you review your current reality and prepare to move forward from where you are right now to where you want to be.

YOUR CURRENT REALITY

You're now at your healthy weight and equipped with habits that will serve you well for the rest of your life—a life that may indeed be longer and of higher quality as you align with your fundamental choice. Let's review these habits:

- You're eating smaller portions at regular intervals (every three hours).
- You're eating lower-glycemic carbohydrates, healthy proteins, and healthy fats and oils.
- You've learned how to plan meals in advance so you're no longer just reacting to hunger and your environment.

As a result, you've gone from an overweight fat-storing state to a healthy fat-burning state and have reset your body weight. You've also turned up the heat making it easier to maintain your healthy weight. Now it's time to move forward by solidifying your healthy eating strategies and continuing your journey toward optimal health.

Your Current Reality

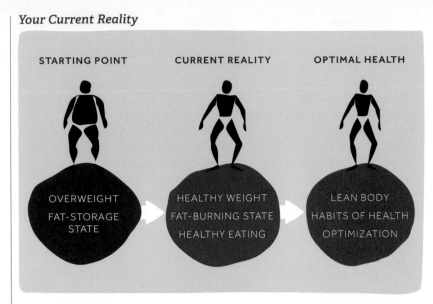

As you enter Phase II, your current reality has shifted from your starting point. This transition brings you closer to optimal health.

OVERVIEW OF YOUR TRANSITION

The transition to your lifetime healthy eating strategy consists of two parts:

- Adding calories until you reach your body set weight point (calories in = calories out), which is a key part of keeping insulin at a healthy level and leptin working effectively
- Introducing a full range of foods to support optimal health and maintain your healthy weight

First, let's figure out your body set weight (BSW) set point, which is determined by two different measurements. First is the insulin/leptin balance, which you will know is dialed in because you will not be hungry and you will have lots of energy. The second measurement will be your response to adding calories—the point at which the number of calories you take in is equal to the number of calories you use and at that point your weight will stop fluctuating. The best way to reach that point is to figure out how many calories you burn in the course of a day. That will allow us to know how many calories you should eat daily to maintain your healthy weight.

What is transition?

In Phase I, we focused on decreasing your weight and eliminating the extra fat in your body, which will dramatically improve your health and fitness. We have taught you a series of new eating habits that have lowered your total energy consumption and improved the quality of food you are now eating. As a result, we have specifically limited the types and amount of food you ate by burning the extra fat stored by your body.

So, you're at a point where you have modified your body weight set point and accomplished your first major desired outcome.

Your body is much healthier and, by protecting your muscle from being cannibalized (because we flipped the metabolic switches), you are generally much healthier. In order to continue making progress, we need to transition your body to the full range of healthier foods that will allow you to eat a more exciting variety of meals. And we need to make sure we do not add too many healthy calories or overstimulate insulin in the process of transition from Phase I to Phase II.

Because you have lost weight, it's important that your calorie consumption is reduced—you have lowered your total size, and we need to increase the set point that will allow you to gradually increase more energy in order to increase energy expenditure. It is important to keep the balance of the set point, so that you increase leptin but stop insulin from increasing, which will prevent any transitional weight gain.

We are going to estimate how much energy your body uses by calculating your current energy expenditure to help provide a starting point and target for transitioning calorie intake.

We are going to use a very simple formula now which will give you a great place to start transition, but we will make the formal scientific calculations available at HabitsofHealth.com for those of you who want to be more precise. What follows are the determinants which will help you know how to increase your expenditure.

> *Transition: A process or a period marked by change. The passage from one state to another.*

DETERMINING YOUR TOTAL ENERGY EXPENDITURE (TEE)

Want to figure out how many calories you need to eat in Phase II to keep those jeans fitting just right? The most common method is a simple formula to calculate your total energy expenditure, or TEE. Calculating your TEE as it is right now at your healthy weight will help us determine your optimal caloric intake during this phase. (We'll work on increasing that number in the next section as part of our overall Habits of Health strategy.)

Your TEE is determined by three factors:

- Your basal metabolic rate (BMR)
- Your physical activity level (PAL)
- The thermic effect of the food you eat (TEF)

Together, these show us how quickly your body is burning the fuel you're taking in, day in and day out. Let's begin by looking separately at those three components.

2.8

> *Turn off the TV during meals! Studies show that watching TV during meals increases the likelihood that you'll overeat.[2]*

Basal Metabolic Rate (BMR)

This is the energy you use for your basic bodily needs. Even when your body is at rest, it's using fuel to breathe, grow, circulate your blood, adjust your hormone levels, repair cells, and perform other functions. Typically, BMR is the largest portion of the TEE energy equation. Because the energy required by these basic functions remains fairly consistent, this number doesn't tend to change much.

Physical Activity Level (PAL)

This is the energy you use when you move—playing tennis, walking to the store, chasing after the dog. You have control of this number and can change it quite a bit depending on the frequency, duration, and intensity of your activities.

Thermic Effect of Food (TEF)

This is the energy your body uses to process your food. Digesting, absorbing, transporting, and storing food all take energy— about 10% of the calories you use each day. For the most part, this number stays steady.

Take a look at the following diagram. You'll see that BMR is the largest energy user, accounting for 60–75% of your daily expenditure. PAL ranges from 25–30%, and TEF takes up 10–15%.

Total Energy Expenditure (TEE)

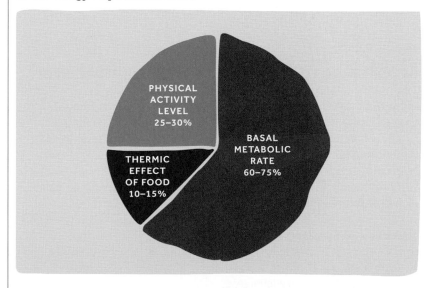

To find out how much energy you use and how many calories you should be eating, we're going use a simple formula that incorporates your basal metabolic rate, your physical activity level, and the thermic effect of the food you eat. Each of these three components accounts for a certain percentage of your total daily energy use.

CALCULATING YOUR TEE

Now that you know what goes into your TEE, let's start figuring out your number. There are a couple of options available to help us, some more accurate than others. If you're not a math major or don't feel like getting out the calculator, you can start with a rough method to calculate your daily caloric needs. This initial number doesn't need to be exact, since it's only a starting point that you'll be adjusting as you monitor your weight throughout transition.

Option 1: The easy way to calculate TEE
To find out your TEE using the easy method, use the following formula:

Your current weight (in pounds) × 11 calories = TEE (daily caloric need)
This formula is based on a sedentary individual, so you'll need to adjust it as you step up your exercise (see below):

Multiply your TEE by:
- 1.2 (for light exercise)
- 1.5 (for moderate exercise)
- 1.7 (for heavy exercise)

For example: 162 lbs × 11 kcal/lb = 1,782 kcal × 1.2 = 2,138 kcal
Remember to recalculate this number as you track your weight over the next several weeks.

Option 2: Formal TEE Calculation
Go to HabitsofHealth.com and you can calculate the individual contribution of each component.

Now that you know how to calculate your TEE, let's find out the best way to add foods and increase your daily calorie consumption to match it.

YOUR TRANSITION EATING PLAN

If you used the portion-controlled meal system exclusively during Phase I, you'll need to introduce new food groups as well as additional calories into your eating system. Read the next section about the process of transitioning from the packaged portion-controlled meal system to learn how to do this effectively.

If you're using the healthy eating system along with the scientifically formulated prepackaged meals, you're already employing many of the principles of your permanent eating strategy and you can skip the next section and go right to *Transitioning to Your Permanent Eating System.*

Journal your weight. If you start to see your weight trending upward, check in with your coach and check in on your choices to see where you can improve.

Don't forget that fuelings are a great way to add calories into your diet during transition and beyond.

TRANSITIONING FROM THE PREPACKAGED FUELINGS

If you've reached your healthy weight using portion-controlled meals, you will need to add the full range of food groups back into your diet as well as calories. You're already used to preparing a healthy lean and green meal along with your fuelings, so this transition should be pretty easy for you.

We're going to introduce these new foods in a logical order that allows your digestive tract to become accustomed to them. Your starting point is five portion-controlled meals and one lean and green meal, for a total of 800 to 1,000 calories a day. For the first four weeks of your transition, you'll increase your daily caloric intake incrementally each week by adding one of the four food groups that you avoided during Phase I.

Below is the schedule we use at OPTAVIA™ to transition from weight loss into maintenance:

- Week 1: additional vegetables
- Week 2: fruits
- Week 3: dairy
- Week 4: whole grains

By the end of week four, you will have added each of these four food groups and will be consuming approximately 1,350–1,500 calories a day.

TRANSITION

Once you've achieved your healthy weight, you're ready to make the transition to lifelong healthy eating. The transition phase gradually increases your calorie intake and reintroduces a wider variety of foods. The calories you need after transition to maintain your weight varies according to your height, weight, gender, age, and activity level. This six-week transition leads to an ultimate goal of fewer than 1,550 calories a day.

	TARGET NO. OF CALORIES	FUELINGS	LEAN & GREEN MEALS	ADDITIONS
WEEK 1	850 – 1,050	5	1	• 1 cup (2 servings) of your favorite vegetables (any kind)
WEEK 2	900 – 1,150	4	1	In addition to your week 1 additions, add: • 2 medium sized pieces of fruit • Or 1 cup of cubed fruit or berries (2 servings)*
WEEK 3	1,000 – 1,300	4	1	In addition to your week 1, 2, and 3 additions, add: • 1 cup of low fat or fat-free dairy (1 serving)
WEEK 4–6	1,100 – 1,550	3	1	In addition to your week 1, 2, and 3 additions, add: • 4 – 6oz of lean meat • And 1 serving** of whole-grains***

*   Fresh or, if canned, unsweetened and packed in juice, not syrup.
**   Grilled, baked, poached, or broiled, not fried.
*** Examples: 1 slice of whole-grain bread, 1/2 whole-grain English muffin, 3/4 cup high-fiber cereal, 1/2 cup whole-wheat pasta, or 1/3 cup brown rice.

Here's how the first four weeks should look.

Week 1: Add vegetables (850 – 1,050 Total Calories Per day)
- Add any vegetable from the green section of the charts.
- You're now eating five fuelings, one lean and green meal, and one additional cup of vegetables.

Week 2: Add fruit (900 – 1,150 total calories per day)
- Drop one prepackaged meal.
- Add any fruit from the green section of the charts. (Fresh or frozen fruit is preferred, but canned may be used as long as it's not packed in syrup.)
- You're now eating four fuelings, one lean and green meal, one additional cup of vegetables, and two medium-sized pieces of fruit or one cup berries or chopped fruit.

Week 3: Add dairy (1,000 – 1,300 total calories per day)
- Dairy includes low-fat and sugar-free yogurt, milk, or lactaid products.
- You're now eating four fuelings, one lean and green, one additional cup of vegetables, two medium-sized pieces of fruit or one cup berries or chopped fruit, and one cup of low-fat or fat-free dairy.

2.8

Week 4: Add whole-grains (1,100–1,550 total calories per day)

- Drop one fueling.
- Whole-grain choices include one slice of whole-grain bread, ¾ cup high-fiber cereal, ⅓ cup whole-wheat pasta, or ½ cup brown rice.
- You're now eating three fuelings, one lean and green meal, one additional cup of vegetables, one medium-sized piece of fruit or ½ cup berries or chopped fruit, one cup of low-fat or fat-free dairy, and one portion of whole-grain starch.
- If you're exercising, add 4 oz of lean meat, poultry, fish, or other protein.

Breakfast:	*½ cup high-fiber breakfast cereal (over 5 g of fiber per serving) with ½ cup skim milk and 1 cup fresh strawberries*
Mid-morning:	*Frothy cappuccino boost fueling*
Lunch:	*4 oz deli turkey; 2 cups salad greens with a cup of diced cucumber, tomato, and green pepper (plus ½ tablespoons reduced-calorie salad dressing if desired)*
Mid-afternoon:	*Chicken flavored and vegetable noodle soup fueling*
Dinner:	*4 oz poached salmon with 1 cup green beans*
Evening:	*Decadent double chocolate brownie fueling with 1 teaspoon fat-free whipped topping*

After the first four weeks, you will have introduced all four of the food groups you avoided during Phase I and will be eating approximately 1,500 calories per day. Over the following weeks, you'll continue to add calories until you reach your TEE, either by adding foods to one of your fuelings as outlined in the transition guide that came with your low-calorie, scientifically formulated meals, or to one of your meals using my color-coded portion-control system.

As an example if your target TEE was 1,900 calories, this would mean adding 400 calories over the next four weeks. An easy way to do this is to add 100 calories each week until you have reached the permanent healthy eating schedule outlined in the next section.

Note: If you've reached your healthy weight using portion-controlled meals, you can skip the next section and move to planning meals.

TRANSITIONING TO YOUR PERMANENT EATING SYSTEM

In Phase I, if you used my healthy eating system to help improve your health, then you learned how to eat every three hours for a total of 1,200–1,300 calories per day. Using your nine-inch plate, you learned the right proportion of foods from the four major food components, and my color-coded, low-glycemic system helped you choose healthy carbohydrates, fats, and lean proteins, and showed you how to select your vegetables and fruits from the darkest green charts for the lowest-glycemic carbohydrates. This put you in a fat-burning state that helped you reach your healthy weight.

Now that you're transitioning to your lifelong eating plan, you no longer need to unload excess fat. Our new priority is to increase your daily calories until we reach a state of equilibrium between energy in and energy out. As part of that plan, we're going to add in some slightly higher-glycemic carbohydrates from the light green section of your color-coded charts. Eventually, you'll be able to choose from any of the carbohydrates on the green charts.

We're going to add calories back into your diet gradually in order to allow your body to adjust to this additional fuel. Let's take a look at your Phase I eating schedule, which taught you the basics of healthy eating.

Dr. A's Healthy Eating Schedule From Phase I

BREAKFAST	300 – 400 CALORIES
MID-MORNING FUELING	100 CALORIES
LUNCH FUELING	100 – 200 CALORIES
MID-AFTERNOON FUELING	100 CALORIES
DINNER	400 CALORIES
EVENING FUELING	100 CALORIES

This is how your daily intake looked in Phase I. Now you're going to add calories gradually until you reach your Total Energy Expenditure (TEE), which is the point where your intake and output meet.

Transitioning into your permanent plan is simply a matter of adding about 100 calories to your daily intake for each week of transition, until you reach your TEE. (If you lost more than 50 lbs, you'll want to go a bit slower, adding an additional 100 daily calories every two weeks of transition.) Here's how your transition might look if your TEE is 1,900 calories per day:

Don't Forget to Monitor Your Weight During Transition!

Your weight may fluctuate during transition as your body gets used to the additional carbohydrates, salt, and calories. Remember to monitor your weight vigilantly and adjust your calorie intake up or down if you fluctuate by more than a few pounds from your healthy weight. If you notice that you're gaining weight, cut back on calories a bit by recalculating your TEE and adjusting your intake accordingly. Give your body time to readjust its lower set point and be ready to catch yourself early!

2.8

As a rule, the more acidic a fruit, the lower its glycemic index because it slows down gastric emptying.

Week 1	add 100 calories to lunch
Week 2	add another 100 calories to lunch
Week 3	add another 100 calories to lunch, bringing it to a full 400 calorie three-component meal (using a nine-inch plate)
Week 4	add 100 calories to the mid-morning fueling
Week 5	add 100 calories to the mid-afternoon fueling
Week 6	add 100 calories to breakfast
Week 7	add 100 calories to dinner
Week 8	monitor weight and adjust as necessary

Note that I haven't added calories to the evening fueling because it's important to minimize the body's workload at night.

Remember, fuelings are an excellent way to add these incremental calories during transition, as well as after you reach your optimal daily caloric intake. Here's an example of what the permanent eating strategy might look like for someone whose TEE is 1,900 calories:

Permanent Healthy Eating Schedule

BREAKFAST	500 CALORIES
MID-MORNING FUELING	200 CALORIES
LUNCH FUELING	400 CALORIES
MID-AFTERNOON FUELING	200 CALORIES
DINNER	500 CALORIES
EVENING FUELING	100 CALORIES

This is how your daily intake might look by the end of transition to Phase II if your TEE is 1,900 calories.

Your own permanent eating strategy may look different, depending on how many calories you need to take in each day for weight maintenance, based on your TEE. Remember, the total number of calories in all your meals and fuelings should equal the TEE you've calculated for yourself. You may need to adjust this number either up or down after the first couple of weeks to maintain your healthy weight and a BMI of under 25.

PLANNING MEALS DURING TRANSITION AND BEYOND

Transition is a great time to add high-quality proteins, nutrient-dense grains (starches), and a full range of fruits and vegetables to your diet. Just remember to continue your healthy eating strategies, including the following:

- Continue to use the prepackaged portion-controlled meals.
- Use a nine-inch plate for all your meals.
- Select healthy options from the three major food groups.
- Choose foods using the color-coded, low-glycemic shopping system. Stay with foods in the dark green sections (GI <30) until you reach your new daily caloric allowance (your TEE), then add foods from the light green sections (GI = 30 – 50). Use foods in the orange sections (GI >50) only occasionally.
- Do not eat anything from the bright red section.
- Utilize the 100-calorie fueling choices from Part 2.6, *Building Healthy Meal Plans for Optimal Health,* to add your additional daily calories.
- Utilize the menus you will find at HabitsofHealth.com to create healthy meals, including the new 400-calorie lunch you'll be building over the first three weeks.

Here are some guidelines to follow as you add healthy foods into your diet from each of the three major food groups.

Adding Calories from the Vegetable and Fruit Group
It's hard to go wrong in this category. All fruits and vegetables are healthy, low in calories, packed with vitamins and minerals, and provide fiber to help fill you up. On top of that, diets rich in fruit and vegetables may reduce the risk of some types of cancer and other chronic diseases.

By the end of transition, you'll have added a portion of fruit or vegetable to each of your six daily fuelings. You should be having at least two servings of fruit and four servings of vegetables per day. The research states that up to 10 servings of vegetables / fruit maximized their benefit to optimal health.[3]

Shopping tips:
- Choose fresh fruit and vegetables when possible, as outlined in Part 2.5, *Choosing Wisely: Dr. A's Color Coded Shopping System.*
- If choosing frozen or canned fruits and vegetables, ensure they contain no added fat, sugar, or sauce.
- Include lots of salad greens in your diet.
- Add higher-glycemic choices such as corn, peas, and other fruits and vegetables with caution.
- When adding corn, keep the glycemic index low by buying corn on the cob with the husk intact.
- Sweet potatoes have a moderate GI of 46 (light green chart) when steamed, boiled, or baked.

Save Your Salad with Salad Spritzers!

Too much dressing can turn a healthy salad into a calorie disaster. In fact, a recent study showed that in most salads, excessive calories are contributed from salsa and dressings! That's why salad spritzers are such a great invention. They deliver just one calorie per spray, helping you coat all of your yummy vegetables without all those calories.

An even better choice is to avoid processed salad dressings and instead used a drizzle of extra virgin olive oil with vinegar instead!

2.8

- **Polluting your body with empty calories from processed foods**
- **Sugar and fat: the non-nutritive agents**

- Yams have a GI of 37 and are high in fiber and nutrient dense.
- The lowest-glycemic fruits—citrus (orange, grapefruit, mandarins)—are great choices, as are stone fruits (apricots, plums, peaches, nectarines).
- Pineapple, watermelon, and cantaloupe can be eaten in moderate amounts. It is important to understand that watermelon has a high glycemic index, but it also has a high water content. Its glycemic load is very low, and it can be eaten in moderation once a healthy weight is reached.
- Berries are very low glycemic and a great choice as you add calories to breakfast, fuelings, and lunch.

As you begin adding your 100 calories per day in the transition schedule, make your selections primarily from the dark green color charts. This will keep your insulin pump turned off and give you some time to increase your energy expenditure as you begin my movement program in the next few parts. Once you have reached your TEE and your weight is stable, you can start adding selections from the lighter green charts, and even a higher-glycemic choice on occasion.

Estimating How Many Calories in Fruit and Vegetables
- 1 cup cooked vegetables contains approximately 50–70 calories.
- 1 medium piece of fresh fruit contains approximately 80 calories.
- 1 cup of cubed fresh fruit contains approximately 80 calories.

Adding Calories from the Grain (Starch) Group
Your grain or starch selections have the biggest effect on your glycemic intake and require special vigilance as you complete your permanent eating plan.

Low-glycemic starches are a great steady source of nutrient-dense calories. You should have four to five servings a day, particularly if you're active. One serving equals one slice of whole-wheat bread or half a cup of cooked brown rice, whole-wheat pasta, or whole-wheat noodles.

Healthy breads: Whole grains are high in fiber, nutrient dense, and contain vitamins and minerals.

Good choices include:
- Pumpernickel
- Sourdough
- Stone ground or whole wheat
- Chapatis or other Indian breads made with chickpea flour

Cereals: Almost all commercial breakfast cereals are processed, which means that the grains have lost their structure and are no longer intact, making them high glycemic and poor choices. Although they are in the orange sections in the glycemic charts I consider them as toxic red chart items because their GI is so high.

Consider them as toxic red chart items.

Good choices include:
- Rolled oats made into oatmeal (the gold standard of breakfast cereals!)
- Barley, bulgur, and wheat bran
- Homemade muesli (fruits, nuts, seeds, rolled oats)

Pasta: Pasta is made from semolina grain. As long as you cook it al dente and serve it with a healthy protein, it's fine to have a cup of pasta. Choose a low-glycemic variety such as spinach rotini.

Rice: Rice is generally very high glycemic and should be avoided except in small quantities on limited occasions. Brown rice, which has a GI over 50, and long grain and basmati, with a GI around 58, are better choices than many other types of rice, which can have a GI approaching 100! Because sushi is served with seaweed, vinegar, and protein, its GI drops below 50.

How Many Calories?
One slice of low-glycemic bread or half a cup pasta or cereal contains approximately 80 calories.

Adding Calories from the Protein Group
As with grains (starches), your protein selections should not come from processed or fatty foods, which not only add health-robbing saturated fats, but also really pack on the calories. It's worth remembering that two slices of bacon or one hot dog a day increases your risk of dying of heart disease by 21%![4]

Remember the tips for choosing healthy proteins that you learned in the healthy shopping guide in Part 2.5, *Choosing Wisely: Dr. A's Color Coded Shopping System.*

- Eat red meat no more than twice a week, and make sure it's lean.
- Eat fish at least twice a week, and make sure it's fresh.
- Choose skinless, white-meat poultry.
- Choose low-fat or non-fat dairy.
- Don't forget nuts, seeds, and legumes.

Today's average male eats almost 3,000 calories a day, and the average female around 2,000 calories a day. The U.S. topped the list as the biggest eaters, according to calorie intake data released by The Food and Agriculture Organization in 2018. Americans eat an average of over 3,000 calories a day, according to the report. This is well above the U.S. Department of Agriculture recommendations. Amazingly, 40% of those calories come from refined, processed sugars and fats—primarily saturated animal fat.[5] But when we fill up on calorie-laden fried foods and desserts, we leave ourselves very little room for the healthy, nutrient-rich foods our body needs.

A Habit of Health: Avoiding Fast Foods

When I talk about dining out, I'm not talking about fast food restaurants. Fast foods make it nearly impossible to maintain a healthy weight. In fact, they're the masters of calorie creep, as anyone who's seen the movie *SuperSize Me* knows.

The bland, grey-looking stuff served in fast food restaurants—made palatable with the help of some synthetics from a fragrance company, no doubt—provides immediate gratification, loaded as it is with salt, high-fructose corn syrup, and animal fats, but it lacks much nutritional value. And the red and yellow color scheme is designed to attract you like a hummingbird to a feeder by stimulating your hunger and creating a stress response that will ultimately have a negative effect on your immune system.

So, if you never enter another red and yellow establishment again, you'll have added another Habit of Health! If you find yourself having no other choice, then make the best of the situation and get a salad with grilled chicken and a low-calorie dressing. If you choose a typical fast food restaurant, you're probably doomed from the beginning. A study showed that having a healthy item on the menu triples the chances of picking something unhealthy. We feel a sacrifice is unnecessary and say we deserve something naughty![6]

Try this tip! Check out menu selections on the restaurant's website before you go to avoid a potentially unhealthy environment or to preselect a healthy choice.

Where are our daily calories coming from? Let's look at a breakdown:

A "Waist-land" of Empty Calories [7, 8]

	DAILY CALORIE INTAKE	FAT CALORIES	SUGAR CALORIES	TOTAL FAT AND SUGAR CALORIES	REMAINING CALORIES
MALES	3,000	1,200–1,500	600	1,800–2,100	900–1,200
FEMALES	2,000	800–1,000	400	1,200–1,400	600–800

This means that the average man gets only 1,200 calories and the average woman only 800 calories per day from foods that contain nutrients!

This dramatic nutrient deficit is a major reason that many of us have a constant desire to eat, despite our ample caloric intake. It also means more cravings, more overeating, and excess weight. It's yet another Habit of Disease taking us down the slippery path to non-sickness and sickness at a breakneck pace.

My healthy eating strategy ensures that you get nearly 100% of your calories from high-quality, nutrient-packed low-calorie meals and whole foods. Eating this way helps you feel pleasantly satisfied and protects you from the onslaught of nutritional pollution, while supporting your goal of optimal health.

Legumes, including chickpeas, beans, soybeans, and lentils, are a wonderful alternative protein source—low-glycemic, loaded with fiber and phytonutrients, and nutrient-dense with vitamins and minerals. I recommend eating them at least twice a week or more as your main protein source.

How Many Calories?

- ½ cup legumes contains approximately 100–200 calories and is very low-glycemic.
- A four-ounce portion of lean meat contains about 250 calories.
- A six-ounce portion of skinless white-meat chicken contains about 300 calories.

CHOOSING RIGHT WHEN YOU'RE DINING OUT

Going out to eat has become a way of life. I certainly look forward to dining out with family and friends. After all, everyone needs an occasional hassle free evening, pampered by great service, with nothing to prepare or wash. You can make this indulgence a healthy one as long as you control your nutritional intake by following a few important guidelines.

Watch for Pitfalls

Look at dining out from the restaurant's point of view. Restaurants are in the business of making money and keeping their customers happy (so they can make more money). They want you to come back and bring all your friends. And fat, salt, and sugar sell.

Restaurants have a secret weapon. What's the first thing that happens when you enter a restaurant? They ask you if you want a cocktail. And why not? After a busy day, a cocktail or glass of wine is the perfect way to relax. But after just one drink, the inhibitory neurons in our brain start to shut off. We begin to lose our ability to remember those primary and secondary choices we made so carefully. And with that, we lose our reason to avoid that 2,400-calorie Bloomin' Onion™. And then there's the alcohol itself, with seven calories per gram, almost double the calories of sugar, and absolutely no nutritive value. Drink sparkling water with a slice of lime or a splash of cranberry juice instead of a cocktail while you wait for your meal. If you must drink alcohol, your healthiest choice is a small glass (five ounces) of red wine. But here's the key—order your food first!

Deciding the restaurant is even more important than deciding what to eat on the menu. Less than one in ten people even claim to be good at resisting the temptation of unhealthy options on a menu.[9]

If you know where you'll be eating out, call in advance and ask the restaurant to either text, fax, or email their menu to you, or look for their menu on the Internet. Decide in advance what you'll choose and stick to it. And try to choose restaurants that offer healthy dishes. In other words, stay away from the pizzerias and "all-you-can-eat" buffets!

If the timing of your dinner reservation means that you'll be exceeding your three-hour time period without eating, have a prepackaged portion control meal or a low-calorie snack before you go out. This will keep your appetite in check while you wait for your table and your food.

Once you're seated, ask for any bread or chips to be removed from the table or placed out of reach. Also, ask for a to-go box and put half your meal in it or share an entrée with your partner or friend! Save your calories for more nutritious foods. And remember to keep that salad healthy by bringing your own low-calorie bottled salad dressing or a homemade dressing of balsamic vinegar, lemon, and a drizzle of olive oil. Restaurant dressings are full of fat, calories, and sugar.

Choose Healthy Cooking Methods

Scampi-style, au gratin, broiled—what does it all mean in terms of calories? Here are some quick tips to help you sort the good from the bad.

Bear in mind that this is just a rough guide and that there's no guarantee that items prepared in the preferred methods are really low in fat, since fats are often added in the cooking process (for example, grilled items may be brushed with oil, poached items may cooked in buttery liquid, baked items often contain oil or cheese, and marinara sauces often start with a base of oil). If the cut of meat, fish, or poultry you choose is high in fat to begin with, it will likely still be high in fat after cooking, even using healthy cooking methods.

Prepackaged Meals: The Healthy Fast Food for Weight Loss and for Life

Scientifically formulated portion-controlled meals are a convenient choice for your three-hour fuelings, especially if you don't have a lot of time to prepare food. These convenient low-fat, low-glycemic foods are loaded with vitamins and minerals, offer a careful balance of protein and carbohydrates, and provide you with a specific dose of calories so you don't have to worry about calorie creep. And because our fuelings are completely portable, they help ensure you're getting a proper fueling when it's not otherwise feasible. That's why I've used them for myself for over 17 years. They really help me to get in my five to six daily fuelings even if I'm in the midst of a busy lifestyle, traveling away from home, or just out and about and hungry. For more information on ordering your fuelings, see the resource list in the appendices.

2.8

Stay away from cream sauces and soups, butter, oil, au gratin, breaded, Alfredo sauce, gravy, and anything battered or fried. Blackened entrees are usually dipped in butter or oil, covered with spices, and then pan fried with a higher probability of AGES and its toxic effects on our health.

Don't be afraid to take charge of your meal. Choose only lean cuts of red meat such as loin and flank. If you're having chicken, remember that white meat contains less fat. Ask for your meat, fish, or poultry to be prepared with minimal oil and butter or prepared "light". Have the chef trim all excess fat before cooking and be sure to remove the skin from poultry before you eat.

Request that vegetables be steamed with no added sugar or butter. Optimal cooking methods are baked, broiled, grilled, poached, or steamed. And of course, fresh is best!

Keep Portions in Check

Restaurant servings have become out of control. An occasional treat is fine, but if you eat out often, you need to develop an overall strategy for portion control. Here are a few tips:

- Visualize the divisions on the nine-inch plate.
- Order two appetizers instead of an entrée, such as soup and a dinner salad, or shrimp cocktail.
- Split a meal with your dining companion.
- Don't rely on the chef or waiter to serve you the proper amount of food. Surveys show that people generally eat everything that's put in front of them, whether they wanted it or not.
- Ask for a leftovers container when you place your order. When your meal comes, eyeball your proper portion right away and put the rest into the box to take home.

Beginning Your Lifetime of Healthy Eating

You should now have a firm grip on the eating strategy that will support you for life. You understand the full range of healthy foods that will help you maintain your weight and set the foundations for optimal health. You've calculated your daily energy requirements and are starting to increase your caloric intake based on those calculations, adding calories gradually according to the amount of weight you lost.

As you learned in Phase I, you're eating every three hours, using my low-glycemic, portion-controlled system to keep a handle on your daily fuelings. You know how to use the system even when dining out, and you're savvier about avoiding the pitfalls of the restaurant environment.

It's not always easy to have a low-fat, low-glycemic, low-calorie meal on hand when you need it. That's why portion-controlled meals have been a lifesaver for many of my patients and others I've coached. As a high-quality, portable fast food, our fuelings are just about unbeatable. It's a great tool as you continue your journey.

A recent study showed that simply by decreasing portion size and energy density by 25%, people were able to maintain their healthy weight.[10] And now, so can you. Combine your new understanding of portion control and energy density with your knowledge of healthy protein, starch, fruit, and vegetables, and you have the Habits of Health to support a lifetime of healthy eating.

Your transition to a sustainable and satisfying eating strategy is now complete. Let's turn our focus to the energy out portion of the equation and get your body moving.

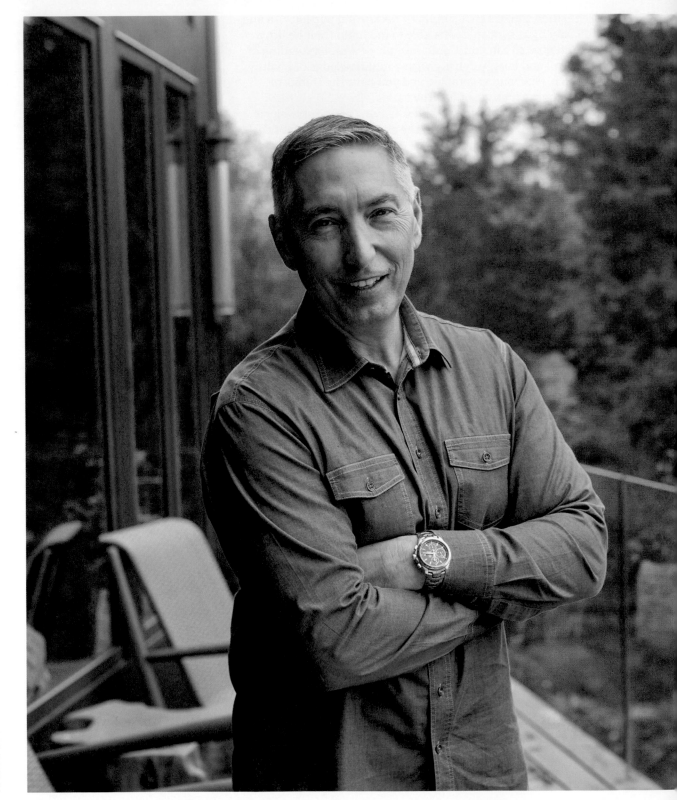

TRANSFORMATION: DOMINIC TARINELLI

I was about 245 lbs* when I was introduced to the Habits of Health. I've lost over 65 lbs,* and I'm keeping my weight off.

I tried all different types of ways to lose weight. I've tried the grapefruit diet and the cabbage diet, and it just never worked. I tried to exercise my weight off. I tried fasting. I tried all these different things, and it just seemed like I got heavier and heavier. It wasn't until I learned better habits and being a little bit more mindful of what I was doing that I was able to adopt these Habits of Health and keep the weight off long-term.

It's the little choices that you make every day. Dr. A talks about whether you have a bacon cheeseburger today for lunch or a healthy salad with grilled chicken, the impact is not going to be dramatic right that day, but each day if you make those choices, you're going to move towards either health or disease. If you're mindful of the choices that you do make, and you make the choices that are going to lead you to optimal health, very simple, small steps will get you there.

In the past, it was always about the short term. I was going to lose weight for a month, two months, three weeks, whatever it was to a specific deadline. But with the Habits of Health, I realized that it's not just short term; it's a lifestyle. It's not so much what you're giving up, it's what you're getting, and that's long-term health.

I like to live an active lifestyle. I grew up playing sports, and as I got older and I put on more and more weight, the ability to do that was really diminishing fast. The Habits of Health helped me get to a healthy weight so I can now be more active. I'm 58, and I'm still skiing, playing golf, and shooting basketball. The things that I really enjoy the most with my family are on ski vacations. This is when we can spend time being active together and it's really important to us.

We have four kids, and the exciting part is to be able to know that if we take care of ourselves and we make good choices, then the odds are in our favor that we will live a long healthy life together, and that's what we've always wanted.

> **"**It's not so much what you're giving up, it's what you're getting, and that's long-term health.**"**

*Average weight loss on the Optimal Weight 5 & 1 Plan® is 12 lbs.

2.8

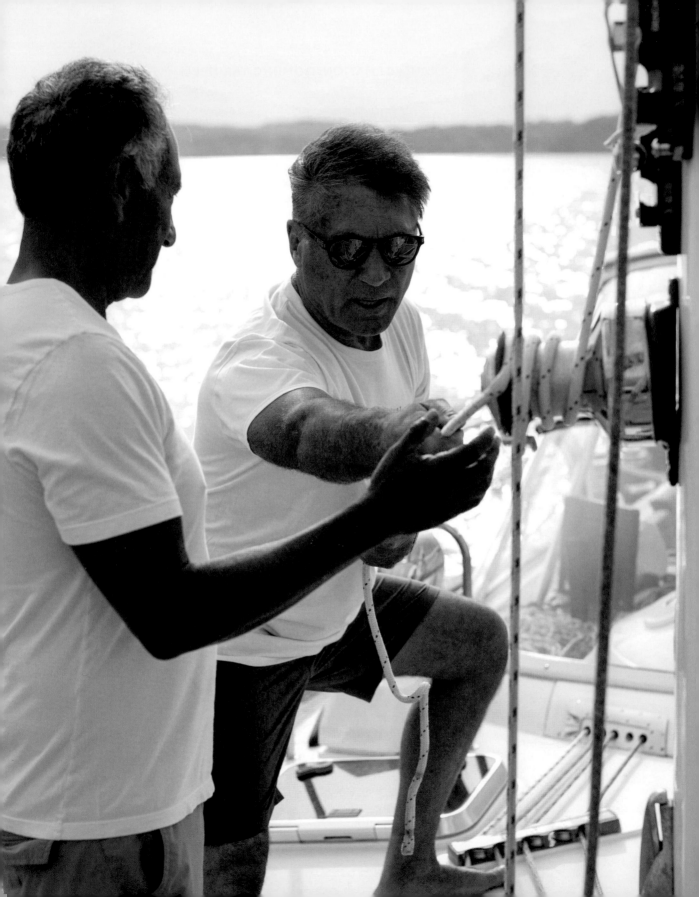

ACTIVE LIVING: INSIDE AND OUT

HABITS OF
HEALTHY MOTION

Our focus in Parts 2.9–2.12 is on transitioning your body into a state of increased energy expenditure. We're going to get you moving more and burning more calories inside and out: inside by building up the mitochondria (the energy users) in your cells and utilizing the natural thermic (energy burning) effect of food; outside by increasing your daily movement.

Increasing your activity level— with exercise as the ultimate if not immediate goal—is essential to disease prevention and optimal health. But exactly what that means day to day is different for everyone. As you'll have gathered by now, I firmly believe that the best way to integrate movement into your life is gradually, using a plan that's tailored to your current state of health, activity level, and weight.

Up to this point, we've targeted the energy-in side of the energy balance equation because that's the most efficient way to reach a healthy weight. But to make your healthy weight last, and to continue your journey to optimal health, we also need to focus on upping your energy expenditure by increasing your physical activity level.

Unlike our ancestors, who had to continually search for food and hold onto every calorie they could, we've become so efficient at obtaining food and storing it away in our bodies that it's hard for us to unload enough energy to keep our weight stable. And, for many of us, the thought of working out in a gym three days a week, as most plans recommend, is far from appealing.

Relax! I know workout gear probably isn't your preferred uniform (despite the popularity of "athleisure" fashions). The truth is that an intense three-day-a-week workout isn't a good starting point for most of us. It's certainly not the easiest, most efficient entry point and, unless you're an exercise enthusiast, you should actually delay formal workouts until we've moved you a little farther up the path toward optimal health.

THE HABITS OF MOTION

My approach to physical activity takes a much broader outlook than exercise-focused plans do. It's based on creating habits of active living. We begin by stabilizing your healthy weight (without a lot of weight lifting and aerobics), then proceed to gradually introduce the foundational principles of the Habits of Motion. Throughout, we ensure that you're using the most efficient means possible to maintain your healthy weight. Fortunately, the most efficient way is also the easiest and safest way for you to start your movement plan!

I'm a firm believer in the motto, "you need to crawl before you can walk." My plan gives you time to build your foundation by assimilating some basic principles of physical activity. When you're ready, we'll move into some more advanced techniques at a pace that makes sense for you.

At the center of my plan is getting you to move your body like you did when you were a kid. Now that we're adults, life just seems to get in the way of getting out, playing, and having fun. Combine that with our terrible eating habits and sedentary jobs, and it's easy to see why we've just stopped moving. So we're going to start with baby steps, based on your current reality, and crawl our way back to energy equilibrium, fitness, and optimal health.

We'll start by looking at all the many little movements that make up your day and put them to work for us. As I teach you the Habits of Motion, I'll be focusing on two major objectives:

1. *Stabilizing your weight by increasing your energy expenditure, primarily through physical activity*
2. *Optimizing your health through carefully paced exercises*

10,000 years ago, we were in perpetual motion throughout our waking hours. It is estimated that we spent in excess of 3,000 minutes a week moving. Consider that if we move 300 minutes a week today, we are considered to be extremely active. How times have changed. And unfortunately, most are getting less than the 150 minutes a week recommended to prevent a steady progression to poor health.[1]

2.9

Obesity and Rigorous Exercise: A Dangerous Combination

Exercise alone is ineffective for weight loss. In fact, it can be downright dangerous for those who are seriously overweight. Asking someone who's out of shape and carrying an extra 50 lbs or so to go jogging, lifting weights, or do circuit training is a recipe for disaster, leading all too often to back, neck, and knee injuries that can set them up for long-term failure. The added stress on an already overworked cardiovascular system can have serious, even deadly, consequences.

Our approach, by contrast, features a movement plan that can be customized to all levels of health, weight, and fitness. It begins with activities that help you maintain your healthy weight and progresses to ones that move you toward optimal health.

We'll accomplish our first goal by teaching you how to become more active through movements centered round your job, your chores, your plans, and your activities. But. in order to help you understand how to harness your body's own energy, we're going to revisit our old friend: TEE.

INCREASING YOUR TOTAL ENERGY EXPENDITURE (TEE) THROUGH THERMOGENESIS

Activity and exercise have different roles in our system. Introducing each of them correctly and in the right sequence is critical to making your new energy plan a permanent Habit of Health.

Habits of Motion

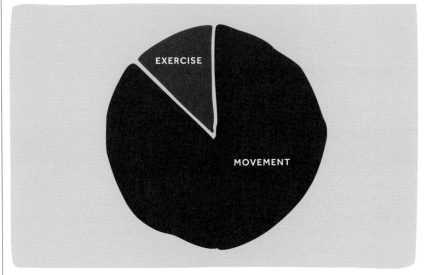

One big difference between exercise and physical activity is that exercise is generally done for a short period of time, usually just a few hours a week. However, physical activity can be integrated into your daily life in a much more organic and complete manner (see *The Three-Day-a-Week Workout,* page 349). Our main objective in increasing your activity is to put all your waking hours to work by upping your energy expenditure. By tapping into the thousand different ways your body is active, we'll start increasing your total energy expenditure (TEE) even if your current activity level is minimal. Our goal is to turn you into a perpetual motion machine.

In the last part, we figured out how to find your energy equilibrium point or body set weight point by calculating your TEE. By learning how many calories you burn in a day, you established a starting point. What that tells you is how many calories you are able to ingest in order to maintain your healthy weight.

Now we're going to take another look at the three components that make up TEE and find out how to increase each one. After all, we're energetic creatures. Together, we're going to turn up your metabolic furnace and increase your ability to burn calories in a whole variety of simple ways you probably never even thought about. It's simple, it's scientific, and it's called thermogenesis.

Remember the TEE equation? TEE = BMR + PAL + TEF
Let's break that down into parts and show you how to turn up the heat!

Total Energy Expenditure Components

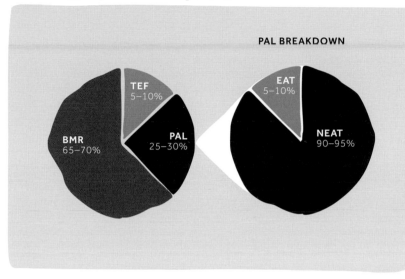

BASAL METABOLIC RATE (BMR)

As you may recall from Part 2.8, *Healthy Eating for Life: Your Transition to Permanent Health,* Basal Metabolic Rate (BMR), which measures our body's basic functioning, accounts for the majority of the calories we expend—on average between 65 and 70% of TEE. It's calculated at a point when the body is in a neutral, resting state—after a night of restful sleep, in a temperate environment, on an empty stomach. It's the point at which our organs are using the least amount of energy. Because many people think of this as a passive measurement, it's assumed that BMR is difficult to change. Nothing could be further from the truth.

As the biggest component of our metabolic pie, BMR offers us a wonderful opportunity to tap into a thermogenic energy source that burns energy 168 hours a week. How? By ingeniously increasing the activity level and even the size of our organs to boost energy

> *NEAT (Non-Exercise Activity Thermogenesis) can have a huge effect on your daily TEE (and therefore on your daily calorie consumption). In fact, even minor changes in daily non-exercise physical activity can increase TEE by 20%.*

A Habit of Health: Lowering room temperature to 68°

Being in a cooler environment is another way to increase your BMR and help you burn more calories. And the added benefits are that you'll probably sleep better, suffer from fewer respiratory issues and burn less fuel—so you'll be helping the planet while you help yourself!

ACTIVE LIVING: INSIDE AND OUT

After age 20, we begin losing muscle cells at an ever-increasing rate. They're replaced with fat cells, which burn far less energy.

Physical activity? Exercise? What's the difference?

You may think of the terms physical activity and exercise as one and the same, but it's important to make a distinction. Physical activity happens anytime your body's in motion. As you'll see later in this part, motion can be voluntary or involuntary. Exercise, however, is planned movement that's more vigorous and leads to improvements in overall fitness.

consumption. Let's look at two organs that are open to this process and have the biggest appetite for calories—our muscles and our brain.

MUSCLES IN THE BASAL METABOLIC STATE

When we think of energy that is consumed when we use our muscles, we're usually thinking of working out or performing some sort of physical activity. That's the type of energy use we'll discuss in the Physical Activity Level (PAL) section. Right now, we're talking about the energy your muscles use even when you're lying in bed in the morning, dreaming about sleeping in.

Unlike your bones, immune system, lungs, and other organs whose energy requirements are fairly fixed, the basal metabolic contribution from your muscles varies. And most of that variation—75%, in fact—is based on how much lean body mass you have.

How does it all work? It really comes down to tiny mitochondria, which are the little energy factories of our cells. Mitochondria work very hard taking the nutrients we consume and converting them into energy to power the machinery of our cells. In the case of our muscle cells, mitochondria are influenced by the type of work the particular muscles are performing.

Our bodies generally have the highest proportion of mitochondria when we're in late adolescence, after which point they start to diminish. Beginning at age 20, we lose about a pound of muscle each year. And what do those muscle cells get replaced with? You guessed it—fat cells.

Here's the kicker. Each pound of muscle consumes around 50–70 calories a day. Fat, on the other hand, consumes much less energy—less than 10% of the energy that muscle uses. That means that as we lose muscle over the years, our energy expenditure decreases. And when energy expenditure decreases, our accumulation of fat increases.

That's why this loss of muscle mass and muscle strength—known as sarcopenia of aging—is linked to pre-obesity and obesity and contributes to a decrease in both BMR and PAL. Having weak, flabby muscles also plays a large part in our downward spiral to non-sickness and disease. The good news is that this muscle deterioration is reversible.

In Phase I, we shed a whole bunch of those inefficient fat cells by decreasing your fat stores, especially around your vital organs. In Phase II, we'll focus on increasing your lean muscle mass and go to work on increasing the size of the mitochondria in each cell through specific techniques you'll learn in Part 2.12, *Dr. A's Habits of Healthy Motion Part 2: EAT System*. In doing so, we'll tap into an energy expenditure system that stays at work 24/7.

This behind-the-scenes increase in BMR sets the stage for long-term weight maintenance and permanent health. And, as an added bonus,

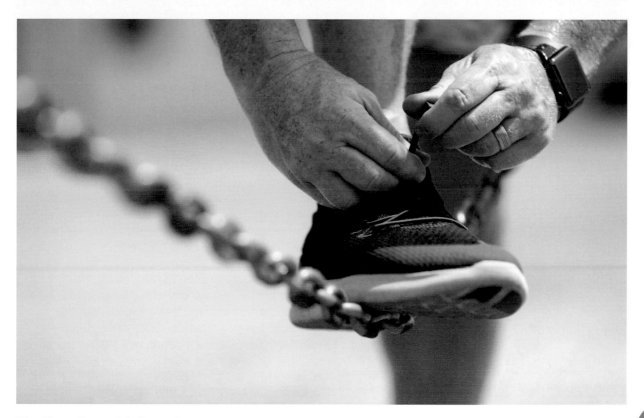

The Three-Day-a-Week Workout: Inefficient for Weight Loss, Great for Health

What's wrong with intense, muscle-burning workouts? As long as you're in shape and can do them, nothing at all—they're just not very efficient at creating weight loss. Think of it this way: there are 168 hours in the week. The average three-day-a-week workout uses just two percent of those hours. However, our energy management program will help you tap into all 168 as we turn you into a perpetual motion machine!

A lot of weight-loss programs tout intense workouts as an essential part of fitness. Unfortunately, this type of vigorous exercise leaves most overweight people discouraged and believing they just don't have what it takes to maintain a healthy weight.

Remember, if the degree of effort is too high, as we showed in Part 1.5, *The Bedrock of Transformation: Successful Habit Installation,* it becomes unsustainable.

Intense exercise can be a valuable tool if it's introduced properly and customized to meet each person's ability. Otherwise, it's unlikely to succeed long term. In the next part, we'll create a functional plan to increase your exercise level at a pace that makes it easy to incorporate into your life and easy to sustain. That's the way to ensure that these health-giving activities become permanent Habits of Health.

Already exercising? You've got a great head start on creating optimal health! By adding my motion plan to your regular routine, you can harness those 100+ hours you're not already using for exercise. You'll pick up some great ideas to improve your fitness levels and see a dramatic boost in your energy expenditure!

"

Thermogenesis: The body generates heat, or energy, by increasing the metabolic rate above normal. Thermogenesis can be activated by a variety of mechanisms, including supplements, nutrition, exercise, and exposure to cold.

"

Swap your office chair for one with better back support or switch to a yoga ball to promote good posture.

in addition to benefiting from increased energy expenditure during rest (BMR), your newly enhanced muscles will burn more energy when you're in motion too.

YOUR BRAIN AND BMR

You may not think of the brain as a calorie burner but, in fact, our brains consume an incredible amount of energy (which explains why more than a few minutes without oxygen can have catastrophic consequences).

In fact, our brain accounts for about 25% of our BMR. What's more, the amount of energy consumption decreases with age as our brain atrophies—just like our muscles. To prevent this, we need to do some active intervention.

Researchers are systematically revealing the hidden secrets of the brain, including what it takes to keep our brain healthy and our memory intact. One of the most important discoveries they've made is that our brain cells and neurons have an amazing ability to develop in size and connectivity as we age. That's why activating new pathways and engaging in new activities are important ways to exercise your brain.

By learning the Habits of Health, you're already stimulating your brain by exchanging previous behaviors with new, healthy cognitive activities. And that's just the beginning. Even changing the way you do simple everyday activities—brushing your teeth with the opposite hand, for example, or driving home using a different route—stimulates the brain and actually increases your metabolic rate.

Another important way to stimulate brain waves and increase energy consumption is to tap into music and motion. In fact, combining music and rhythmic movement such as dancing or rowing, can improve many aspects of our health, even helping to decrease systemic inflammation.

So, hopefully you can see that BMR is far from fixed. By focusing on the Habits of Health, you can actually increase the size, capacity, and metabolic function of your brain and muscles, even when you're resting. You'll learn how to give your body a workout in the next few parts and then, in the longevity sections, we will increase your muscle and brain gym time once you are optimally healthy.

PHYSICAL ACTIVITY LEVEL (PAL)

Your Physical Activity Level (PAL), which accounts for 25–30% of TEE, is the part of the TEE equation that's easiest to change. That's why PAL has such a central role in helping you control your weight—both directly, through movement, and indirectly, by increasing the amount of calorie-burning muscle in your body.

PAL is made up of two parts: planned physical activity (what you probably think of as exercise) and the voluntary and unconscious movements you make as part of your everyday life. As we plan an activity program customized to your age, fitness level, and lifestyle, it's helpful to consider these two categories separately. One handy way to break it down is through the acronyms EAT and NEAT.

EAT AND NEAT

EAT (Exercise Activity Thermogenesis) consists of the planned physical activities we perform in order to increase our energy expenditure and improve our overall fitness. It's what we do when we say we're "working out". These may range from the minimal task of going for a brisk walk to Herculean feats, like in professional cyclist Chris Froome expending over 9,000 calories a day during the Tour de France. But despite all our talk of exercise today, for the vast majority of us, EAT is actually negligible. In fact, even exercise enthusiasts will find that EAT's contribution to daily calorie consumption pales by comparison to the power of NEAT.

NEAT (Non-Exercise Activity Thermogenesis) consists of the voluntary and unconscious movements we make as we go about our daily lives—by working, doing chores, and the combined effect of all the silly little motions we make. As I sit here writing, for example, I'm consuming extra calories just tapping my foot. It's easy, and it happened naturally as a result of getting into the beat of a great song on my iPhone. NEAT is highly variable, ranging from about 15% of total daily TEE in very sedentary people to more than 50% in people who are highly active.

Let's focus on two areas that contribute to your daily NEAT: work time and non-work time.

Our society's decreased activity levels—and resulting decrease in NEAT—has been blamed to a great extent on a shift from manual labor to sedentary desk jobs. This is certainly a major contributor, but beyond the workplace, our cars, remote controls, snow blowers, elevators, and a myriad of other labor-saving devices add to the impact. No wonder we're turning into the sort of muscle-atrophied creatures that appear in *Star Trek* with their huge heads and marshmallow bodies!

In the end, the compounding effects of those small daily choices have much more impact on weight maintenance than any exercise program. Formal exercise, including weight resistance training, circuit training, and aerobic exercise, is great for your health, and we'll introduce it to your life as you aim for the summit of optimal health, but in terms of weight maintenance, it's just the icing on the cake.

10 years ago when I introduced my Habits of Motion system, I challenged the conventional wisdom. My view was it was the total daily motion that mattered with a shift in focus to each of us

Even astronauts (generally some of the fittest people on the planet) can lose 20% of their muscle mass after five to 11 days in space. This muscle atrophy occurs at a surprisingly fast rate when we are not subjected to gravity. Sitting at a desk for an extended time simulates this effect because we take away the antigravity muscles, which include the quadriceps, as well as the back, neck, and calf muscles.[2]

2.9

Did you know that having responsive, lean muscle is critical to maintaining healthy levels of insulin and glucose? Did you also know that unhealthy insulin and glucose levels are big contributors to a whole range of diseases? That's why reversing sarcopenia—the loss of muscle mass and strength—is a big focus on our journey to optimal health.

becoming a perpetual motion machine where most still felt that the two to three days a week of exercise was all that was needed to stay healthy. Very few people outside of scientists were even familiar with NEAT.

In the last 10 years, hundreds of studies are now confirming that our sedentary lifestyle and many hours of working at our desks is having an extremely negative on our health. And the three hours of treadmill and exercise a week does not offset the negative impact of sitting.[3]

That is why in in Phase II we'll focus on all those everyday ways to increase daily energy expenditure—things that are available to each of us, all the time. But first let's spend a few moments finding out how to increase energy expenditure by selecting foods that actually boost your TEE from the inside.

THERMIC EFFECT OF FOOD (TEF)

Like BMR, this third component of TEE—the energy we use digesting and processing our food—is usually considered a fixed quantity that's not easy to change. But like BMR, it can be modified to boost your total energy consumption. The timing of your meals, the amount of food you eat, and the content of your food all have a big effect on energy expenditure.

Let's start putting this forgotten component to work! Here are just a few ideas:

Eat Every Three Hours
While further documentation is needed, this great Habit of Health may actually contribute to an increased TEF by causing your body to start up its metabolic machinery more often.

Choose Lean Protein
Protein is a complex fuel that must be broken down into amino acids before it can be used. That takes energy—almost twice as much energy as your body uses to process carbohydrates and fats.

Drink Cold Water
Switch to ice water and up your TEF. Drinking just one eight-ounce glass of ice water burns 9.25 more calories than drinking a glass of room-temperature water.[4]

Seek Out Naturally Thermogenic Foods
Several naturally occurring substances increase your energy expenditure, including caffeine, polyphenolic compounds (found in green tea), and capsaicin (found in red pepper, mustard, ginger, and cinnamon). Other substances with a thermic effect include selenium, chromium, alpha lipoic acid, L-carnitine, L-tyrosine, and calcium

carbonate. We'll discuss these types of substances in greater detail later in the book, when you enter Phase III.

You now understand how these three components—BMR (your body's metabolic rate), PAL (your activity level made up of your NEAT and EAT), and TEF (the energy you use to burn food)—can be modulated to increase your total energy expenditure (TEE).

In the next three parts, we'll outline a progressive plan to increase your daily energy expenditure, incorporating each of these important components. Our primary focus will be to incorporate the Habits of Motion into your life, slowly but steadily, to help you tap into a new life of motion.

The Mortality of Being Seated

The old school stated we could maintain our health by getting on a treadmill for 30 minutes a day and then be motionless for the other 23.5 hours. They were dead wrong. Working out three days a week doesn't keep you healthier either. Being active throughout the day is what keeps us healthy. In fact, many studies are now showing that sitting for hours independent of our weekly exercise is lethal.[5]

A recent survey in juststand.org showed that 86% of all Americans sit all day. Daily sitting ranges from 9.3 hours on average to as high as 15 hours in some individuals.[6] We are literally sitting down more than we sleep in a day. Another large study including 125,00 participants showed excessive sitting increased mortality and decreased lifespan across the board.[7]

A study evaluated the amount of activity of overweight versus lean people and discovered that obese individuals sat 2.5 hours more than lean people. They estimated that by adopting the NEAT behaviors of their lean counterparts that these obese individuals could expend an additional 350 calories a day.

Reducing chronic inactivity is even more essential than brief periods of intense exercise. Even seven hours of moderate to vigorous physical activity was not enough to keep people alive. A study of over 240,000 adults who were the most active with over seven hours a week exercise but who also spent the most time sitting had a 50% greater risk of dying from any cause. They doubled their risk of dying from heart disease.[8]

We must help you find more time to become a perpetual motion machine. Your life depends on it.

"We've all heard of exercise, and many of us talk about exercise, but the reality is that 60% of Americans don't take part in any kind of regular physical activity and 25% do no activity to speak of at all![9]"

2.9

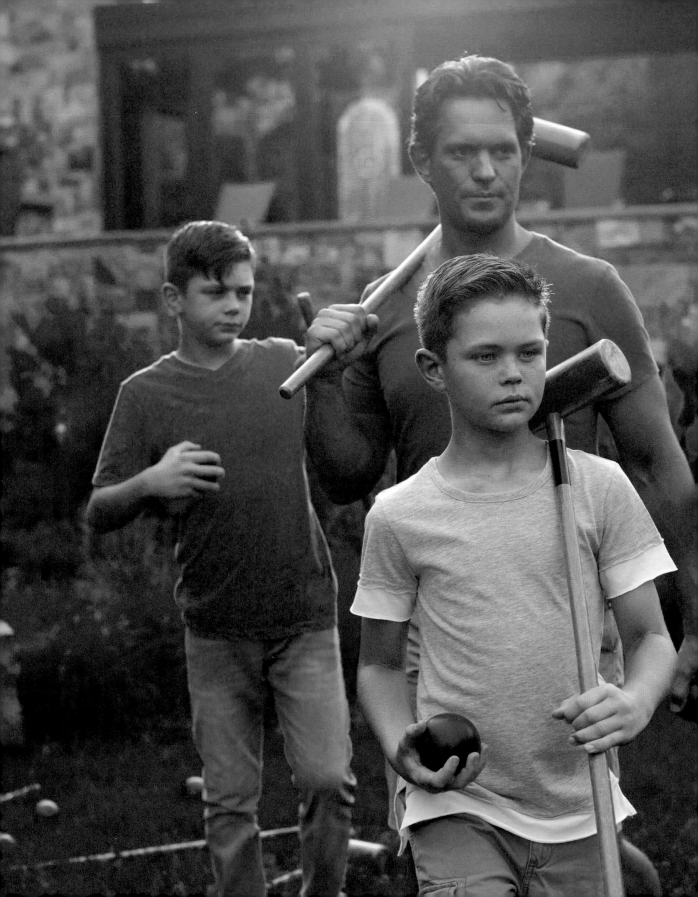

FIRST STEPS: INTRODUCTION TO DR. A'S HABITS OF MOTION SYSTEM

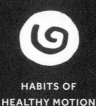

HABITS OF
HEALTHY MOTION

The numbers speak for themselves: 60% of us get no regular physical activity; 25% of us get no activity at all; 50% of those who begin exercising quit within six months; 90% of all exercise equipment is unused and relegated to a coat rack or a cat perch one year after purchase.

What do these statistics tell us? That until you have your weight under control, increased your flexibility, developed a more active lifestyle, and organized your daily choices to support health, the honest truth is that launching yourself into a full-blown exercise program just isn't likely to be successful.[1-4] That's why, in this section and the next, we're going to focus on simple movements and activities that you can incorporate into your daily life right away, regardless of your current health, weight, or fitness level. They're easy, they'll help you maintain your weight, and they serve as the transition to a more healthy and active lifestyle. These Habits of Motion are the foundation of a total movement program—a program that you can use for life.

THE PROBLEM WITH EXERCISE

When I was about five years old, my dad, following the belief system of the time, introduced me to swimming by throwing me into the deep end and proudly shouting, "Swim!" This wasn't uncommon back then and you may have even gone through a similar experience.

It's not unlike what happens when an out-of-shape, overweight individual starts an intense exercise program. Millions of people who are convinced (mistakenly) that they must undergo vigorous exercise to lose weight suffer the same fate I did 60 years ago when I was thrown into deep water.

The aerobics revolution of the 1970s didn't help either. The idea of running a marathon to become "aerobically optimized" simply creates too high a barrier for most people. 30 years later, we're still trying to overcome the notion that you have to exercise intensively in order to be healthy and fit. As you can tell from the bleak statistics above, the vast majority of us simply can't keep up.

And, of course, many of us just don't like the gym experience and will find any excuse to avoid it—not enough time, too hard, or just boring. Many of these excuses are the result of our own, sometimes mistaken perceptions, but just as many are logical and real. In the end, if we can't overcome our psychological and logistical barriers to exercise, any success will be fleeting at best.

> *Exercise: Planned movement that's vigorous enough to improve overall fitness.*

Barriers to Exercise

TIME	GYM EXPERIENCE	OTHERS
• Not enough time	• Intimidating	• Afraid to aggravate old injury
• Feel guilty for time away from family	• Inconvenient	• Too hard
• Unable to work out five times a week, so why bother?	• Expensive	• No results
	• Makes me feel self-conscious	• Boring

There are plenty of reasons to avoid exercising—some based on our perception and some based on logistics. Unless we can overcome each of these barriers, we won't stay fit.

OVERCOMING THE LOGISTICAL AND PSYCHOLOGICAL BARRIERS TO LIFESTYLE CHANGE

Logistical Barriers

We have designed the whole *Habits of Health Transformational System* around making our habit installation easy and minimizing the time requirements so it fits into a chaotic lifestyle. Our prepackaged fuelings, the easy to read color-coded *Green to Stay Lean* charts, the

2.10

Can Lifestyle Changes Cure Obesity?

The answer from medical science is a resounding "yes!"—if we can overcome the barriers in our way. Dr. Michael Dansinger of Tufts–New England Medical Center is a diet researcher. His views are clear: "Most able-bodied persons who can find a way to overcome the monumental logistical and psychological barriers that prevent the full application of lifestyle change can reverse obesity within months."[5] It might sound simplistic, but the solution to the obesity crisis may actually depend on finding a way to implement lifestyle recommendations in just the right dose to foster meaningful and permanent change.

microHabit of Health system with structural tension, and our habit loops make it really easy to create sustainable transformation. In the area of Habits of Motion, you will find the microHabits of Motion particularly useful to create permanent patterns of progressive movement, which we will install in baby steps to create permanent fitness and weight management.

Psychological Barriers

As a species, we were designed to conserve and store energy. 10,000 years ago, we moved 3,000 minutes a week because we had to for our survival. We were either foraging for food, evading predators, or seeking shelter and better weather.

Today, we do not have those same imperatives in our lives. There is no natural driver to activity at this level. If we want to become more comfortable with the idea, there are three key areas specific to enhancing our psychological experience with exercise in general.

First, it is important to connect with our "why" for increasing activity and exercise and it is critical to connect to immediate effects versus long-term benefit. There are many obvious long-term benefits to moving more, such as weight management, creating optimal health, and preventing disease.

Studies have shown that those that are most likely to initiate and sustain an increase activity and exercise are those that can connect immediate benefits to their exercise.

In the following diagram (we introduced it in Part 1.6, *You in Charge of Yourself: Setting Up for Success* , we talked about connecting the long-term benefits of the Habits of Health to immediate rewards in order to initiate the daily activity.

Building Your Future Health and Wellbeing

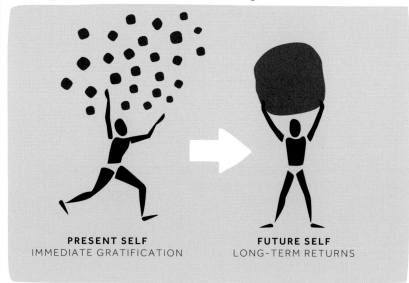

PRESENT SELF
IMMEDIATE GRATIFICATION

FUTURE SELF
LONG-TERM RETURNS

Below are some of the immediate benefits of added activity and exercise. It has been said that the immediate effects of exercise on our mood, attentiveness, performance, and creativity are the equivalent of taking a Prozac in terms of serotonin and mood enhancement, and a Ritalin in terms of attentiveness and alertness. And if the activity is intense enough, your body also releases endorphins and dopamine that lights up the nucleus acumbens: the brain's reward center.

Immediate Effects of Exercise[6]

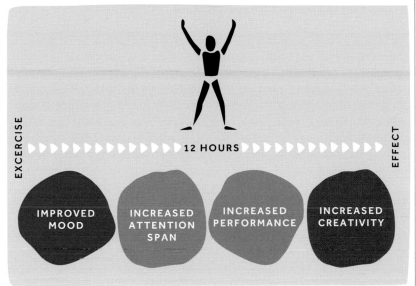

Exercise is a Key Player in Advanced Energy Balance

While exercise comprises only a small part of our daily activity (if it's done at all), its ability to build muscle can help increase your calorie-burning potential. In Part 2.12, *Dr. A's Habits of Healthy Motion Part 2: EAT System*, we'll look at some specific EAT activities that build more and bigger muscle cells to fan your metabolic fire.

These benefits are immediate and may last as long as 12 hours—all without any side effects. Then we need to talk about how you think about the prospect of increased activity and exercise. Do you think of it as a chore or something you dread?

Let's reframe that attitude to one of giving yourself a gift. Think about the immediate benefits you are giving to yourself and the long-term benefits of sustained weight control, optimal health, and the potential to live longer in a healthy state.

Remember that your own care—I call it "self-care"—is the best gift you can ever obtain in the process of creating optimal health and wellbeing. And beyond the improvement of just about every health marker, it may also help you sleep better, improve your sex life, and increase your energy levels and confidence!

And finally, with the growth mindset that you are developing, you'll be more open, more curious and want to learn more about how to evaluate how you are feeling in the morning, afternoon, and evening after different intensities of activity. These will be things you will want to record in *Your LifeBook*.

EAT: Your Graduate Degree in Optimal Health

The exercise that makes up EAT is critical for reaching optimal health. It builds muscle, increases energy expenditure, boosts your immune system, and is especially effective at lowering inflammation. It's sometimes said that if we could put exercise in pill form, it would be the world's most prescribed medicine. In my opinion, it's the best longevity medicine there is, if it's properly introduced in a schedule and at a dosage that makes sense.

EAT is like your graduate degree in health. First, you need your prerequisites and that's where the small, daily movements of NEAT come into play. Once you've incorporated NEAT into your life, we'll begin to block out some time for planned exercise. But even at that point, sessions of moderate length and intensity will do the trick. In fact, on most days, a 30-minute brisk walk is all you need to achieve the same benefits that the rigorous exercise enthusiasts of the past would have had you do! We will, of course, teach you many ways of adding exercise to your habits.

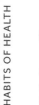

Add an extra 1,000 steps to your routine with the goal of building up to a total of 10,000 steps per day.

So you now have a strategy, tactics, and processes in place to overcome the logistical and psychological barriers to help make the Habits of Motion become an integral part of your transformation.

Now, we're going to show you how to lower the threshold to the addition of new activities and increase your energy expenditure to reverse the sedentary lifestyle that so many have fallen victim to in the epidemic that history might record as "The Great Sit Down".

THE HABITS OF MOTION: THE KEY TO ENERGY EXPENDITURE

Our plan is about simplicity. It's about weaving movement into the tapestry of your everyday life, ramping up at your own pace and within your own comfort level. It's about finding little nooks and crannies in your routines that lend themselves to movement. And it's designed to be incorporated into your busy schedule without any additional time commitment. Whether you're 200 lbs overweight and currently inactive or a weight lifter with eight percent body fat, the Habits of Motion can profoundly and permanently enhance your health and your life.

Sounds good, right? But exactly how can we achieve this? Just look around at today's environment. Our jobs are sedentary. Energy-saving devices are robbing our bodies of flexibility, energy expenditure, and muscle. But by tapping into your daily movements, even incrementally, you can create enough additional motion to offset the obesigenic effect of an automated world. Working within your existing daily routine, my plan taps into all your myriad natural movements, enhancing their quality and quantity to increase their contribution to energy expenditure.

Think of it as a basic course in movement. It's the way children go about their day. They don't go to the gym or lift weights or think about how many calories they're burning. They just play! That natural motion is just what we're going to restore. But don't worry, I won't make you get onto a set of monkey bars!

ACTIVITY THERMOGENESIS (AT): YOUR DAILY ENERGY BURN

You may recall from that Physical Activity Level (PAL)—the part of Total Energy Expenditure (TEE) that has to do with your body's motion—is the key modifiable area of energy expenditure. That's why we'll be focusing on PAL as we boost your calorie-burning mechanism and convert you from an energy-conserver to an energy-user.

Another term that's used to describe this process is "activity thermogenesis" (AT)—the process by which the body generates heat or energy as it moves. AT is the energy used by our muscles to move and support our body. From the time you get up in the morning until you go to sleep at night, every movement you make requires energy. Our movement plan teaches you how to enhance your energy expenditure by adding movements that increase thermogenesis. Combined with your new healthy eating plan, this movement plan (in which, you may be pleased and surprised to learn, active exercise plays only a small role) provides a total system of healthy, balanced energy management for a lifetime of health.

Now let's revisit the two components of activity thermogenesis—EAT and NEAT.

EAT: THERMOGENESIS THROUGH EXERCISE

EAT (Exercise Activity Thermogenesis) consists of those activities performed expressly for the purpose of improving fitness—in other words, exercise. EAT activities—such as sports, workouts, and jogs—usually take place at a specific, planned time, and may range in intensity from a walk in the park to a grueling triathlon.

As you may recall, EAT takes up less than two percent of our weekly time, making it a less-than-effective way to burn energy. In addition, exercise stimulates several metabolic pathways, a process that may actually make you want to eat more. This state, known as compensation, is particularly prevalent among women when they start exercising.

What it comes down to is that the scheduled exercise that makes up EAT simply can't be counted on as a reliable way to maintain energy balance—at least not in the beginning, when successful weight loss leads to a corresponding drop in daily energy use (because less mass means less calorie consumption).

Now, that's not to say that EAT doesn't play an important role in long-term health. In fact, exercise is a critical part of reaching optimal health and, in Part 2.12, *Dr. A's Habits of Healthy Motion Part 2: EAT System*, I'll teach you some simple, easy ways to make exercise a part of your busy life. The problem is that EAT only works if you do it, and few of us actually do.

Think of it this way: EAT is like going to graduate school for your advanced degree in health. First, you need the prerequisites, and that's where NEAT comes in. NEAT forms the basis of the first part of my movement plan, setting the right foundation for a progressive movement plan that's easy to learn and apply, which prepares you for your climb to optimal health. After all, if you're going to continue moving forward, a mobile, flexible body and an active lifestyle make great starting points.

Exercise for Long-Term Health

Once you've got the basics of NEAT (daily, non-exercise activities) under control, we'll slowly but surely integrate EAT (planned exercise) into your life in ways that are easy, simple, and fun to do. Why? Because along with helping you maintain your healthy weight, regular moderate exercise can:

- **Help prevent heart disease, strokes, diabetes, and other chronic diseases[7]**
- **Boost your overall mood**
- **Lower high blood pressure**
- **Reduce stress**
- **Strengthen muscles, bones, and joints**
- **Improve metabolism and increase your energy level**
- **Strengthen your immune system while decreasing inflammation and CRP levels (C-reactive protein—a way of measuring the level of inflammation in our blood and body)**
- **Help prevent depression**
- **Increase bone density and help prevent osteoporosis**

2.10

Can Standing for One Hour a Day Cure Obesity?

A team of researchers at the Mayo Clinic, led by Dr. James A. Levine, spent ten days studying groups of mildly obese and lean volunteers—all self-proclaimed couch potatoes. They discovered that the obese group stayed seated for about 2.5 hours longer per day than the lean group, burning on average 350 fewer calories per day.[1]

The team's groundbreaking research showed that as humans overeat, the activation of NEAT burns enough excess energy to keep us lean. When NEAT fails to activate, however, the result is weight gain. And as we've learned from the work of James Hill,[3] a mere 100 to 200 calories per day of excess intake may well account for today's obesity epidemic.[9]

NEAT: THERMOGENESIS THROUGH EVERYDAY MOVEMENT

NEAT (Non-Exercise Activity Thermogenesis) is made up of all of the movements your body makes outside of planned exercise. Compared to EAT, it's actually a much more efficient way to fight calorie creep and a more important contributor to energy expenditure. It's also much easier to do. In fact, you're already doing it.

Think of NEAT as your exercise training wheels or as the movement version of the portion-controlled meals—an easy way to begin offloading excess calories and get your energy in balance without making a big time commitment. I'll start by giving you a short undergraduate class on NEAT before introducing the Habits of Motion system.

HARNESSING NEAT

What do sitting, standing, walking, talking, toe tapping, guitar playing, dancing, singing, shopping, gum chewing, and fidgeting have in common? They're all part of NEAT. As we search for solutions to the real energy crisis in our lives (offloading the excess energy we eat), something as simple as changing our posture can have a dramatic effect on our energy balance.

But NEAT can be hard to measure, especially since it's made up of so many diverse activities. Unlike the exercises of EAT, which are limited in duration and can be measured using metabolic equivalents (METS)—a technique I'll introduce in Part 2.12, *Dr. A's Habits of Healthy Motion Part 2: EAT System*—the many little movements that comprise NEAT are going on all the time. So how do we know if they're having any effect?

When Dr. James A. Levine and his innovative Mayo Clinic team did their groundbreaking research on NEAT (see sidebar, *Can Standing for One Hour a Day Cure Obesity?*), they outfitted their test subjects with an array of equipment, including an inclinometer and a triaxial accelerometer, to continually measure body posture and movements. They also had their subjects drink radioactive water to track NEAT'S contribution to energy expenditure. This painstaking work gave us a good indication of just how much energy our daily low-level movements consume in comparison to inactivity. Some of their results are shown in the following chart.

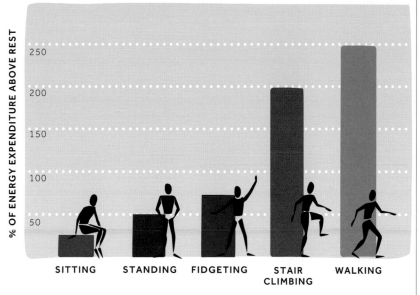

When Dr. James A. Levine and his team of Mayo Clinic researchers measured the non-exercise (NEAT) activities of their subjects (see sidebar, last page of this part, Can Standing for One Hour a Day Cure Obesity?), they found out which ordinary activities generate the greatest energy expenditure.

Measuring NEAT in this way is all well and good, but not very practical for everyday life—unless you're prepared to get hooked up to lots of wires and wear space-age undergarments! Luckily, there's another, simpler way to measure NEAT, which I'll teach you in the next part when I introduce the NEAT System as part of my Habits of Motion.

But first, let's look at the various kinds of NEAT we'll be tracking as we work on upping your daily energy expenditure.

OCCUPATIONAL NEAT AND LEISURE NEAT

Work makes up a big portion of our day and presents a very different set of obesigenic conditions and challenges.

According to the Bureau of Labor Statistics, the average person spends 44 hours a week at work. Add the transportation to and from our workplace and one-third of our time is spent in some way connected to work.[10] Although what we do when we're working isn't always under our control, there are a number of potential openings for our motion plan even during working hours. This is particularly important today, with the advent of the computer and a resulting reduction in manual labor, which has cut movement out of our

DR. A SAYS…

"*Find out whether you're pushing yourself too much by taking the "talk test" during your workout. If you can't say the Pledge of Allegiance without huffing and puffing, you may be exercising too vigorously.*"

2.10

Staying Safe While You Move: Evaluating Your Heart Rate

Your heart is the most important muscle in your body. As you increase your physical activity, your heart will be working a bit harder, just like your other muscles. That's why monitoring your heart rate is so important. If you have a heart rate monitor, just strap it on and read the results.

If you're measuring your heart rate by hand, sit down in a quiet place and measure your heart rate by counting your pulse for one minute (alternatively, count your pulse for 10 seconds and multiply by six, though this measurement may be slightly less accurate). To take your pulse, place your index finger and third finger on your radial artery (located on the inside of the wrist below your thumb).

Warning: Do not use the carotid artery (side of the neck). Doing so can cause a stroke in individuals with occult plaque.

working lives dramatically (we'll discuss ways to "sneak" movement into your work day in the next part).

What about leisure time? That's an area where we do have control. But an increasing number of energy-saving devices have become increasingly central to our lives. Far from making our lives better, most of these so-called "advancements" are actually robbing us of our daily activity and, consequently, our health. In fact, experiments have shown that the energy costs of non-work automation are between 100 and 200 calories a day. That alone could account for the entire obesity epidemic!

Given what we now understand about the importance of normal, daily motions and weight control, it's all the more important to say no to excess automation in your life. In other words, don't let the machines steal your health.

The good news is that even an act as trivial as chewing gum can increase your energy expenditure 20% above your resting level and that means 20% more calories burned. What a great ad for sugar-free gum that would be! A mindless motion like fidgeting can raise energy expenditure 20–40%. And strolling along while shopping at the mall, even at a slow pace of one mile per hour, doubles your energy expenditure. Pick up the pace to two or three miles per hour and you'll nearly triple your expenditure.

Movements like these are key components of my Habits of Motion system. Making it easy for you to measure, track, and increase the calories you burn is all part of my long-term plan to make motion in all its forms an integral part of your life.

Just one word of warning: it is very important that you consult your healthcare provider before beginning this program. The instructions and advice presented here do not substitute for medical consultation. As with any exercise program, if at any point during your workout you begin to feel faint, dizzy, or have physical discomfort, stop immediately and consult a physician.

DR. A'S HABITS OF MOTION SYSTEM: A MOVEMENT PLAN FOR LIFE

Before introducing this active living system, I need to put on my physician's coat and take a moment to fill you in on your responsibilities.

Any time you change your level of activity, it's important to be evaluated beforehand by your healtchare provider. This is why I suggest you get a complete physical at the outset, taking into account any pre-existing health conditions like knee or joint problems, arthritis, or high blood pressure. You need to discuss how these conditions may be affected by an increase in movement. Heeding this warning is particularly important if you've just lost a lot of weight and are out of shape.

Tools for Success:

Before you get moving, it's worth investing in a few simple devices to help you monitor your activity, track your progress, and stay safe. If you're looking for a top fitness tracker—be it a activity band, fitness watch or a clip-on tracker—there's no shortage to choose from. There are many leaders in the game, with bands to suit every budget and fitness level. And fitness trackers are becoming more feature rich and affordable for people who want to stay fit and healthy. No longer just pedometers, they now focus on heart rate monitoring, sports tracking, sleep statistics, and even help you to feel less stressed during the day.

The right fitness tracker will be based on your individual needs and how active your lifestyle is. Some will just look for step counting and reliable sleep tracking, while others want built-in GPS for running and a heart rate monitor to deliver advanced resting heart rate data. The good news is that there's something out there for everyone, even without breaking the bank. Don't get too hung up about getting the best fitness tracker for iOS or Android—all of them play nicely across both operating systems.

If you do not want to invest that much, you can buy a simple stopwatch or pedometer.

Heart Rate Monitor

Heart rate monitors are usually worn on the wrist (more accurate ones have a monitor around your chest) and they provide an easy way to measure your heart rate automatically, though a watch with a second hand can be substituted. We'll be using a heart rate monitor to evaluate your physical response to increasing levels of movement, setting a target heart rate to guide us as we slowly condition the most important muscle in your body.

Stopwatch

Most heart rate monitors also function as stopwatches. We'll be using this device to measure your NEAT activity and other movement routines.

Pedometer

A pedometer enables you to count your steps as you begin your movement program and allows you to monitor your progress as you move forward. As part of my movement plan, you'll strap a pedometer on from the moment you get up out of bed until you hit the pillow at night. That way, we can tally your total steps per day and use that figure to determine how many calories you're burning through NEAT.

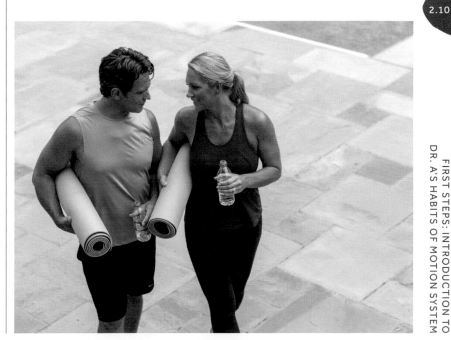

Three Important Heart Rate Measures:

- **Resting Heart Rate (RHR):** the number of times your heart contracts per minute, measured when you're at rest.
- **Maximum Heart Rate (MHR):** the highest number of times your heart can contract per minute during maximum physical exertion. MHR is most accurately determined with a cardiac stress test but, for our purposes, we'll use the following formula: MHR = 220 - your age. For example, the MHR of someone 50 years old is 170 beats per minute (220 – 50).
- **Target Heart Rate (THR).** Between 50% and 85% of your maximum heart rate. As we increase your movement using NEAT, we'll check your THR to make sure we're not raising your heart rate too quickly. Once you're on track and adding NEAT, we'll also use your target heart rate to maximize your cardiovascular fitness level.

Take the time to make that visit to your healthcare provider your first step. I also suggest you go slow at the beginning and, as I've already mentioned, pay attention to any signs of discomfort. You can be assured that in the first part of my movement plan, we'll only be adding mild activity in order to keep your heart rate in a safe range.

So, if you've got the green light from your healthcare provider, we can go over the basics of my Habits of Motion system and prepare to add movement to your life.

And just to allay any anxiety you may have, the actual risk is very low. A study tracked 4,846 coronary heart disease patients performing all types of exercise and, in 129,456 hours of moderate exercise, there was only one case of exercise induced cardiac arrest. Even with intense exercise, the number only went up to two cardiac arrests. In both cases, these were cardiac patients who benefited greatly from exercise and lived longer as a result.[11]

ON YOUR MARK, GET SET...

We're going to equip you with the knowledge and skills you need to add movement to your life in baby steps, through a logical schedule that slowly but surely builds Habits of Motion to last you a lifetime. We'll start at the beginning, with a plan that's slow and easy, yet flexible enough to suit the needs of even a more advanced mover. It's a plan that's safe for all ages, that minimizes time commitment, that's effective, and most important is sustainable over time— and by that, I mean for the rest of your life.

Thank goodness a plan like this exists because, until now, we've had nothing like it.

In the next two parts, I will outline a system that will give you all the Habits of Motion you need to maintain a healthy weight and move up the path to optimal health. We'll begin in Part 2.11, *Dr. A's Habits of Healthy Motion Part 1: NEAT System,* by putting NEAT movement into your daily life, and continue in Part 2.12, *Dr. A's Habits of Healthy Motion Part 2: EAT System,* by adding EAT—progressive, scheduled movements that fit your lifestyle. By the end, you'll have a complete system that will enable you to develop muscle and fitness at a pace and schedule you can stick with.

So, if you're ready, let's take our first steps.

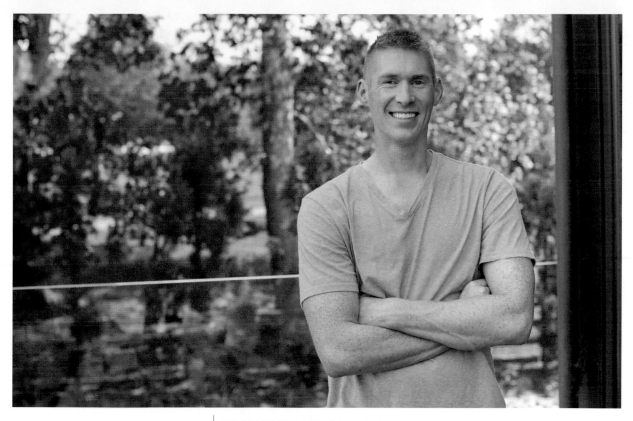

TRANSFORMATION: BRAD MILLER

> "
>
> *The foundation of our marriage and our family was set up on microHabits.*
>
> "

I was in high school when I was starting to form unhealthy habits. After I graduated, I started in construction and put on about 30 lbs after getting married.

This is my first weight loss endeavor. I never really thought about nutrition, because when you're a three-sport athlete in high school, they just tell you to eat everything you can; they don't tell you anything about nutrition.

At first, I started this as a diet. I saw my family lose weight, so I was planning on losing weight, but the process is about the Habits of Health. I started recognizing that I was feeling better and sleeping better.

I dove into Dr. Andersen's book and started recognizing things he was talking about were happening to me as I was taking care of myself.

The coolest thing about the Habits of Health is that it's a lifelong journey, so it's not, "Hey, I got to be perfect today." It's, "I'm starting a journey, and as I go through it, I'm going to start figuring out what works in my favor and what doesn't work in my favor." And you can start working on that, because nothing gets done in one single day. The microHabits make all the difference.

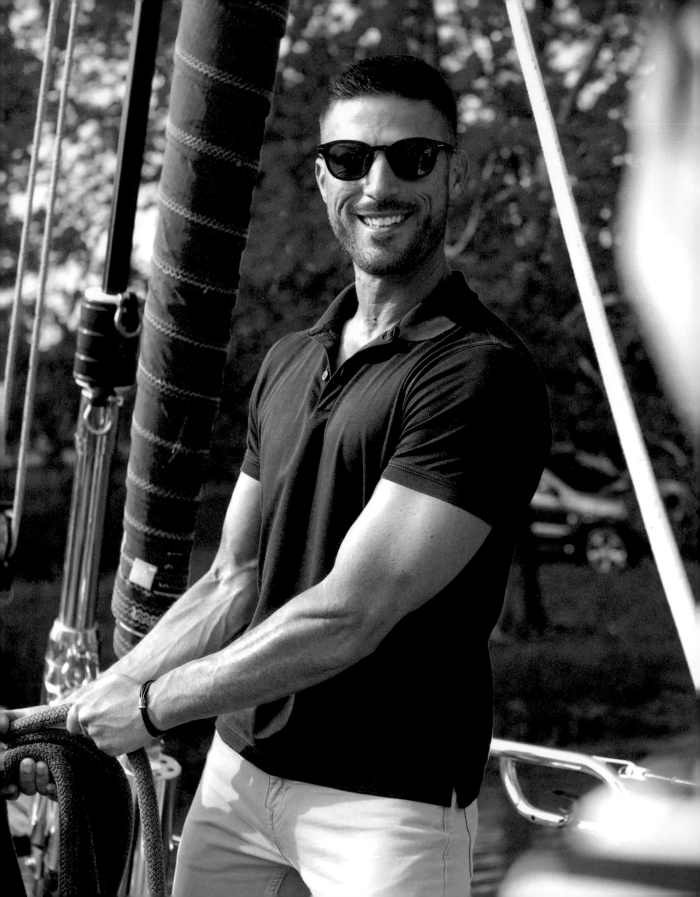

DR. A'S HABITS OF HEALTHY MOTION
PART 1:
NEAT SYSTEM

**HABITS OF
HEALTHY MOTION**

The NEAT System is designed for everyone. It's easy, it's effective, and you're already doing it—we're just going to make you NEATer!

NEAT is a bit like the story of the tortoise and the hare. By making small daily choices, you can win the race of weight management and set the stage for exercise at your own pace. My NEAT System adds motion to every aspect of your day, but does so gradually so that it won't seem like much effort at all. That makes it particularly helpful for people who aren't used to exercising, for those with a BMI (body mass index) above 30, or those with medical conditions (don't forget, if you have a medical condition, you need to be cleared by a healthcare provider first). NEAT is a system you can do right now and continue doing into your 90s and beyond.

Just by making these little NEAT motions a part of your daily routine, you'll soon accomplish your primary goal of offloading a couple of hundred calories each day, and that's going to help your energy management system function flawlessly and indefinitely. Best of all, it's safe. There's no intense exertion involved (though we'll keep a close watch on your target heart rate just to be extra sure). It's important that you feel comfortable and protected as you start creating a more mobile and fitter world for yourself. And now that you've lost some weight and are feeling better, you're ready to go!

MANAGING NEAT: THE SIX S'S OF SUCCESS

The NEAT System helps you take control of your body's energy balance by harnessing the movements you make in the course of your daily activities— the way you move your body, for example, or the way your perform everyday tasks at work and at home. To help you keep track of these motions, I've divided NEAT into six categories that represent the movements and postures that typically fill our days. Together, they serve as a training system to help you transform NEAT into an integral Habit of Health.

The Six NEAT Categories:

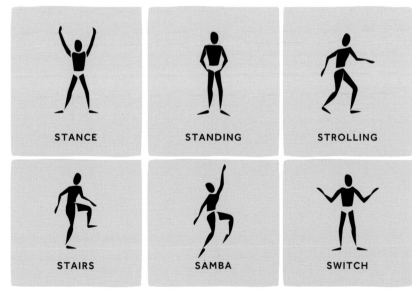

These six categories cover the full range of muscle energy expenditure in your everyday life (outside of the scheduled exercises that make up EAT, that is). As part of this system, I'll teach you to track each one individually so you can be sure you're doing the most you can to increase your daily calorie burn. We want to make sure, especially

"

Boost your motivation! Paint or decorate your office stairwells to make them more attractive to walk up.

"

Exercise and Your Heart: The Benefits of Taking It Slow

It's a well-known medical fact that an unfit, sedentary lifestyle causes cardiovascular disease. Combine that with too much excess weight, and jumping too quickly into exercise can be a recipe for disaster. Although the risk is low, sudden death and heart attack are more likely to take place during exercise. That's why it's so important to ramp up slowly using the NEAT System and to continue monitoring your heart rate. By the time you progress to the active exercising of EAT, your heart will be stronger than ever.

DR. A'S HABITS OF HEALTHY MOTION
PART 1: NEAT SYSTEM

By making small changes in each of the six NEAT categories, you're making secondary choices that support your primary goal to increase healthy movement.

<u>NEAT: It's in the Genes</u>

Some people just have naturally high levels of NEAT. They're more active by nature, and usually thinner as a result. But luckily, environment is more critical than biology when it comes to NEAT, and that's why the NEAT System arms you with the knowledge and techniques to augment your daily motion.

in the beginning, that you're targeting behaviors from all six categories.

STANCE (POSTURE)

When the muscles that support your body's core axis—the chest, shoulders, back, legs, and abdominals—are aligned properly, they create balance throughout your body. Focusing on these foundational muscles helps you burn more calories and provides great training for your transition to the EAT exercises that follow.

This focus is particularly important when you're sitting: a position we find ourselves in a lot in our automated world, especially at work. As you proceed through the six S's, you'll find some great ways to get up and move, starting by simply reminding yourself to get out of your seat whenever you can. But as this first NEAT category shows, even if you are stuck sitting, you can still increase your energy expenditure and enhance your health.

In fact, sitting is one of the best times to work on your posture and core axis alignment. Start by using a proper chair that helps you sit up straight. Now flex your stomach muscles and take deep, slow breaths (we'll discuss deep breathing more thoroughly in Element 04, of *Your Lifebook, Building a Healthy Mindset*).

NEAT Ideas
At work: Focus on sitting up straight in meetings. Get up and move around as much as possible, but when you must sit at your desk, try using a balance ball chair, which forces you to use your core muscles for strength.
At home: Focus on sitting up straight while watching TV or riding in the car, even better, get up and move any time you can!
MicroHabit: Add two additional minutes of focus on core position per day.
Target goal: 30 minutes of focus on core position per day.
Additional target: use a balance ball chair all day at work.

STANDING

Merely moving from sitting to standing can substantially increase your energy consumption. When you stand, you begin to use weight-bearing NEAT and one of the advantages of this is that the heavier you are, the more calories you expend. That's good news, because it means that if you're overweight, you can start off slow and still receive the benefits of increased movement.

NEAT Ideas

At work: Get out of your chair as much as you can. Stand when talking on the phone and use a mobile phone with an earpiece or a portable headset, even if you have to buy it yourself (remember, you're investing in your health). Get rid of comfy couches and get a "standing desk" either through purchase or improvisation. Start off slow and do not stand all day, or you will regret it. Start with an hour or two and work your way up to half a day. To soften the adjustment, you can buy a fatigue mat, and try to avoid locking your knees. The great thing is since you can walk away easily, you will be more likely to be more active and more creative.

At home: All of the above, plus stand while you prepare meals, wash dishes at the sink, iron clothes, watch TV, and read the paper.

MicroHabit: Add 10 additional minutes of standing per day.

Target goal: Two hours of standing per day.

STROLLING (WALKING)

When I talk about walking in terms of NEAT, I'm referring to anything outside of a formal walking program. That includes going to the water cooler, delivering a memo to your boss, or shopping for that new dress at the mall. Remember, the point of NEAT is that it takes place within your normal routines.

As we get older, we typically take fewer steps per day. After age 60, most people are down to around 4,500 steps. Our goal is to increase your daily step count to over 10,000, which is achieved mostly through NEAT and supplemented, if necessary, through my EAT System walking program, which I'll introduce in the next part.

NEAT Ideas

At work: Walk around the room when you're on the phone, walk to work or park your car farther away, talk to co-workers in person rather than by email or phone, have walking meetings, choose the farthest restroom and water cooler, have your lunch (or fueling) in the park, try out a *"walk and work"* desk.

At home: Take the dog for a walk, meet people face-to-face rather than shouting from the other room, park your car as far as is safely possible from your destination, walk on the beach instead of sunbathing, pass on elevators, escalators, and drive-thrus. Get off the couch!

MicroHabit: Add 100 additional steps per week.

Target goal: At least 10,000 steps per day (a mile is about 2,000 steps).

Start Where You Stand:
Silent NEAT

Want to burn sixty extra calories a day without lifting a finger? You can by paying attention to the first two S's.

The first two NEAT categories (stance and standing) may not seem much like movement at all. In fact, they're really just baseline body positions. But if you could put on a pair of electron X-ray glasses and observe your muscles at the microscopic level, you'd be amazed to see that your muscle cells are in continuous motion. By focusing on your body position and effort, we can put more demand on microscopic muscle fibers and, at the same time, improve your overall health.

mHoH

Invest in a standing desk to cut down on how much time you spend sitting.

"

Stay on track while you're staying with friends or family by asking them to join you on a walking tour or offering to cook a healthy meal.

"

Can a "Walk and Work" Desk Cure Obesity?

Researches at the Mayo Clinic think so. In a recent study, Dr. James A. Levine replaced normal desks with workstations attached to a treadmill. By using the treadmills at a slow pace (around one mile per hour) for two to three hours per day, Levine's obese subjects burned 100 calories an hour. That's as much as 66 lbs in one year![1]

STAIRS

Stairs are a great way to accelerate NEAT. In fact, climbing just one flight of stairs is the equivalent of walking 100 steps. That means that climbing 10 flights of stairs gives you the same benefit as half a mile of walking.

When you climb stairs, you're actually lifting your total mass against gravity, making this one of the most effective NEAT activities available. Speed isn't critical here, so it's a great activity if you're overweight and, since it's a weight-bearing activity, the heavier you are, the more calories you burn.

Just one note of caution: stair climbing is a moderately intense activity. If you're overweight or relatively inactive, see your healthcare provider first, then start slowly and pay close attention to any signs that your body needs to take it easier. The good news is that if you add your NEAT activities in the order I've suggested, you should be fine by the time you begin stair climbing.

NEAT Ideas

At work: Take the stairs instead of the elevator or escalator (especially in bad weather, when you can't walk outside). Use the restroom or water cooler on a different floor. Take a stair break instead of a coffee break.
At home: Walk up and down the stairs at the mall, ballpark, or department store.
MicroHabit: Add one additional flight of stairs per week.
Target goal: 10 flights of stairs per day.

SAMBA (DANCE)

Here, we're looking at movement generated by your body's natural rhythm. What do I mean by that? Put on a song you like and watch what happens. You might start tapping your pencil or your foot or even singing as loud as you can.

For the EAT System activities in the next part, we'll use music to distract you from discomfort and enhance your performance. And as you'll see in Part 2.14, *Inflammation: Dousing the Flame*, music and rhythm can even help decrease inflammation.

For the purposes of NEAT, we'll be focusing on music's ability to enhance motion by amplifying brain arousal—a phenomenon that researchers have shown may actually increase the intensity of your activity—and that means you're burning more calories.

NEAT Ideas

At work: Turn on your music; at lunch, go outside, and get in motion.
At home: Use music to augment everything you do on your own, from gardening to cleaning (avoid music in situations where it would prevent you from interacting with others, though, since talking also increases NEAT). Go dancing! Start with ballroom and work your

way up to tap dancing, square dancing, and eventually more intense dances such as jitterbugging and hip hop.

MicroHabit: Add 10 additional minutes of music per day; work up to an hour or more of dance per week.

Target goal: 90 minutes of music per day; one hour of dance per week.

SWITCH

To switch means doing things by hand instead of by machine. That includes dishwashers, electric knives, snow blowers, remote controls, computers, and all the other automatic devices that steal from your energy-use account at an ever-growing pace. Your goal is to burn an extra 30 calories per day doing tasks by hand that you previously had machines do for you.

> *Warning: Do not extend "switch" to movements that can cause repetitive injury or exacerbate current conditions such as tendonitis.*

NEAT Ideas

At work: Take notes and sharpen pencils by hand.

At home: Put away the appliances and start doing kitchen and other indoor chores by hand. Take out the garbage, rake leaves, shovel snow, wash your car by hand, and mow your lawn with a hand mower (your neighbors will love the peace and quiet and the smell of freshly cut grass).

MicroHabit: Add one or two substituted manual tasks per day.

Target goal: 10 substituted manual tasks per day.

TRACKING NEAT

The NEAT system includes a robust and comprehensive tracking and scoring system to help you measure your progress. The full breakdown of how to track your NEAT points and the calories you have burned is available in Element 17 of *Your LifeBook, How Do You Become a Perpetual Motion Machine?* as well as online at HabitsofHealth.com, which is especially handy as you may need to print out extra tracking sheets as you fill yours in.

If you feel that tracking the NEAT increase is too detailed for you, it's okay to make your life more active in a more impromptu fashion. I want you to have fun and get into perpetual motion.

How often?

Any time you think about it. Just say no to machines. Also, remember if you get up and move every 20 minutes, you dramatically lower your risk of heart disease, especially if you have an all-day desk job.

Some NEAT Pointers

- To maintain your healthy weight, aim to burn about 200–300 calories a day through NEAT activities.
- Be good to your heart! As you add new NEAT activities or increase your level of effort, keep checking your heart rate, especially if you feel lightheaded or weak. Make sure it's in the 50–60% range until you feel comfortable.
- Don't be discouraged if you still have a lot of weight to lose as this can actually work to your advantage. The more you weigh, the more calories you burn with each movement, particularly when it comes to weight-bearing activities such as walking, stair climbing, and dancing. Pretty NEAT, huh?
- Get comfortable with NEAT before you move on to more vigorous exercise.

A Habit of Health:

Increasing NEAT by flexing your stomach muscles while you sit up straight.

"

Keeping track of your daily activity, how you feel before and after working out, and what keeps you motivated can help you learn what works and what doesn't. This means that if you start to plateau, you'll be better able to get yourself out of it and keep moving forward. Make sure you're also using Your LifeBook!

"

You can set a timer on your phone, put up post-it notes to remind you, or drink a lot of water, which will have you getting up more often.

See if you can turn yourself into a perpetual motion machine. Your body's 50 trillion cells need to sense motion in order to optimize your health and to prime your future generations!

Perpetual Motion Machine

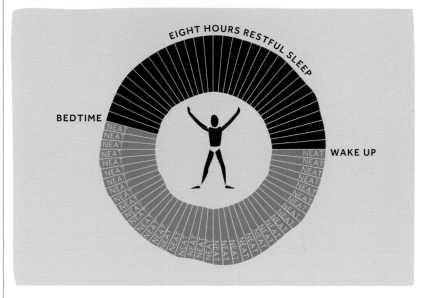

MOVING FORWARD: FROM NEAT TO EAT

By the end of the second month using my NEAT System, you'll be burning 200 more calories each day than you are right now, just by enhancing your normal, everyday activities. And that increase in energy expenditure means you'll be able to offset the natural decrease that occurs as you lose weight, which is the key to healthy weight management! Just as importantly, you'll increase your flexibility, mobility, and total daily motion to make your whole body stronger.

This initial series of activities is the first step in your movement program for optimal health. Now let's look at my scheduled exercise plan, beginning with walking, to help you prepare for your graduate degree in motion.

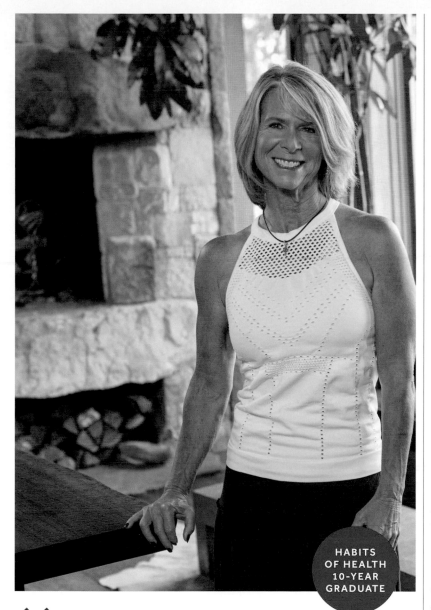

TRANSFORMATION: LISA CASTRO

I was at a place where I really let my health go in so many ways and actually had a mild stroke at 30 years old. Twelve years later, after all kinds of health issues, I finally got the diagnosis of autoimmune disease. I was looking back thinking I probably didn't help my body heal itself and caused a lot of things that created inflammation instead of healing the body from within.

My sister-in-law showed up at my door and introduced me to a way to create health. I thought it was about a way to lose weight. But what I found was I could lose weight by eating properly, and I could start to exercise again without it causing a flare and putting me in bed for days.

When Dr. A introduced the Habits of Health, he wrote it based on people's stories of creating health – not just losing weight, but getting the body moving and nourished, getting good rest, and then working on inflammation.

I've gone from surviving to thriving, from victim to victor, and I'm so grateful for what Dr. A has given us in creating health. I'm so grateful for the healing of my body and even more grateful for the healing of my mind.

HABITS OF HEALTH 10-YEAR GRADUATE

Instead of just losing weight, I started really losing the emotional baggage that went with it.

*Average weight loss on the Optimal Weight 5 & 1 Plan® is 12 lbs. Clients are in weight loss, on average, for 12 weeks.

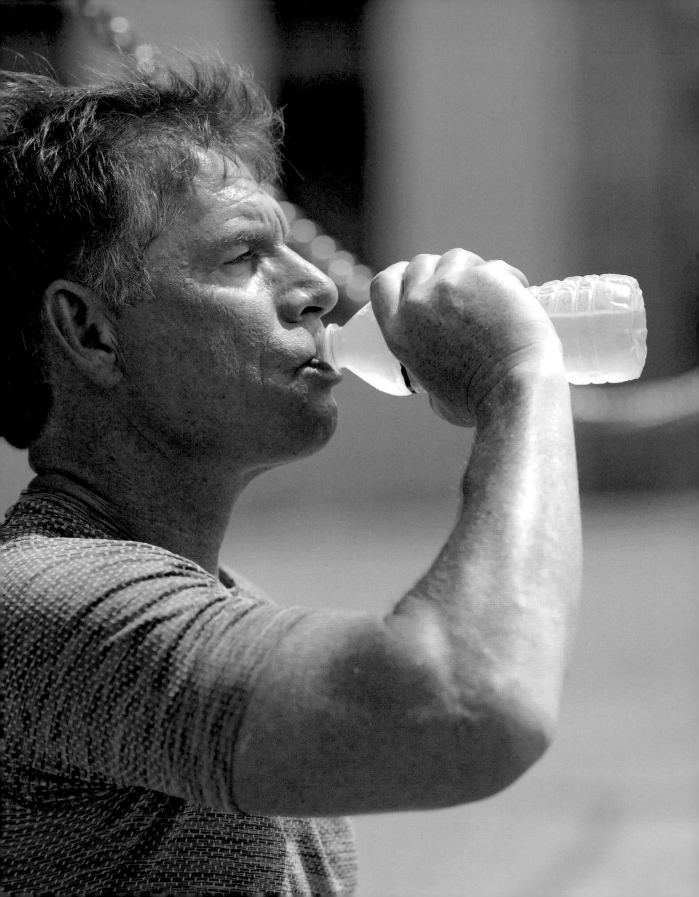

DR. A'S HABITS OF HEALTHY MOTION PART 2: EAT SYSTEM

The NEAT System showed you how to burn an additional 200–300 calories a day without making major changes in your activity level or daily routine. And you were able to put this user-friendly system to work right away to help maintain your weight, increase your flexibility and mobility, and build a healthier lifestyle.

But as you know, we have an even higher goal. We want to create optimal health. That's why you need the second part of my movement plan—the EAT System. Exercise Activity Thermogenesis helps you optimize your health through specific, regularly scheduled exercises that boost your energy expenditure and significantly improve your all-around health, from your heart and immune system to your mental aptitude and sex life. As a result, you'll work better, feel better (EAT can decrease your need for medication and arrest the progress of disease), and even live longer. In fact, EAT is our most important predictor of longevity. It's the type of movement we didn't want to rush you into, but now that you're well on your way to a healthy weight and have increased your daily movement, it makes sense to add this powerful health-enhancing plan to your life.

BUILT TO LAST

My philosophy is that it's best to incorporate activities of moderate intensity based on the premise that you're going to use them until you reach the end of a full, thriving life.

And although the EAT System will take a bit of time out of your day, it's specifically designed to minimize your daily commitment by giving you the most effective results in the least amount of time possible.

Best of all, its part of a long-term strategy to reach and maintain optimal health for the rest of your life. It helps you rehabilitate, condition, enhance, and protect the very organs that help your body move: your musculoskeletal and cardiovascular systems. Optimizing these two systems through exercise ensures that you can enjoy great health into your 90s and beyond!

In fact, exercise becomes even more important as we age. By the time we reach our 60s, the average number of steps we take in a day declines by as much as 25%.[1] One tragic result is an increased prevalence of hip fractures among the elderly due to falls. These fractures, which are much more common in people whose balance and strength are diminished from lack of physical activity, lead to death within a year in up to 30% of sufferers.[2]

But it doesn't have to be this way. By optimizing your body systems and making use of the advances in life extension that you'll discover through the Habits of Health, you should be able to increase your shelflife and support your health for as long as possible.

That's why I don't recommend aggressive exercise programs for the majority of people and especially not for senior citizens. They're just not sustainable. Either they're too difficult to keep up, or worse, they cause injuries that put your future capability at risk. Instead, the EAT System, like all the Habits of Health, is designed to teach you small steps you can do right now, which you will want to continue doing for life. Think of it this way: if you want your car to offer you reliable transportation, you treat it with loving care by warming it up before

"

Exercise Activity Thermogenesis (EAT): Planned movement that's vigorous enough to improve overall fitness. Any activity performed deliberately to enhance the body's conditioning, ranging in intensity from a brisk walk in the park to a triathlon.

"

What Can We Learn from Cuba?

Several years ago, I was invited to Cuba to speak about nutritional intervention. One thing that struck me while I was there was that the streets were full of 1950s American cars, all in pristine condition. How so?

Well, the Cuban people, knowing they can't replace their old cars, treat them with extra loving care. Just think! They're helping themselves while protecting the planet from overconsumption. We would do well to learn this lesson in proper maintenance, beginning with taking better care of our bodies and, as an added benefit, lessening the tremendous burden on our medical care system.

AHA Recommendation

For overall cardiovascular health: At least 30 minutes of moderate-intensity aerobic activity at least five days per week for a total of 150
Or:
At least 25 minutes of vigorous aerobic activity at least three days per week for a total of 75 minutes; or a combination of moderate- and vigorous-intensity aerobic activity
And:
Moderate to high-intensity muscle-strengthening activity at least two days per week for additional health benefits.

you drive it and changing the oil regularly. It's really no different for your own body!

30 MINUTES A DAY, A LIFETIME OF HEALTH

That's all it takes! 30 minutes a day of moderate activity for a lifetime of health and longevity. And that's because the NEAT System is already contributing the lion's share of your daily energy expenditure through your 10,000 steps a day and the other S's. The EAT System builds on this foundation by increasing your energy expenditure even more as you train and optimize your cardiovascular and musculoskeletal systems. And our system meets all the American Heart Associations recommendations for overall cardiovascular health (see sidebar).

By adding EAT into the picture, you position yourself to achieve the three core goals of the Habits of Motion system:

- Increasing energy expenditure to create a consistent balance between energy in and energy out
- Optimizing cardiovascular health so that your heart, lungs, and blood vessels can deliver enough oxygen to keep your cells functioning properly, especially your brain cells
- Building a strong, healthy support system of bones and muscles to help you stay active, keep fit, and maintain a healthy weight

Goals of Dr. A's Habits of Motion

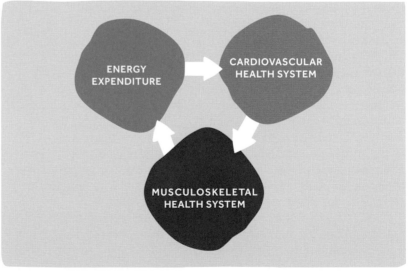

Our movement system has three goals: energy expenditure, cardiovascular health, and musculoskeletal health. These three components work together to support each other and help your entire body achieve optimal health.

CARDIOVASCULAR HEALTH

In the 20 years I spent as a critical care physician, I helped patients with wounded cardiovascular systems do what healthy systems do naturally: deliver oxygenated blood to all the cells in the body.

Just 20–30 minutes of walking a day at a moderate pace is all you need to keep your heart, lungs, brain, and blood vessels healthy so they can support your entire body indefinitely. You can reach that goal by walking about one and a half miles at a pace of three to four miles an hour, or by doing other things you enjoy, such as riding a bike, swimming, skiing, or walking nine holes with a pull cart for your clubs. That's a far cry from Richard Simmons' *Sweatin' to the Oldies®* (though aerobics are fine too, if that's what gets you going)! The important thing is to find things you enjoy so that doing them is fun, rather than a chore you dread. The best exercise is the one that you will actually do!

MUSCULOSKELETAL HEALTH

Sarcopenia, the degeneration of muscle mass and strength (sometimes referred to as osteoporosis of the muscles), is a serious condition that affects people who don't use their muscles regularly for lifting and moving. It creates flabby, weak muscles that then lead to more inactivity, ultimately stressing all the organ systems. But, by devoting just a little time each week, you can recondition your muscles and increase both their number and size. That's why the EAT System includes two 30-minute weight resistance sessions each week to support healthy weight, physical appearance, and overall fitness.

BEFORE YOU BEGIN: STAYING SAFE

Before you start your EAT program, make sure you know the ground rules for protecting your body from injury and staying safe. In research done with cardiac patients, the risk to your heart and brain are low, but we still want to start slow and only after you have been evaluated by your healthcare provider. Musculoskeletal injury is more likely if your overdo exercise and activity until your body has acclimated to more strenuous activity.

- **Keep it slow.** Use slow, careful movements for weight training and other strengthening exercises. At the beginning, keep your heart rate at 50–65% of your maximum heart rate. For example, if you're 50 years old:
  220 - 50 = 170
  170 × 0.5 (in other words, 50%) = 85 bpm (beats per minute)
  170 × 0.65 (in other words, 65%) = 110 bpm

Weight Training:
The Calorie-Burning Gift
That Keeps On Giving

There's a lot more to muscle building than meets the eye. Not only does weight resistance training burn calories both during and after exercise, but the long-term results of weight training (more muscle) help you to continue burning extra calories 24/7. That's because muscle is the most important modifiable determinant of basal metabolic rate (BMR), the rate at which your body processes food and burns it for energy. Adding a pound of muscle can increase your daily BMR (the number of calories you burn in a day) by 50–70 calories.

Post Workout Benefit

In a recent experiment, participants rode a stationary bike at a high intensity for 45 minutes and burned 420 calories. More interesting was that over the next 14 hours, the participants burned an additional 190 calories![3]

Swimming and other water exercises are great ways to meet your movement goals and are especially beneficial for the elderly, those who have arthritis, or anyone who's recovering from an injury. The buoyancy of water reduces your weight by about 80–90%, minimizing the amount of stress on your weight-bearing joints, bones, and muscles, while still giving you a workout in all three key areas of our movement system: cardio, strength training, and flexibility.

Healthy Heart Zone: 50–60% of your maximum heart rate. This is an easy and comfortable zone to exercise in. You will be able to carry on a full conversation. This is the lower end of the moderate-intensity zone.

Fitness Zone: 60–70% of your maximum heart rate. In this zone, you are attaining moderate-intensity exercise. You are breathing heavier but can still speak in short sentences and this should be your goal for most of your walking workouts for fitness.

Aerobic Zone: 70–80% of your maximum heart rate. At this intensity, you are breathing very hard and can only speak in short phrases indicating that this is a vigorous-intensity exercise.

So, your target heart rate range is between 85 and 110 bpm throughout your daily activity.

As you progress and begin to feel more comfortable, you can aim toward 65 or 75%, and eventually 85% once you're optimally fit.

- **Stretch it out.** Help prevent injury by stretching your major muscle groups, preferably directly after your daily EAT activity. Add some extra stretching for a few minutes each day to keep your muscles flexible, improve your balance, and increase your range of motion.
- **Cool it down.** After each session, allow your musculoskeletal and cardiovascular systems to return to their baseline state. I'll teach you some great stretching techniques to add to each workout on HabitsofHealth.com.

The EAT System has three progressive levels of difficulty. It is designed to take you at a pace that allows you to build self efficacy and install the habits that create long-term success into your exercise program. If you are ready, then let's start at Level One with our EAT Walking Program.

LEVEL ONE: EAT WALKING PROGRAM

Since you're already walking as part of your NEAT System activities, adding this natural, low-impact, safe, and simple activity in a more scheduled way should be a breeze. All you need is proper clothing, comfortable shoes, and your pedometer, and you're on your way!

You may be wondering how the NEAT walking you're doing differs from the kind you'll be doing in EAT. Basically, while adding steps through NEAT helps you burn more calories, it's not intense enough to produce fitness. The EAT Walking Program, however, is designed with fitness in mind, so you get essential cardiovascular benefits. And because walking is convenient and easy to do, you're more likely to keep at it so it can become part of your long-term plan for sustainable health.

Here are a few general guidelines to make your first experiences with the EAT Walking Program pleasant and successful:

- **Where to walk:** choose a route that's safe and avoid busy roads. Walking outside will enable you to get fresh air and sunshine, but if you prefer, you can walk indoors on a track or treadmill. Upbeat music or television can help combat boredom. See _Forest Walking_ on page 386.
- **What to wear:** wear comfortable, loose-fitting clothing, preferably layered to respond to changing weather conditions. Avoid plastic or rubberized fabrics that trap moisture and heat. When walking in low light, wear bright clothes or clothing with reflective tape.

- **Shoes:** invest in walking shoes that give you the proper support and traction to maintain good balance and posture.
  A well-fitting shoe should allow your feet to roll inward and outward slightly to absorb impact. It's a good idea to get professional advice from a store that specializes in exercise footwear to be sure the shoe matches your individual motion and keeps your musculoskeletal system in the proper position for pain-free walking. Remember, you'll be walking over 1,500 miles a year, for many years to come, as part of your Habits of Health.

STEPPING OUT: YOUR FIRST DAY

The best way to build success is to start slow. Clear your pedometer and set a goal for your first walk. It doesn't have to be long, just five to 10 minutes.

As you walk, pay attention to any discomfort you may be feeling—perhaps in the fit of your shoes, and especially any shortness of breath or chest discomfort. If you find yourself unable to carry on a conversation without catching your breath, slow down or stop until the feeling passes. Don't worry, you'll be able to pick up the pace soon. In the meantime, signs such as these will help us monitor and guide your progress. For some extra help finding your comfort zone, try a handy self-evaluation tool called the Rate of Perceived Exertion scale (see box, page 387).

Keep at a slow pace until your muscles feel warm and relaxed. If your heart rate is at the low end of your target zone (say, 65%) and you're not experiencing shortness of breath, you can begin to pick up the pace.

Here's a goal to set for your initial walking sessions. You can use either the amount of time or the number of steps to keep track.

Warm up	5 minutes at 1 mph	about 160 steps
At pace	10 minutes at 2 mph	about 665 steps
Cool down	5 minutes at 1 mph	about 160 steps

This 20-minute session of around 1,000 steps (about a half mile) will consume approximately 50 calories if your BMI is 30.

Once you finish, spend about five minutes stretching. As you practice these, make sure to follow my rules for stretching (see box, page 392).

Walking: A Wonder Drug?

Studies have shown that walking just 30 minutes a day can have a dramatic positive effect on your health by:

- Lowering your risk for depression
- Eliminating your need for medications
- Reducing breast cancer risk by 30% and increasing survival rates by 70%
- Lowering your blood pressure and preventing injury to your cardiovascular system by keeping blood vessels open and flexible
- Increasing survival rates from heart attack by 80%[4]

EAT Walking Program Key Points

- Begin by walking 20 minutes a day, including five minutes for warm up and five minutes for cool down.
- Add five minutes each week, or as much time as you're comfortable with.
- Work up to a brisk pace of around four miles per hour.
- Work up to around 20,000 steps per week by week 10 (depending on your level of fitness and weight-loss goals).
- Your long-term goal is to walk for 30 minutes a day, five days a week.

Note: Playing an active sport for an hour will add 8,000 to 10,000 steps.

Just 30 minutes of moderate physical activity each day—say, walking one and a half miles at three to four miles per hour—supports cardiovascular health.[5]

Feel Better, Feel Good, Feel Wonderful Walking in the Forest

Time in forests seems to significantly improve mood in countless studies replicated in a variety of cultures. Many studies have compared the psychological effects of urban walking versus nature walking and have found that nature walks tend to correlate with greater mood improvements.

Shinrin-yoku is a term that means "taking in the forest atmosphere" or "forest bathing". It was developed in Japan during the 1980s and has become a cornerstone of preventive healthcare and healing in Japanese medicine. Researchers in Japan and South Korea have established a robust body of scientific literature on the health benefits of spending time under the canopy of a living forest. Now their research is helping to establish shinrin-yoku and forest therapy throughout the world.

The idea is simple: if a person simply visits a natural area and walks in a relaxed way, then calming, rejuvenating, and restorative benefits will be achieved.

Physical activity in the form of a 40-minute walk in the forest is associated with improved mood and feelings of health and robustness. Levels of the stress hormone, cortisol, decreased in test subjects after a walk in the forest, when compared with a control group of subjects who engaged in walks within a laboratory setting. Forest bathing seems to significantly mitigate the root cause of a multitude of ailments.

Excess stress can play a role in headaches, high blood pressure, heart problems, diabetes, skin conditions, asthma, and arthritis, among many other ailments. Forest bathing catalyzes increased parasympathetic nervous system activity that promotes rest, conserves energy, and slows down the heart rate while increasing intestinal and gland activity.

Lower cortisol concentrations are also a signal that the body's stress-response system isn't being triggered as often.

When this system is triggered, cortisol and other stress hormones are released into the body. Overexposure to these chemicals in response to chronic stress can increase the risk of anxiety, depression, heart disease, weight gain, and memory and concentration impairment. However, the natural chemicals secreted by evergreen trees, collectively known as phytoncide, have also been associated with improvements in the activity of our frontline immune defenders.[6]

RATE OF PERCEIVED EXERTION (RPE)

Have you ever felt uncomfortable while exercising, or have you pushed beyond what seemed like an appropriate level? The Rate of Perceived Exertion (RPE) scale is a handy self-evaluation tool that helps you determine your comfort zone, so you can keep your exercise sessions at a level that's more likely to prevent injury and promote long-term success.

Rate of Perceived Exertion

BORG SCALE	RATE OF PERCEIVED EXERTION
0	NOTHING AT ALL
0.5	VERY, VERY LIGHT
1	VERY LIGHT
2	LIGHT
3	MODERATE
4	SOMEWHAT HARD
5-6	HARD
7-8	VERY HARD
9	VERY, VERY HARD
10	MAXIMUM EXERTION

Adapted from Borg, G. V., "Psychological Basis of Perceived Exertion", Medicine and Science Sports 14 (1982): 377–81.

To use RPE: using a 0–10 scale, rate how much exertion you feel while exercising, with 0 being the equivalent of sitting quietly in a chair and 10 being akin to running up a steep hill. The recommended RPE range for most people is usually between three and five. Remember, you're rating how hard you feel you're working, not how fast your pace actually is.

GETTING IN STRIDE: MOVING INTO YOUR PROGRAM

You've just completed the initial part of what may well be the first successful long-term exercise program you've ever done. Now let's talk about progressing at a pace that builds a lifetime of health. Your goal each week is to add five minutes of moderate walking (three to four miles per hour), until you're walking five days a week for 30 minutes each day. That's around 20,000 steps, or 10 miles each week.

To keep track of your progress, use the EAT Walking Program Daily Tracking Sheet, which you can download from www.HabitsofHealth.com. Just enter your daily minutes, steps, miles, and calories burned in the appropriate boxes.

To figure out how many calories you've burned, locate your Energetic Step Value (ESV) on the following chart and divide your total number of steps by your ESV. For example, according to the chart, the ESV for a woman with a BMI of 35 is 18. If she takes 20,000 steps in a week, she'll divide 20,000 by 18, for a total of 1,111 calories.

DR. A SAYS...

Schedule one of your fuelings for within 60 minutes after exercising to replenish your system, repair muscles, and give your immune system a boost.

Warning: Do not begin the EAT program until you've lost weight and have become comfortable with the NEAT program. As with starting any new activity, consult your healthcare provider first.

You'll complete the EAT Resistance Program on the two days each week that you're not walking as part of the EAT Walking Program. Together, these two programs provide a complete cardiovascular and strength-training system in just 30 minutes a day.

Use the EAT Walking Program Tracking Sheet to track your progress and to challenge yourself.

That's 222 calories for each day of walking, on top of the extra 200 calories burned through NEAT!

Energetic Step Value: Steps Required to Burn One Calorie

BODY MASS INDEX		ESV: FEMALE	ESV: MALE
18–24.9	HEALTHY	36	28
25–29.9	OVERWEIGHT	30	24
30–34.9	CLASS 1 OBESITY	24	20
35–39.9	CLASS 2 OBESITY	18	16
40+	CLASS 3 OBESITY	12	11

Locate your BMI in the left-hand column of the chart to find out how many steps you must take to burn one calorie. This number is your Energetic Step Value (ESV).

As you progress through the program, track your progress. *Your LifeBook* can be a good place to start, and the website includes a preformatted EAT Walking Program Tracking Sheet, and you can go online to HabitsofHealth.com to print out as many copies as you need!

PICKING UP THE PACE: ADVANCING YOUR PROGRAM

The goal of the EAT Walking Program is to boost your cardiovascular and musculoskeletal health now and for years to come. It's a solid program that you can stay with for life just as it's outlined above. But, you can also adapt the program to increase your level of fitness by adding hills, distance, and speed.

You can boost your workouts either by increasing the intensity or the duration of your movement. My 30-minute guideline is merely the baseline required to maintain fitness without cutting too much into your daily commitments. If you have time for more, that's great. You'll see that by increasing the intensity, you will be more effective at burning fat. We will explore that in more detail a little later when we talk about High Intensity Interval Training (HIIT).

If you'd like to intensify your workout, burn more calories, and strengthen leg and buttock muscles, try walking up hills or raising the incline on your treadmill. It will help as you walk uphill to lean forward, shorten your steps, and pump your arms. Or to increase your cardiovascular fitness, try carrying lightweight dumbbells or wearing ankle weights or a weighted vest. However, please don't attempt this until you're up to 20,000 steps per week and at a point where walking has become a Habit of Health.

As you step up your intensity, remember the basic principles of cardiovascular fitness:

- If you're unable to carry on a conversation, slow down.
- Keep your Rate of Perceived Exertion (RPE) below a six.

Once you've reached your EAT Walking Program goal of 20,000 steps per week (on top of the steps you're taking as part of the NEAT System) and have been walking five days every week for at least a month, you're ready to advance to Level Two and add the other essential component of the EAT System: resistance training.

LEVEL TWO: EAT RESISTANCE PROGRAM

Does the thought of weight training conjure up images of sweaty, grunting meat-heads in tank tops spending hours at the gym lifting ridiculous levels of weight? This type of boot-camp workout is not only unnecessary, it's downright unsafe. It has no place in a sustainable health plan.

The EAT Resistance Program is something else entirely—two 30-minute sessions a week specifically targeted to add strength to your musculoskeletal system (bones and muscles). The goal is to turn your underused, sarcopenic muscles into lean, efficient, healthy tissue that can support you for a lifetime. Despite the negative effects of years spent in an environment of "*labor-saving*" devices, you can improve your muscle and bone strength in just a few months if you approach it correctly.

The EAT Resistance Program, like all the Habits of Health, is easy to learn, doable, and sustainable. This makes it very different from programs that expect you to spend hours in the gym trying to learn difficult exercises. And because the program only takes two days a week, it's a perfect complement to the five days you spend on the EAT Walking Program. Together, these two components provide you with a complete cardiovascular and strength-training system that takes only 30 minutes a day.

THE SCIENCE OF HEALTHY MUSCLES

Creating healthy muscles begins with the sarcomere: the microscopic muscle cell unit that creates all motion. As the functional unit of the muscle, a sarcomere works like a ratchet. When you contract your muscles, the filaments slide together, shortening the muscle. When you relax your muscle, the ratchet is released and the filaments move back to their original position, returning the muscle to its original length. By doing this over and over, you create little micro-tears that the body then repairs, thereby making the muscles stronger and larger.

This is traditionally accomplished by lifting weights repetitively until the muscle grows fatigued and tears occur. To facilitate this,

Boosting Your Walking Workout

- **Lean forward slightly from your hips to increase momentum, pace, and intensity.**
- **Tighten your abdominal muscles and buttocks to burn more calories.**
- **Flex your toes to engage your leg muscles and increase your speed.**
- **For a more energetic stride, swing your arms with your elbows bent 90 degrees, shoulders rounded and relaxed.**
- **Keep your focus about 20 feet in front of you to straighten your posture to help you walk tall.**

Music: Your Secret Weapon for Long-Term Motivation

You already know that music can boost your energy expenditure as part of NEAT as a legal ergogenic aid. It's also a great motivator for workouts and can even help your muscles heal faster. In fact, it's been shown that the people who listen to music during exercise have a better chance of staying with their program, thus enjoying such long-term benefits as enhanced quality of life and lower incidence of coronary heart disease, not to mention that music reduces the pain and discomfort from stress and anxiety.[7]

Healthy Eating, NEAT, and EAT: Working Together for Total Health

Most exercise programs try to do too much. They promise weight loss, cardiovascular performance, and muscle enhancement, and deliver none of these very effectively. The Habits of Health, on the other hand, focus on a variety of small daily choices to create first healthy weight, then optimal health. We're not relying on exercise for weight loss as you're already doing that through the fat-burning healthy eating system. Energy expenditure is taken care of through the NEAT System, the EAT Walking Program covers cardiovascular health, and the EAT Resistance Program completes the picture by serving as a muscle and bone reconditioning program to help you retain your full range of movement for life!

I know I am repeating myself, but remember: the best exercise program is one that you will actually do!

some schools of thought have you lift more weight, and some have you do more repetitions. The time, degree of effort, and results of these techniques are all massively variable.

My goal was to develop a safe, effective technique that anyone could use and sustain long term. This led me to the University of Florida, my alma mater and home of my beloved Gators. In the 1980s, researchers at the University of Florida School of Medicine discovered that moving a muscle group slowly through the full range of motion improves strength, bone density, and overall function. It's the slowness that's particularly important, as it eliminates gravity and momentum, causing the muscle to work more completely. As a result, the muscle is forced to develop more fibers and grow more quickly. Holding the muscle just as it's reached its point of maximum contraction reinforces the effect. And, as an added benefit, slow and controlled movement minimizes the chance of injury, making it ideal for long-term practice.

PUTTING SCIENCE TO WORK

The EAT Resistance Program uses this science of slow contractions and relaxations, along with maximum hold time, to help you build muscle quickly and maintain it indefinitely. We'll focus on working your core muscles to improve your overall stance and posture, maximize energy consumption, and provide you with a platform to carry you into old age in excellent shape.

To create complete musculoskeletal health, we're going to work your core muscles and upper and lower extremities in rotation through slow, continuous repetitions that also work your cardiovascular system. That means you'll be getting cardiovascular benefits even on the days you're not walking! You'll then stretch each muscle group to maintain your full range of motion and flexibility.

This program is easy to learn and safe to do because it requires only moderate weights, when it uses weights at all. In fact, I've used these very techniques my whole life, both through everyday movements and through isometric exercises, and I can attest that they've enabled me to maintain my strength without ever setting foot in a gym. And if they work for me, they'll work for you too!

Before we begin, let's go over the core principles of the EAT Resistance Program:

- Muscle groups are moved slowly through the full range of motion in order to eliminate gravity and momentum and work muscles more completely. *Improves strength, bone density, and overall function.*
- Movements are held at the point of maximum contraction just before lockout to enable the muscles to grow fatigued and

encourage them to recruit more muscle fibers. *Builds muscle.*
- Focus is on the core muscles. *Improves overall stance and posture and maximizes energy expenditure.*
- Movement is continuous. *Boosts cardiovascular health.*
- Muscles are stretched to the full range of motion after each muscle group movement. *Promotes long-term flexibility.*

EQUIPPING YOURSELF

Ready to go over the equipment and weights you'll be using? Take a look in the mirror. That's right, the most important piece of equipment is you!

By putting you at the center of your workout, I hope to eliminate any excuses you might have about driving to the gym, buying exercise equipment, or being short on space in your home. In fact, all I suggest you buy in the way of equipment is a mat, a balance ball and, as your fitness increases, a pair of dumbbells.

Why don't I want you to use exercise machines? My program teaches you a complete system that you can use anytime, anywhere, for many, many years to come. And since my goal is to give you better balance, strengthen the muscles that stabilize your spine, and equip you to perform the movements you need for everyday life, it just makes sense to make you the principal piece of machinery!

Once you've made some initial progress, a few simple free weights—dumbbells, medicine balls, and vest and ankle weights, for example—will help you a lot more than machines and cables that isolate muscle groups and move your body on just one plane. After all, that's not how we move in real life. The movements you'll practice through the natural form of resistance training that I teach are much better preparation for unloading the groceries, taking out the trash, lifting your kids, and walking the dog.

If you do want to use weight-training machines, by all means give them a try but just make sure you stay safe by getting in great shape first. However, if you want to increase your coordination and strengthen your core, stay with the basics.

WHAT ABOUT JOINING A GYM?

The EAT Resistance Program is designed to be completely doable from your home, with you, this book, the Habits of Health website, and the accompanying *Your LifeBook* as the principal equipment. In fact, you can do these exercises anywhere that provides you with 30 minutes of uninterrupted private time.

That being said, there can be advantages to going to a gym. You'll be surrounded by fellow exercisers whose motivation and knowledge

DR. A SAYS...

"

Before walking outdoors, remember to put on sunscreen and a high-SPF lip balm. Wait 15–20 minutes to allow the ingredients to be absorbed.

"

Avoiding "Lockout": A Key to Effective Exercising

It's common to "lockout" your joints during an exercise, for example by straightening your elbows during a push-up or your knees during a squat. But this transfers the weight onto your bone structure and away from working muscles, and is not recommended. Avoiding lockout helps you increase tension and maintain a high level of intensity throughout your repetitions. In fact, the key to effective long-term muscle development is moving the muscle slowly through the full range of motion and holding it at the point of maximum contraction just before lockout.

Important Rules for Stretching

- The best time to stretch is directly after your walk.
- Never stretch cold muscles.
- Problem areas may be stretched prior to your walk, but only after you've warmed up.
- Don't bounce when you stretch.
- Ease into a stretch slowly and hold gently. Stretch to the point where you feel a gentle pull, but never to the point of pain.
- Hold each stretch for 30–40 seconds. If you have problems with a particular area, stretch that area twice. Hold for 30–40 seconds, release, then stretch again.

Choosing a Trainer

A certified personal trainer can help you get the most out of your exercise program by speeding up your learning curve, ensuring you're performing each exercise correctly, and adding a measure of accountability. If you do choose to hire a trainer, just make sure they're a full-time professional certified by a reputable organization such as one of the following:

- American College of Sports Medicine (ACSM)
- National Association of Sports Medicine (NASM)
- American Council of Exercise (ACE)
- The National Strength and Conditioning Association (NSCA)

can be helpful if you're new to working out, and many gyms provide professional trainers who can help you get started and ensure you're doing the movements correctly. In fact, hiring a trainer—either at a gym or in your home—is an investment that I highly recommend if you haven't been exercising regularly or received training in the past. A trainer can really be helpful if you want to take your workout to the next level. Then, once you're comfortable with exercising at the level that you desire, you can continue on your own.

A gym also gives you access to cardiovascular equipment that you can use to fulfill your EAT Walking Program requirements in bad weather or when you'd just like a break from your routine. I recommend doing 30 minutes on an elliptical cross-trainer, which gives a great workout to the cardiovascular system as well as the upper and lower body. Other equipment can be used to complement your EAT Resistance Program once you've reached a more advanced level.

All in all, there's much to gain from an EAT-friendly facility that gives you time to exercise away from distractions. That being said, I don't use a gym myself and manage to stay in shape in the comfort of my home. And so can you. It's whatever you prefer and whatever gets you exercising.

YOUR EAT RESISTANCE PROGRAM

Each EAT Resistance Program session works either your upper body or your lower body, along with your core muscles. Our major areas of focus are as follows:

Upper Body
- Core (upper)
- Chest
- Latissimus dorsi (back)
- Shoulders
- Arms

Lower Body
- Core (lower)
- Thighs
- Gluteals
- Hamstrings
- Calves

The exercises you choose to engage these muscle groups is up to you. Traditional routines are a good place to start, but you can also adapt your routine to account for a previous injury or to adjust the difficulty level. Go slow at first, and gradually increase the intensity from session to session.

To get you started, we created a sample Level Two program, as well as EAT tracking sheets that you can find online at HabitsofHealth.com.

YOUR COMPLETE HABITS OF MOTION SYSTEM

To create and maintain optimal health, you need to be active every day. My Habits of Motion system is designed to make sure you get enough activity to keep your weight under control while moving you toward optimal health. You'll get most of this healthy activity through the NEAT System and the EAT Walking Program. The EAT Resistance Program takes you the rest of the way by helping you maintain your cardiovascular and musculoskeletal systems for the long term. If you want to take it even further, a fitness trainer can help you create a more advanced program tailored to your goals (I've started using a trainer regularly myself). Now that you've put the Habits of Motion system together, let's take a look at the program in its entirety. Here's what a single week might look like once you're in the swing.

A Typical Week on the Habits of Motion System

	NEAT SYSTEM	EAT SYSTEM	CALS BURNED
MONDAY	Walked four flights Walked to lunch	30 minute EAT upper body	450
TUESDAY	Walked four flights Cleaned closet	30 minute EAT walk	425
WEDNESDAY	Walked four flights Washed car	30 minute EAT walk	375
THURSDAY	Walked four flights Raked lawn Washed dishes	30 minute EAT Lower body	450
FRIDAY	Walked four flights Walked to lunch	30 minute EAT walk	400
SATURDAY	Walked four flights Mall shopping Dancing	30 minute EAT walk	650
SUNDAY	Climbed stadium Upper deck	30 minute EAT walk	400

By reviewing your activity and total calories burned for a week on the NEAT and EAT systems, you can see how effective these activities are at upping energy expenditure without taking a lot of time from your day.

Up to this point, we have talked about endurance training such as an aggressive walking program, some running, or swimming and, of course, the Habits of Healthy Motion weight resistance training. Now we're going to discuss a different method for fitness training.

EAT Resistance Program: Key Points

- Before you begin, make sure you've got the EAT Walking Program down and have been racking up 20,000 steps per week consistently for at least a month.
- Choose two days each week for your resistance workouts, leaving at least two days between sessions to let your body recover. I recommend doing the upper body session on Monday and the lower body session on Thursday.
- Find a spot where you can focus without distraction, and use an exercise mat for support and cushioning. Take it slow and review each new exercise before you try it out; limit yourself to one rotation for the first week; and add new exercises slowly, letting your body become accustomed to the new movement.

LEVEL THREE: BOOSTING YOUR WORKOUTS
HIGH-INTENSITY INTERVAL TRAINING (HIIT)

In the previous edition of this book, we reserved the introduction of High Intensity Interval Training (HIIT) until the Ultrahealth™ section of the book because of the conditioning that is required to perform this level of CV fitness. Recent studies and growing evidence is showing that HIIT is highly effective at removing that stubborn resistant fat once you are in shape and have aerobic fitness. So, when you have reached the level of fitness described below, you might want to consider using at least some HIIT. I recommend starting with a fitness instructor.[8]

Aerobic Fitness: Target Heart Rate Zone

The target heart rate zone is an increase in your heart rate—50–75% of the maximum heart rate for your age—which is significant enough to give your heart and lungs a good workout. You can use the target heart rate zone as a guide to make sure your exercise is intense enough. If you are not reaching your target zone, you may need to increase the intensity. If you are achieving a target rate in the lower end of the target rate zone, you can set goals to gradually increasing your target. If you already exercise regularly, you can stop to check your heart rate periodically during an aerobic workout. If you do not exercise regularly, you can do a simple test by checking your heart rate after a brisk 10-minute walk.

Target heart rate zone

AGE	TARGET HEART RATE ZONE: BEATS PER MINUTE	MAXIMUM HEART RATE: BEATS A MINUTE
25	98–146	195
35	93–138	185
45	88–131	175
55	83–123	165
65	78–116	155

Recent research shows that HIIT exercise is the best form of movement for burning fat, especially in our belly area. A 15-week program of HIIT was nine times more effective than a 20-week endurance program for reduction of visceral adiposity.

An astonishing study in 2011 compared two groups. One group ran 30–60 minutes three times a week on a treadmill. The other group ran four to six 30-second sprints with four-minute recovery times between sprints three times a week. Both groups had significant fat mass decrease. The endurance group with 90–180 minutes of exercise lost 5.9% fat mass while the sprinters six to nine minutes a week had a fat loss of 12.4%.[9]

It sounds crazy, but it can be a very effective way of removing extra visceral adiposity once you are fit! And it is important to have recovery time. It is effective in burning fat in a short amount of time. But it only works if you are in good enough shape that you will actually do it. It can be progressed as a microHabit and requires just a small amount of time.

Take a look at Element 18, *Exercise is Your Gift to Yourself,* in *Your LifeBook* where I describe six ways to boost your EAT resistance training. Then I present two HIIT routines which will get you in amazing shape in no time at all.

> *Note: In order to both support you and ensure that you remain fully autonomous, I want you to decide what EAT program you want to use. As I mentioned earlier, I am a firm believer that the best exercise program is the one you will actually do, and my system of EAT is just one of many options available to a trainer who can then help you decide which one is best for you and your surroundings.*

I am partial to EAT as the system combines the antidote to the sitting disease as well as being designed so that you can do it for the rest of your life. You can see how well the Habits of Motion system increases your daily calorie expenditure without causing a lot of disruption to your day or schedule.

You now have the knowledge you need to take control of your energy management system. These Habits of Motion, combined with the Habits of Healthy Eating you've already learned, will have a dramatic impact on your journey toward a healthy weight and optimal health.

We're now going to look at an area of your life that's equally important, but all too often brushed aside in our time-starved world. Yet, nothing has the ability to age you faster or extend the quality of your life more than our next essential habit: the Habit of Healthy Sleeping and Energy Management.

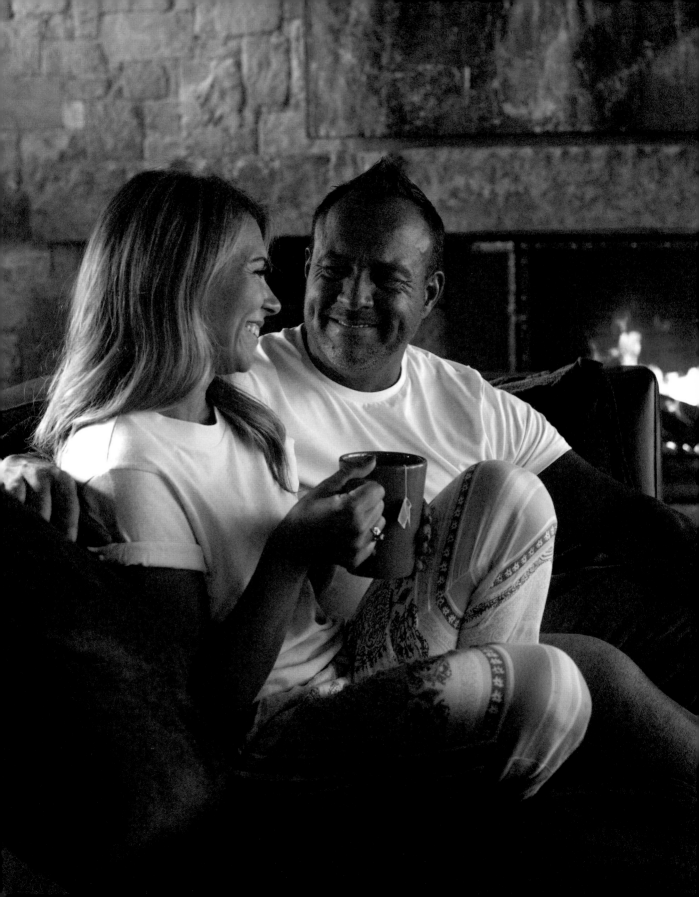

PART 2.13

HEALTHY SLEEP AND UNLIMITED ENERGY: CORNERSTONES OF AN OPTIMAL LIFE

The right amount of high-quality sleep—once thought to be unimportant in your life—has been properly elevated to an essential role in our health and wellbeing. Sleep is your body's way of restoring organ function, stabilizing chemical imbalance, refreshing areas of the brain that control mood and behavior, and improving performance. Without it, the rest of the picture of health cracks and fades, but with it, the energy of life is yours to spend as you wish.

In this part, we will explore the full MacroHabits of Healthy Sleep, giving you the fundamental understanding you need to recognize the importance of sleep and to understand how you can harness its power in your favor, so that you can reach optimal health and fill your days with vibrancy and unlimited energy.

With 45% of the population struggling with sleep, the new knowledge we are about explore may change your life.[1]

In *Your LifeBook,* you will customize, prioritize, and help plan for your day to maximize your sleep and energy relationship. You will use personalized logs to help you install the key elements and track and adjust your sleep and energy habits until they are optimized.

The Stages of Sleep: One Sleep Cycle

SLEEP LATENCY	• Time to fall asleep • Starts when you turn out the lights
STAGE 1	• Light sleep
STAGE 2	• Brain waves slow down resting the parts you use while awake, body temperature drops
STAGE 3	• Deeper sleep; restorative • Delta waves dispersed with smaller fast waves
STAGE 4	• Especially recuperative; restores and recharges the body • Delta waves almost exclusively • Essential to sleep process
REM	• The deepest sleep • Characterized by rapid eye movements • Body (arms and legs) otherwise motionless • Dreaming; active brain waves similar to when thinking

It may seem like nothing's happening while you sleep, but your brain is actually going through a series of important stages that make up a complete sleep cycle. We typically experience four to six 90-minute cycles a night. The daytime equivalent, called ultradian cycles, help determine your energy levels; we will discuss these a little later.

WHY IS IT SO IMPORTANT?

Adjusting your sleep and napping rituals so we have you running on an optimum schedule that effortlessly supports your energy and strength will allow you to thrive. It's the human equivalent of your smartphone's optimum status: five bars of service and 100% charge. These powerful habits will provide you with more energy, better mood, better focus, and a supercharged mojo! Living in these times, it is our energy level rather than our time management that really sets up the success we will have in installing our Habits of Health.

Sleep Apnea and Obesity: A Vicious Cycle

Sleep apnea—a sleep disorder characterized by snoring and airway obstruction that results in 10 second or longer periods of non-breathing during sleep—is caused by excess weight, primarily fatty tissue in the neck. Because it interrupts the sleep cycle, sleep apnea can actually spur further weight gain, which then exacerbates the sleep apnea, creating a vicious cycle of increasing weight and deteriorating sleep.

Sleep deprivation, a form of psychological torture, is often considered worse than going without food or water. It rapidly erodes emotions and self-confidence, resulting in erratic behavior.

When your energy and sense of wellbeing are high, you are in a position to begin your day on the right trajectory: early to rise, excited to be up and about, and ready for an optimal day (a highly engaged and productive day of accomplishing what is important to you which concludes with a day of deep satisfaction). As the day drifts into its natural conclusion, it does so with a sense of calm and contentment and in anticipation of a night of restful, deep sleep. Doesn't that sound wonderful? It is, and you will own this new and vital element in your story.

We will design your rituals and routines, and the new habits that will permit your body and mind's operating system to run at its highest efficiency to propel you to become the highest version of yourself.

Everything in my life that has allowed me to flourish is predicated by starting each day with an incredible level of energy that makes the day a joy to live. And it is all set up by the quality of my sleep and supported by my naps when needed. It is my secret weapon. On the days when my previous night's sleep suffers and I lack the time to have a recovery nap, my productivity in my work, my relationships, my choices, and other MacroHabits suffer.

In this part, we are going to explore some of the preemptive things we can do to create unlimited energy and a calm, rested state (and it is not a B12 shot!).

WHY WE SLEEP

10,000 years ago, everything we did was determined by our circadian rhythm. During the daylight, we were highly productive at the full-time job of surviving. Like a squirrel in the fall, we were busy scurrying around to build a shelter, securing abundant fuel for the coming winter.

Yet once the sun went down, our light-sensitive pineal glands released melatonin making us drowsy between sunset and sunrise. This powerful hormone sets us up for sleep by cooling our body temperatures, lowering our metabolic rates, and moving us into the sleep latency stage.

Feeling drowsy, we would find a safe spot to rest and acquire restorative sleep to be ready for the next day. 98% of our programing and our DNA is tied to this rhythm, and it kept us rested, highly fit and strong, with unlimited energy.[2] Our alertness kept us from wandering out and becoming prey.

Artificial light changed everything. Gaining control of natural light with our discovery of fire and our ability to control it extended our waking hours, but it was Edison and the development of the light bulb that started disturbing our natural sleep and energy patterns. Then came televisions, computers, and smartphones.

Today, our sleep debt (the amount of sleep we sacrifice, hour by hour each night) is also having a profound effect on our work performance. The level of depression in those that have sleep issues is five times greater than those that are healthy sleepers.[3]

Just 30 minutes less than the ideal minimum sleep of 7.5 hours might not seem like much, but the effects of this amount of sleep deficit were notable. Survey responders have reported poorer workplace performance due to tiredness, with over half admitting to struggling to stay focused in meetings, taking longer to complete tasks, and finding it challenging to generate new ideas. Along with a lack of focus and diminished creative capacities, participants also indicated a reduced motivation to learn and were less able to manage competing demands.[4]

Along with emotional impact, sleep deprivation can take a toll on your cognitive abilities including perception, judgment, reaction time, and decision-making. In fact, 17 hours of sustained wakefulness, such as a long day in the office, has been shown to result in behavioral changes equivalent to drinking two glasses of wine.[5] If wakefulness continues for 24 hours, you may act as if you have drunk four glasses of wine. Diminished cognitive performance can have huge repercussions for professionals whose jobs demand critical attention to detail, such as surgeons, pilots, and drivers.

Unfortunately, it has become evident that the effects of a sleep-deprived workforce can be disastrous. The Three Mile Island nuclear meltdown, the Chernobyl nuclear explosion, the Exxon Valdez oil spill, and the Challenger space shuttle disaster were all the result of human error caused by sleepiness. Whether it's improving workplace productivity or averting large-scale disasters, better sleep is clearly better for business.

What we can say is that scientists have observed, over longer periods of time, that a chronic lack of sleep can:

- Lead to weight-gain
- Adversely impact learning and memory
- Compromise your immune system
- Elevate your blood pressure
- Increase inflammation
- Shorten lifespans
- Create symptoms of ADHD
- Contribute to mental and emotional health issues[6-10]

As we are helping you make the transformations that will create lifelong wellbeing, it should be clear that your quality of sleep, your attention, focus, and energy are dependent on building the Habits of Healthy Sleep and Energy Management.

Hopefully, you can see that to accomplish our journey your purpose must be bigger than your nightly entertainment.

It turns out that sleepy driving plagues about 60% of adult drivers (168 million Americans have driven a vehicle while feeling drowsy in the past year alone). Alarmingly, 37% of adult drivers, or 103 million people, have actually fallen asleep at the wheel. 13% of those who have actually fallen asleep at the wheel have done so at least once a month. 11 million drivers admit that their sleepiness has caused an accident or near-accident.

According to the National Highway Safety Administration, 100,000 police-reported crashes per year are the result of driver sleepiness (and this is severely under-reported since it is currently very hard to assess sleepiness as the cause of a crash). Drowsy driving could be as dangerous as driving while intoxicated.[11]

"People who do not sleep well are over five times more likely to develop a cold! [12] *"*

mHoH

Eliminate all sources of light in your bedroom (such as all electronics) to get more restful sleep.

ARE YOU GETTING ENOUGH SLEEP?

First things first, are you getting enough sleep? Answer the following questions to find out. Do you:

- Wake up tired in the morning?
- Lack purpose when you get up to start your day?
- Need a nap in the afternoon?
- Fall asleep watching TV?
- Have frequent small accidents at home, or large ones on the road?
- Have trouble focusing on the job?
- Find yourself sleepy after lunch?
- Feel irritable or depressed most of the time?
- Feel like you're not getting anything done?
- Drink alcohol to get to sleep?
- Drink several cups of coffee or energy drinks to stay awake?
- Eat big or sugary meals in the later evening?
- Have difficulty falling asleep?
- Have difficulty staying asleep?

If you answered yes to more than three of these questions, you're probably not getting the kind of sleep you need to support health. But don't worry because the Habits of Healthy Sleep are going to help change all that, and not a moment too soon!

To go even deeper into your Habits of Healthy Sleep assessment, fill out the sleep log and sleep assessment located in *Your LifeBook* and online at HabitsofHealth.com. The results will help you to better identify which specific behaviors are affecting your sleep.

BRIGHT LINE CURFEWS

In order to manage some of the behaviors and habits which may be having a negative impact on our sleep and energy, it is important to create bright lines.

In legal jargon, bright lines are the boundaries we create and enforce by drawing a line in the sand of what can and cannot done. They are lines that cannot be crossed. In terms of the behaviors listed in the following table (such as drinking caffeine), it is usually better not to do these if you want to be best prepared for sleep. But if we are unwilling to eliminate them at this time, we need to set hard curfews to help create a cue for the time we will stop this behavior in order to support our best sleep.

Note that in terms of highly caffeinated products like coffee, espresso, and others with over 50 milligrams (mg); these should be suspended eight hours before you expect to be in bed. All lower level caffeinated items should stop being consumed within five hours of sleep to make sure the level does not interrupt your induction into deep sleep.

Bright Line Curfews: When to Stop Activities by

HOURS BEFORE BED	
8 HOURS	• COFFEE
5 HOURS	• CAFFEINE
4 HOURS	• EXCERCISE
3 HOURS	• ALCOHOL • HEAVY MEALS
2 HOURS	• WORK AND SERIOUS CONVERSATIONS
1 HOURS	• DIGITAL SUNSET
IN BED	• LIGHTS OUT

GOING FROM FULL-OUT-GO TO TRANSITIONING TO SLEEP MODE

In our modern world, we seem to be moving non-stop from the time we get up in the morning until we collapse on the couch in the evening and then we mindlessly watch TV, browse the internet, or gaze at some other distracting device. We really leave so little time for a transition from full-out-go to a more relaxed mellow state: the phase required to move into the conditions necessary for our best night's sleep. It is no wonder that over 80 million Americans have poor, unhealthy sleep patterns. But it isn't just the U.S. that is chronically affected by insomnia. This non-stop go state it is having a significant impact on the whole world.

New data has now shown that on average, no citizens of *any developed country* in the world manage to achieve eight hours of sleep on a regular basis. As the recommended range of sleep for an adult is at least 7.5 hours a night, this highlights a worrying lack of sleep worldwide.[13]

In order to effectively design a transition routine, to create the high-quality energy critical to optimal health, we again turn to structural dynamics and the creative process.

CREATING HABITS OF HEALTHY RHYTHMS OF SLEEP AND ENERGY

We are now going to overlay the chronological clock that runs the world with your biological clock (the one that runs you) so that we once again synchronize and reconnect you to a world which was once orchestrated with the rise and set of the sun.

We will focus on establishing your new rituals and routines that, once installed, will help you reestablish the key behaviors that should be controlled by your circadian rhythm. We are, in essence, designing and engineering an ideal energy rhythm to allow you to have more optimal days.

Let's look at the 24 hours in a day and how we can create time cues to help make adjustments to our behaviors that were once in sync

DR. A SAYS…

"

Losing 90 minutes of sleep reduces daytime alertness by almost a third![14]

"

Lack of Sleep Worse for Women, Studies Show

Sleeplessness is not good for anyone, but it takes a particularly heavy toll on women. Researchers at Duke University who studied 210 healthy men and women found that while sleep quality was comparable for both genders, the women exhibited greater psychological stress, depression, hostility, and anger, as well as higher levels of substances that increase heart disease risk, including insulin, C-reactive protein, and interleukin 6.[15]

That's not all because a large study of 71,000 female nurses found that women who sleep only five hours or less a night are 45% more likely to have heart problems and that even those who sleep six hours a night have a 20% higher risk.[16]

The general consensus at the time of writing, is that we need eight hours sleep on average for optimal health, but it's essential that those hours include rotations through several healthy cycles of REM and non-REM stages.

with our circadian rhythm. In other words, we are creating a Habits of Healthy Sleep and Energy clock to guide you throughout your day and evening. If this idea sounds familiar, that's because we used this concept to reignite your inner perpetual motion machine with the NEAT System.

Let's start with the fundamental Habit of Health (and the physical reality) that most of us need at least 7.5 hours and optimally as much as nine hours sleep to function at our most effective level.

In the following illustration, we have a band of dark blue that represents where sleep should be placed on our biological clock starting at 10pm. You may remember that research supports this period of time as producing the deepest and most amount of REM sleep.

Depending on your age and chronotype (AKA whether you prefer to go to bed and wake up early or late), you may have to shift your bed time. But the main idea is to make the decision to go to bed at a time that allows you to get the recommended range of 7.5–9 hours of sleep.

I have used eight hours in this example as your target—a reasonable and practical duration considering our modern lifestyle requirements. In *Your LifeBook,* we make additional evaluations to help you tweak these timings in terms of start time and length of sleep to adjust to your ideal as you dial into this vital sleep zone.

As you can see in the Habits of Health Sleep and Energy Clock, the behaviors that, if we obey the "bright line" stopping points, can use our natural programming to get a great night of sleep. In the light blue are behaviors that will support your energy, sleep, and overall health and wellbeing throughout the day. The rest points are potential points we can use throughout the day when we feel our energy leaving the building. They can help you maintain a healthy and restorative state throughout the day that keeps you effective at work and in balance with your health.

Rituals will play an important part in your Habits of Healthy Sleep, and we will return to those shortly.

Habits of Health Sleep and Energy Clock

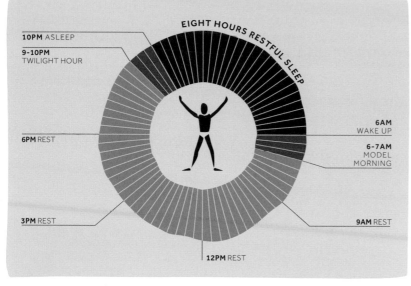

Rest can be Active or Passive, which we will unpack in the Energy section, and may vary daily in the time and length.

The Habits of Health Sleep and Energy clock shows how we should plan and conduct our own 24 hours and how we must make adjustments to our behaviors.

Now let's zoom in and look at the two most vital areas in your biological clock to help you harness your energy, recovery, and set the pace, productivity, and optimal day for supporting your journey to optimal health and wellbeing.

First, it's important to realize that the evening and the morning are the times where we have the most control over our day. Once we are out of the door on our way to work, we become much more limited over being able to create our own schedule.

Most people spend all day tied to a schedule that is usually designed, directed, and accountable to someone else—a world in which you are not the central focus. If we look at our day you can see how we have control over some of our time. In the hours surrounding our sleep, we have more potential control than any other area.

Work: 8 hours, 8am–3pm
Most have little control.

Non-work: 8 hours, 3pm–10pm, 6am–8am
We are mostly in charge, but may have lots of commitments to take care of.

Healthy Sleep: 8 hours, 10pm–6am
Once you decide sleep's importance in making everything work, you can decide to have total control.

"

Why is that young people can sleep under almost any circumstances while older people wake up at the crack of dawn? Because our body secretes less melatonin—a naturally sleep-inducing substance—as we age.

"

"

The word "ritual" came from the Latin word "ritus". In Roman times, ritus were followed religiously because they were a proven way of doing something.

"

EVENING RITUAL AND TWILIGHT

Since your evening ritual is what will set up those uninterrupted hours of healthy sleep, let's dive into how to create the best possible conditions to assure great sleep.

Evening Ritual: From Go to Slow

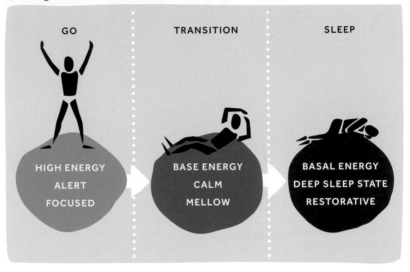

As you create your own personal transition, you need to put an intentional focus on finishing chores and work-related tasks, or resolving any family issues earlier in the evening. The closer you are getting to your hour-before-bedtime ritual, or twilight hour, the more mellow you will become. Dimming the lights and turning off the computer and putting on some soothing music is helpful as well.

As you get better in planning your transition time, you will feel your Go System and stress level decreasing, preparing you for the twilight hour to get your body ready for sleep.

The following is an example of what a twilight hour—defined as one hour before you put your head on your pillow—should look like to initiate the sleep sequence.

Example of a Bedtime Ritual in the Twilight Hour

1 HOUR	30 MINS	15 MINS	IN BED	HEAD ON PILLOW
All pets, children asleep	Out of bath or shower	Last minute entry in *Your LifeBook* or journal	Use the restroom then get in bed	"I love you"
Run hot bath with salts, or shower	Loose-fitting lightweight clothes	Reading with bluelight suppression glasses	Pillows and sheets organized	Hug or goodnight kiss
Thermostat below 68°f	Self-care, teeth brushed and flossed	A few minutes of meditation	Prayer	Mind off
Clean up any clutter	Cool down starts	Deep breathing	Flip the swtich	
All blue light off: TV, computer, phone	Place chamomile, jasmine, lavender on pillow and sheets	Gratitude	Cuddle, partner massage or foot-rub	
Take your medications		Room cold, dark and quite		
Avoid any additional water intake other than a cup of tea		Sleepy-time tea		

If all of this seems a little bit over-structured, that's because it is.

With 80 million people in the U.S. not getting enough quality sleep, we want to make sure you are no longer part of this statistic.[17] With technology overwhelming our body's natural circadian rhythm, we need to create a safe, effective way to shut off our racing mind and induce a restorative sleep. If you do not embrace the kind of structure I have outlined here, you will quickly find yourself reaching for your phone and swiping away what could have been a restful night of healthy sleep.

THE PATH TO HEALTHIER SLEEP

You can go to *Your Lifebook*, Element 19, *How Do You Create Healthy Sleep and Unlimited Energy?*, after reading this and write in the blanks provided. Follow these steps to begin taking back control of your pillow:

Step 1: Find Your Chronotype

Are you a lark or an owl? Your chronotype reflects whether you wake up early and are active and alert in the first part of the day, or prefer to stay up late and are most alert in the evening. Most people aren't wholly one or the other, but somewhere in between.

If most of your sleep occurs at the wrong time of day for your chronotype, it's harder to get the rest you need. Optimally, two circadian markers—maximum amount of melatonin and minimum core body temperature—should occur after the middle of your sleep hours and before you wake up.

Scientists have found that in the morning people's melatonin

Our Caffeine Society

Caffeine is arguably the most robust and popular self-administered drug known to man, with almost 90% of North Americans consuming some form of it on a regular basis.

2.13

Most people aren't harmed by moderate doses of caffeine—say 200 to 300 mg, or about two to three cups of brewed coffee a day. In fact, there is growing research that coffee actually has some powerful health benefits for those that drink it. But it should be consumed in the morning hours to give the drug time to clear from your body. Remember, with a half-life of six hours, caffeine lingers in your body all day and into the night if you've had an afternoon pick-me-up.

Don't alter your bedtime (or wake time) even on the weekends. If you find that you need extra sleep on the weekend, it means you're not getting enough quality sleep during the week.

declines rapidly after it peaks, which may account for their ability to get up early. It declines more slowly in night owls. As far as body temperature, morning types reach their minimum temperature about 4:00 a.m., and evening types at 6:00 a.m.—closer to the time they usually have to get up (and why they are still a little sluggish when they wake up!).

While morning types and evening types both seem to need about the same amount of sleep, knowing which one you are will help you determine which habits and behaviors suit your needs and are, therefore, more likely to succeed. If you're a lark, you might want to get to bed earlier, complete your task list in the evening, and exercise in the morning (actually, this is the ideal time). If you're a night owl, see if you can rearrange your work schedule so you can arrive and leave work later.

The most recent research also reveals that it really does matter when you go to bed, with the ideal time for being asleep being between 10pm and 6am. It appears that we can more easily reach REM sleep in this time, so although you have a built-in tendency, if you can move over time to an early time it will probably enhance your overall sleep and health.

Step 2: Set a Bedtime

Whichever type you are, there's a good chance you have to get up for work in the morning, so in order to set your bedtime, you should first decide what time you need to get up. Count eight hours back from that time which is the range of healthy sleep time. That's when you should be asleep. Your bedtime—the point at which all lights (and other electronic devices) are off—marks the beginning of the sleep latency period or falling-asleep time.

We will have a much more detailed schedule for you to customize your twilight and sleep time in *Your LifeBook:* Element 19, *How Do You Create Healthy Sleep and Unlimited Energy?*.

What's important is establishing a uniform pattern that sets a rhythm and puts your pineal gland back in charge.

Remember that the optimum sleep length—7.5 hours to nine hours—is a guideline. You need to find out what's optimal for you. We will help you tweak that time and amount. A good time to do this is on vacation, when you've left behind the hustle and bustle of your everyday routine (yes, that includes the kids) and can say goodbye to the alarm clock for a while.

You should reach a point when you're going to bed at the same time each night and waking up the same time each day feeling rested. Even cutting back by one hour can decrease your alertness by 35% and move you to a non-sick state. And, just as a reminder, being non-sick isn't being in a good condition.[18]

You'll know you've hit it right when you wake up just before the alarm clock was set to go off.

Also set a specific bedtime for your kids. It can make a profound difference in their performance in the classroom, activity levels, and healthier eating. Remember, honoring the importance of great sleep and installing this habit when they are young can make all the difference. Make sure no digital devices are allowed in their room within an hour of sleepy time and thereafter until the morning.

Step 3: Set Your Routine
Today's chaotic schedules mean that, for the most part, we sleep only when our inability to function forces us to. But, with a little planning, you can change the behaviors that are sabotaging your sleep. In fact, from the moment you wake up, you can start preparing to sleep better the same night.

During the day:
- **Get out of bed:** once you wake up, get up. Limit your in-bed activities to sleeping and lovemaking to avoid sending the wrong signals to your brain.
- **Limit caffeine:** you don't have to give up coffee or caffeinated tea—just savor them in the morning. Once noon rolls around, limit or avoid anything caffeinated, and have absolutely no caffeine within three hours of sleep time.
- **Eat responsibly:** avoid eating within three hours of sleeping. If you really need something before bed, try a small glass of skim milk or chamomile tea. For optimal sleep, eliminate high-glycemic foods throughout the day, and avoid large, energy-dense, or fatty meals in the late evening (a small fueling or portion-controlled meal is fine).

In the Evening:
The evening is your time, and it's important to plan for it wisely. As you head home from work, make a mental note of any tasks or activities that need to be done. For instance, plan to complete your EAT exercises and any other activities that make you break into a sweat at least four hours before bed and even earlier if it seems to interrupt your latency. Here are some guidelines to help you prepare for what I like to call twilight time—the hour before lights out.

- **Decrease stimulation:** since the pineal gland is light-sensitive, it's a good idea to lower your home's ambient light several hours before bed. Turning on a bright light to look for something you need the next day can startle your "third eye". 60 minutes before you plan to hit the pillow, shut off the TV, stop emailing and surfing the Internet, and eliminate any other blue light that raises havoc with your circadian rhythm. In addition, understand that your skin has light receptors, so it is critical that the whole room is dark. A sleep mask will help, but a dark room is much better.
- **Eliminate cell phone use:** recent research indicates that in addition to the blue light from your phone, radiation emitted from your phone may actually stimulate your brain and interrupt sleep. A study at Wayne State University concluded that people who used their cell phones in the evening took longer to fall asleep and

Start Your Day Right:
Say Goodbye to the Alarm Clock
and Hello to the Dawn Simulator

Being startled into alertness by your alarm clock doesn't exactly set you up for a balanced stress-free day, does it? To minimize this morning trauma, try a dawn simulator, a light that increases in intensity gradually at a time you pre-set. As the light falls on your eyes, your brain gets the message to reduce melatonin, preparing your body to wake up naturally.

HEALTHY SLEEP AND UNLIMITED ENERGY: CORNERSTONES OF AN OPTIMAL LIFE

Creating an Environment for
Sleep: Make your bedroom a
comfortable, sleep-inducing
cocoon. Here are some tips:

- Color: Choose a color that soothes you to encourage sleep. Soft pastels such as light blue, green, pink, lavender, yellow, and ivory are calming colors, but so are rich, warm, dark colors such as medium to dark green, chocolate brown, or any rich tans.

- Light: Put your lights on a dimmer and use the lowest setting and avoid fluorescent bulbs in the bedroom. You can buy special night lights that do not have blue light. Apple can actually geo-locate your position and can turn down the blue light after sunset. Also, if you need to read something, there are special glasses you can buy that are inexpensive and will filter out the blue light. Scented candles are fine as long as you remember to blow them out before you get too sleepy. Once the lights are out, make sure your room is completely dark, free of moonlight, streetlights, or glowing clocks and other electrical devices— especially the TV. If necessary, invest in blackout curtains, blinds, or shutters.

- Scent: Try aromatherapy scents like chamomile, jasmine, lavender, neroli, rose, sandalwood, or sweet marjoram. Add essential oils to a dispenser or a hot bath, or just put a few drops on a handkerchief and slip it into your pillowcase.

- Sound: It is very important for your bedroom to be as quiet as possible. You can add an air purifier to create white noise and additionally purify your room. Also, you can buy a sound machine that plays ocean waves, forest noise, or other relaxing sounds.

- Your bed: Take your time choosing a mattress that's the right level of firmness for you. Make sure your spine is aligned neutrally with your pillow— not too high or too low.

- Your temperature: Make sure your bed doesn't get too hot or too cold during the night. Far-infrared quilts, sheets, and pillows can help keep your body temperature neutral. Avoid electric blankets, which can interfere with sleep. Also, wear light comfortable clothes and avoid down quilts that can overheat you.

- Ventilation: Cool the room to 68°F or lower, and maintain adequate ventilation.

- Clutter: Put things away before you make your pre-bedtime bathroom stop, so you're ready to relax once you hit the pillow.

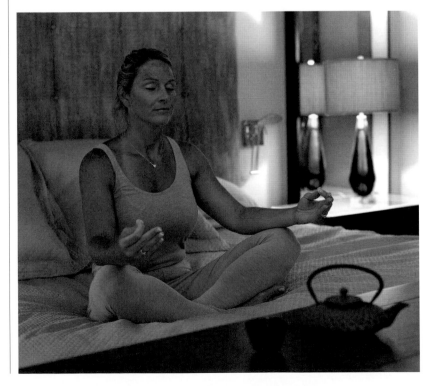

experienced more headaches.[19] If you must talk on your cell phone in the evening, use a headset and turn it off at least two hours before you plan to fall asleep.

- *Minimize liquid intake:* getting up to go to the bathroom is a common sleep disruption. If you find this happening to you, avoid drinking anything two hours before bed and make sure to empty your bladder just before turning in.
- *Avoid exercise within four hours of bedtime:* any other time of day, exercise is a good thing as it helps to increase the body's natural chemicals that induce sleep, but it's too stimulating right before sleep. And make sure you're not sacrificing sleep time for exercise by getting up too early. Giving up some TV time instead leaves you with room in your schedule for exercise and no negative consequences! Morning exercise gives you about 12 hours of improved mood and focus but not at the expense of a lack of sleep.
- *Omega-3 fatty acids:* DHA may improve the length and quality of sleep in children and adults. Refer to the supplementation guide at HabitsofHealth.com for more.
- *Take your medications:* if pain or allergies keep you up, make sure you take any medications an hour before bed so they have time to reach effectiveness. A hot bath can help pain relievers such as ibuprofen get to those sore muscles quicker. Of course, check with your healthcare provider before taking any medication.
- *Avoid alcohol within three hours of bedtime:* alcohol can suppress normal sleep patterns. When it is used to induce sleep, it can cause you to wake up in an arousal state and make healthy sleep difficult to come by.[20]
- *Resolve family issues:* arguments with your spouse, logistical concerns about getting the kids to school, to-do lists for the next day—all these issues should be resolved before bedtime.

Still Can't Sleep?

If you can't get to sleep after 20 minutes, don't lie in bed getting frustrated! Get up and do something else. Go for a walk around the house, take a bath, or read a relaxing book, then reboot and try again. And, even if you're tired the next day, get up at the scheduled time. A day or so of being tired may be all you need to get a good night's rest next time and get back in the habit of healthy, deep, restful sleep.

THE TWILIGHT HOUR: YOUR SLEEPY TIME RITUALS

Let's dive in a little deeper how you can make this sacred hour prepare you for your next optimal day.

This is your time to leave the rest of the world behind! By developing your own personal sleep ritual—one that stays the same each night—you create a conditioned response that tells your body, your brain, and everyone else that you're going off duty. You send the message that, just like a closed ticket window, you and your neurons are simply no longer available (unless the house is on fire, that is).

1. *Preparing your bedroom:* Aim to make your bedroom as visually calming, mentally relaxing, and stress free as possible (see box, page 410, *Creating an Environment for Sleep*). That means that pets, children, and other critters should be in their proper places—

Prepare for Tomorrow, Sleep Easy Tonight

Put your mind to rest before bed by making a to-do list of tasks and priorities for the next day. You'll go to sleep confident that you won't forget something important once your busy day gets going (or wake up in the night worrying about it). Just be sure to make up your list early enough in the evening so you're not thinking about tomorrow's' concerns right before bed.

usually their own beds (I love my Lab, but he's a bed hog and on a different biological clock to mine). And if your significant other snores or has restless legs, get them to their healthcare provider. You'll be helping them out and increasing your chances of a good night's sleep.

2. *Preparing yourself:* Take some time in the bathroom to wash your face, floss, and brush your teeth. If you have time, take a hot bath or shower because research indicates that as your temperature comes down, your body gets sleepy. Then head into some comfy, loose-fitting PJs that don't overheat you—flannel in the winter and cotton in the summer usually does the trick—and maybe even a pair of socks to dilate the blood vessels in your feet and help you relax.

3. *Getting into bed:* Once you're in bed and ready to get sleepy, keep things calm. Some people like to meditate, do breathing exercises, or even a little yoga (for more information, see the sections on stress reduction in Part 3.4, *Brain and Mind Longevity: Protecting and Enhancing Your Future,* and Element 04 of *Your LifeBook, Building a Healthy Mindset*). You may choose to read a relaxing book (set a time limit), cuddle with your partner, or relax with a scalp, neck, shoulder, or foot massage—or whatever else comes up. Or you could just turn off the light and share a goodnight kiss. You can even count sheep! The most important thing is to just let go and let your body drift off naturally without forcing or obsessing. Forget about the outside world and drift into sweet dreams!

THE STRESS AND ANXIETY FACTOR

Research confirms that stress and anxiety are the number one reasons responsible for poor sleep.[21]

In future parts, we will address in detail how we create a healthy mind and flourish in a systematic way in our relationship, thinking, emotional coherence and much more. Here, I want to outline some ways you can immediately lower your stress and anxiety. By now, I hope you are familiar with and using the Stop. Challenge. Choose.™ approach to help put you back in control of your emotions and your response.

The following are some of the best and easiest ways to consciously calm your mind.

1: *Take control of your breath:* if you feel anxiety or stress entering into your day, it is important to use your breathing as a way to calm yourself. First, catch yourself when you feel that icky sensation in the pit of your stomach and take a deep, centering breath. Inhale to six seconds, hold for two, and exhale to seven. Do this four to five times and feel the stress or anxiety leave with each breath.

2: *Use Stop. Challenge. Choose™:* this helps you shake off negative self-talk or break the non-productive loop that you're obsessing over.

*3: **Take five to 10 minutes to meditate:** bring yourself back to the present moment and a calming state. See HabitsofHealth.com for more ways to reduce your stress and anxiety.*

These can be used all day long to help you gain better control of your stress, anxiety, and thoughts. With practice, you can enjoy a calmer mind overall. Also, do all the exercises in Element 23 of *Your LifeBook, Master Your Thoughts and Emotions.*

Beyond that, you will become a master of sleep, flipping that switch, taking that centering breath, shutting your mind off, and entering the right state totally prepared for sleep.

As we mentioned earlier, there are two times during our day when we have almost total control of what we do (depending, of course, on the age of our children). We spent a considerable time on our evening rituals, in moving from full-out motion through transition and slow down to deep, restorative sleep. Now let's move to the time you wake up after eight hours of restorative sleep.

MORNING RITUAL AND JUMP START

The morning provides us the best time to set the tempo, focus, and energy for the coming day. In this period, we are moving from deep sleep and have ingrained the habit to awaken naturally, eager to start the day. I am a firm believer that each morning, you have the opportunity to set the tone for the whole day, and research supports this notion.

As we awaken, we can decide that today will be a day that becomes a little better than yesterday in the key areas and habits we are working on.

HOW DO YOUR MORNINGS START?

Do you wake up in the morning in a calm, relaxed, fully invigorated state, ready to attack the day? If so, congratulations, you're ahead of the game.

For most, it is a little more like a fire drill, with a hectic scramble, filled with a varying degree of stress and chaos. For others, it feels like coming out of a coma with lethargy—a sense of clearing the fog and dreading the day.

As we are rushing to get ready for the day, our minds are plagued with inner thoughts of what we have to do, where we have to go, what we have to accomplish, worrying that we are already running late.

Or maybe there is an unresolved issue with our partner, or our kids. Stressed and rushed or slow and unproductive, we are starting the day on the wrong foot, and it will make it difficult to create an optimal day.

Just like it was critical in the twilight hour to create a ritual to habitualize a routine to align your biological clock to establish high-

Lose the Snooze

For those that use the snooze button, please note that this is a Habit of Disease. In some, this unhealthy habit may last over an hour. Research shows it does not count towards deep restorative sleep. And it sets up a negative precedent to start you day. If you want to break this bad habit, set your alarm clock the night before to the last possible time you can actually get up and make everything happen. Getting up immediately by necessity will help you break this habit in a hurry!

Make Your Bed: It Starts Your Day off Right

It might be a small accomplishment, but it sets the tone for the entire day. No one has extolled the virtue of making your bed each morning as well as Naval Admiral William McRaven, the commander of U.S. Special Operations. In a 2014 commencement speech at University of Texas at Austin, Admiral McRaven said:

"If you make your bed every morning you will have accomplished the first task of the day. It will give you a small sense of pride and it will encourage you to do another task and another and another.

1. It gives you a feeling of accomplishment.
2. It creates a positive state of mind as you go to bed.
3. Make your bed, lower your stress.
4. It prevents embarrassment.
5. It leads to other good habits.

By the end of the day, that one task completed will have turned into many tasks completed. Making your bed will also reinforce the fact that little things in life matter."

Powerful words, and you don't have to be able to bounce a coin off your military-style-made bed to benefit from the act of making it.

quality sleep, the early morning ritual is equally important to establish the optimal physical and mental state to energize and power your day.

Morning Ritual: From Slow to Go

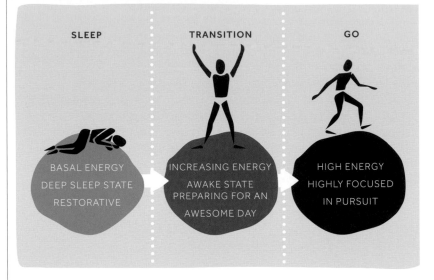

I like to think of the Morning Ritual as a model morning. It is the morning version of the twilight hour in the evening.

By planning and executing a specific routine or ritual in the morning, you are equipped to handle whatever the day throws at you. Our goal is to give you eight solid hours of sleep followed by a model morning that creates a whole transformation of your level of health and wellbeing on which to build your future and assist you on your journey in crafting your new life.

Example of a Ritual for Your Model Morning

AWAKE	CALM	DESIRED OUTCOME	MOTION	SELF CARE	READY WORLD
1 hour before facing the world	Meditate, prayer, reflect 1-10 mins	Focus on what is most important to me	Do 5-10 mins of activity	Shower	Off to work
Get out of bed	Deep breathe	Write down in *Your LifeBook* or journal 3 things I will accomplish today	Walking	Brush and floss teeth	Create an optimal day
Thermostat to normal	Gratitude		Exercize	Other personal hygiene	Fully conscious
Open all blinds to let in sunlight		Visualize your optimal day	Stretch	Fueling	
Use restroom		Possible 10 mins reading			
Weigh		Fuelings, motion, relaxation goals			
Drink glass or two of water					
Put on workout clothes					

If you give yourself an hour just for yourself from awakening until you have to start working with the family, pets, others or leave your home to go to work, you can prepare you mind and body for an optimum day. Let's review this model hour:

Awake

First it is important to adjust the time you go to bed so that in a relatively short time, you are awakening without the alarm. The difference is when we awake without someone or something controlling you it is supports your wishes versus someone else's. I resented having to get up at 5am to go make my rounds every morning before surgery. I have used an alarm less than a dozen times in the last 15 years and wake up naturally, and it really starts my day off right.

But until you get that figured out, you can use a Natural Dawn Simulator Alarm Clock that will simulate the lighting in the morning and wake you up gently.

Once you are awake, get out of bed and do not use the snooze feature. This is critical to create the habit of starting the day every morning with eager anticipation and that the next hour is going to be like Christmas morning and you are going to give yourself a gift before you are available to others. Again, you have to work around family logistics to make this happen.

Open up the blinds or drapes immediately, as the bright light will help your brain turn off any residual sleep chemicals and turn on awake chemicals. Raise the room temperature, go to the restroom, weigh yourself to record your current weight reality, and then put on your workout clothes that you have made conveniently available the night before.

Calm

This is the period of time you align your body and your mind to a state of peace, calm, and clarity of what your purpose is, why you are improving your habits and relationships, and setting the right tone for your day.

Desired Outcome

Once you have yourself centered and in control, you can start visualizing what your day will look like, what you will accomplish, and the priorities you will focus on. Depending on how much time you have, it's always good to read something that will help you with your personal or spiritual growth.

Also, make sure you are focused on your habit installation. The Habits of Health App can help you.

Motion

As we discussed in the section on motion, active movement will give you up to 12 hours of improved focus, mood, and energy. As little as 20 minutes is the equivalent of a hit of Ritalin and Prozac in improving your mental and physical state!

In his renowned 1993 study of young violinists, performance researcher Anders Ericsson found that the best ones all practiced the same way: in the morning, in three increments of no more than 90 minutes each, with a break between each one. Ericsson discovered the same pattern among other musicians, athletes, chess players and writers. This is the same study that established the 10,000 hours of deliberate practice for mastery. On another note from that study he found that another factor significantly influenced peak performance. Guess what it was? Sleep! The best performers on average slept eight hours and 36 minutes. On average, the USA gets just six hours and 51 minutes of sleep on weekdays![22]

Self-Care

This is the time you conclude your model hour with a hot shower directed to your neck and back, as well as brushing and flossing your teeth. During this period, I visualize and smile as I anticipate an amazing day ahead of me as well as express gratitude for everything around me. Then I shave, dry off, put my clothes on and, presto, I am ready to interact in an attractive and successful way with my surroundings.

And the final step is to prepare and fuel yourself with a high-quality first meal of the day.

Ready

At this point, I have preemptively prepared my thoughts, emotions, energy, priorities, and direction to have an optimal day.

> *Note: contact with the outside world isn't part of this ritual. If you are using the recommended times of optimal sleep, this morning model will have you ready to interact with your family by 7:00 am. I focus on my family and my dogs but, most importantly, I have prepared myself with the model morning to create an optimal day for myself before I let the outside world in.*

Depending on your individual needs, such as tending to your children and other family members or other early morning requirements, you can expand or shrink these 60 minutes to fit your obligations.

Developing Habits of Health and rituals that fuel the start of your day and having proper direction can change everything.

YOUR OPTIMAL DAY: ENERGY LEVEL

If everything went well and your evening ritual and twilight hour went without a hitch, you should have had 7.5 hours or more of high quality sleep. Your model morning will place you in the best possible position to have an optimal day. If you have installed the rituals and they are now your Habits of Healthy Sleeping, I will bet you have increased your energy and you'll be in great shape to create better health and wellbeing.

Unfortunately, this does not prevent you from occasionally having a bad night of sleep. Your child may be sick, a bad storm keeps you up, you do not feel well, or you just had a nightmare. And we all have times during the day where we become fidgety or drowsy and just need to take a break.

All is not lost. I will explain how your body cycles its energy throughout the day. And yes, we have this marvelous device called a nap to fall back on. When I wrote the first version of this book 10 years ago, it was thought that napping would actually cause harm. Since then the research has been corrected.

If you go back to Roman times, they had a ritual of napping called Sexta. Sexta means the sixth hour, which was around noon. The siesta, or afternoon nap, was derived from this Latin ritual. It appears that modern man is one of the only animals in nature that attempts to get all its rest at the same time. My labradors remind me of that all day long!

What we are finding is that naps are essential for maintaining our brain, emotional, and overall physical energy throughout the day. Naps can help reestablish our level of energy optimization.

OUR REST AND ENERGY WAVES

It seems that within our waking hours we have 90-minute cycles called Ultradian rhythms, which are similar to our nightly circadian rhythms.

The ultradian rhythm is the equivalent daytime cycle needed to have effective attention and focus.

During the day, we move from higher to lower alertness. When we need a rest, our body signals us by hunger, drowsiness, fidgetiness, or loss of focus. We generally override this need of the body for rest with caffeine, foods high in sugar, and simple high glycemic carbs, and our bodies produce stress hormones like adrenaline, noradrenaline, and cortisol.

In the following diagram the red area illustrates when these stress hormones and are released and the effect they have on both our productivity and our health.

Ultradian Cycle

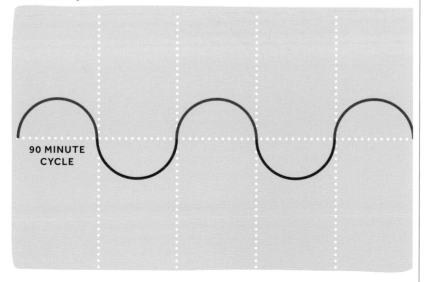

90 MINUTE CYCLE

Advantages of Napping

- Greater alertness
- Better memory and learning capacity
- Increased creativity and sensitivity
- Better health
- Better mood
- Monetary savings[23]

If we work at high intensity for more than 90 minutes, we begin to draw on these emergency reserves to keep us going. Effectively, that means we move from parasympathetic to sympathetic arousal—the physiological state we have discussed several times known as "fight or flight".

The problem is that many of us have become addicted to the adrenalin rush generated by our own stress hormones. Being digitally connected 24/7 also keeps us wired physically and emotionally.

We've convinced ourselves (and we've been convinced by the cultures we work in) that this is how we need to work to get it all done. The problem is that seeking more, bigger, faster generates value that is narrow, shallow, and short-term.

One consequence of relying on our stress hormones as a source of energy is that the prefrontal cortex begins to shut down in fight or flight mode. We become more reactive and less capable of thinking clearly, reflectively, or imaginatively.

These extended periods without rest are not only counter to our productivity, but also our health. So, how can we create the necessary rest waves or napping needed for daytime recovery and optimization?

There are two different recovery methods: Passive Rest and Active Rest. Both are important to boost energy, re-establish alertness, create focus, and improve selective attention.

Ultradian Cycle

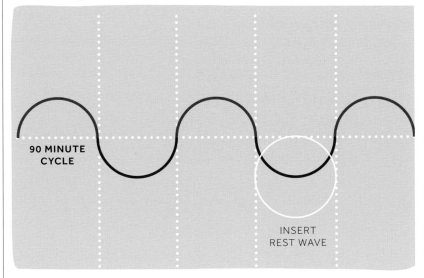

90 MINUTE CYCLE

INSERT REST WAVE

PASSIVE REST

These are true sleep naps and can be divided into two categories based on the length and depth of sleep: power naps and REM naps.

Power Naps

These are six to 20 minute naps that are short and partially replenish our neurotransmitters. Because they are short and create quick recovery, they are ideal for your work day when time is usually limited. If they extend longer than 20 minutes, they can leave you in a groggy state.[24]

REM Naps

These are longer naps that actually place us in a complete sleep cycle including the REM state. Because they need approximately 90-plus minutes, they are not practical for most during the work week. They are deeply restorative and, as long as they do not occur less than three hours before twilight hour, can help keep your energy high when it is needed.

ACTIVE REST

These are methods you can employ throughout the day that help boost your energy, calm your mind, and also help you sleep better that night by keeping your mind from over-racing. There are four key areas that can help restore and balance you energy and alertness:

1. **Physically:** deep breathing, stretching,
2. **Mentally:** meditate, gratitude, listen to soothing music
3. **Socially:** family, friends
4. **Spiritually:** prayer or meditation

As a result of insertion of either active or passive rest waves, you can see we are able to recover much quicker and be much more effective, alert, and productive, as well as take the stress burden and negative health consequences out of the equation. This is the true power of the Habits of Health Sleep and Energy restoration—taking suboptimal days and having them aligned with your health and wellbeing.

Passive Rest Naps activate the sleep version of the rest-activity cycle, which works differently than the waking rest-activity cycle. If you are so fatigued that you need a nap, and a nap is available to you, then by all means take a nap.

Passive Rest:

If you are sitting, close your eyes and listen to your breath and sense your pulse. If you are walking, listen to your breath and sense your pulse but pay attention to where you are walking. Ease into these biological rhythms.

HABITS OF HEALTH

Rest Waves Allow us to Recover

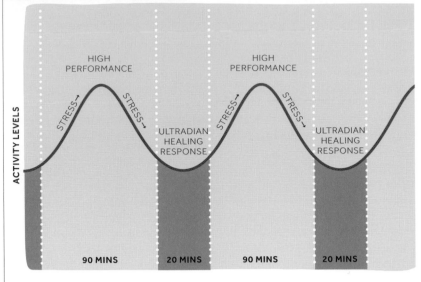

SLEEP DEBT

Another misconception was that you can't make up lost sleep. The incredible advancements in sleep and energy management show that this is not accurate. Inserting naps when you energy level is low or you have had a bad night of sleep can actually help you recover quicker, as seen above in the process of ultradian healing.

In addition, you can decide to go to bed earlier, which will allow you to recover quickly. You will know that you have recovered once you wake up in the morning without the need of an alarm clock.

In *Your LifeBook* in Element 19, *How Do You Create Healthy Sleep and Unlimited Energy?* we provide some questions and a log sheet so you can track your debit and create a plan to recover, putting you in the best position to be an ultradian energy master.

A GOLDEN HOUR

As we conclude the section on sleep, you may still be saying to yourself that you would love to sleep more and add these rituals but you just do not have time. My advice to you is make time. That golden extra hour of sleep (or whatever is needed to get to eight hours) is so crucial to helping you create optimal health and wellbeing. And hopefully now you understand that when you have eight hours of quality sleep, your model morning, and use active and passive rest, your ability to deliver on your work and your habit installation will become easier and more effective.

Here is an idea that might help you find time. In *The Productivity Project*, efficiency expert Chris Bailey talks about the fact that in the age of knowledge it is not time that matters but what we accomplish. This book is all about working smarter by measuring and optimizing your energy and your attention.

The good news is that we just showed you many ways to optimize your attention and energy. By using these principles and by adding a concept he calls Biologic Prime Time (BPT), you can become much more effective at using your most valuable time to do the deep work that requires your highest level of attention and energy. In essence, he shows you how to find the period during the day when you have the highest level of attention and energy and accomplish the most. Knowing when this time falls will allow you to accomplish more in a shorter period of time so you will have more time for sleep and recovery. It's easy. You just pick a three-week period where you:

- Cut out all coffee and alcohol from your diet
- Eat as little sugar as possible (Habit of Disease)
- Eat small, frequent meals throughout the day for fuel
- Wake up and fall asleep naturally without an alarm

Then over the three weeks, you just need to track when you have the highest level of energy in your body and your mind and use these BPT to accomplish the projects that require your higher level of executive function.

In addition, once you know exactly what you want for your future self (which we have been building in *Your LifeBook*), you are becoming more disciplined at only doing the things that move you toward that future. As we discussed earlier, you will be eliminating anything that is not serving you or moving you toward your desired outcome.

Off-purpose activities such as the Internet, social media, TV, and other distracting media and devices that waste your time will lose their power over you. You will jump out of bed in the morning and design your whole day and into your evening around becoming more productive.

The Golden Hour that will increase your ability to do everything better will be yours.

It's time to go beyond the fundamentals and begin optimizing all areas of our health for longevity.

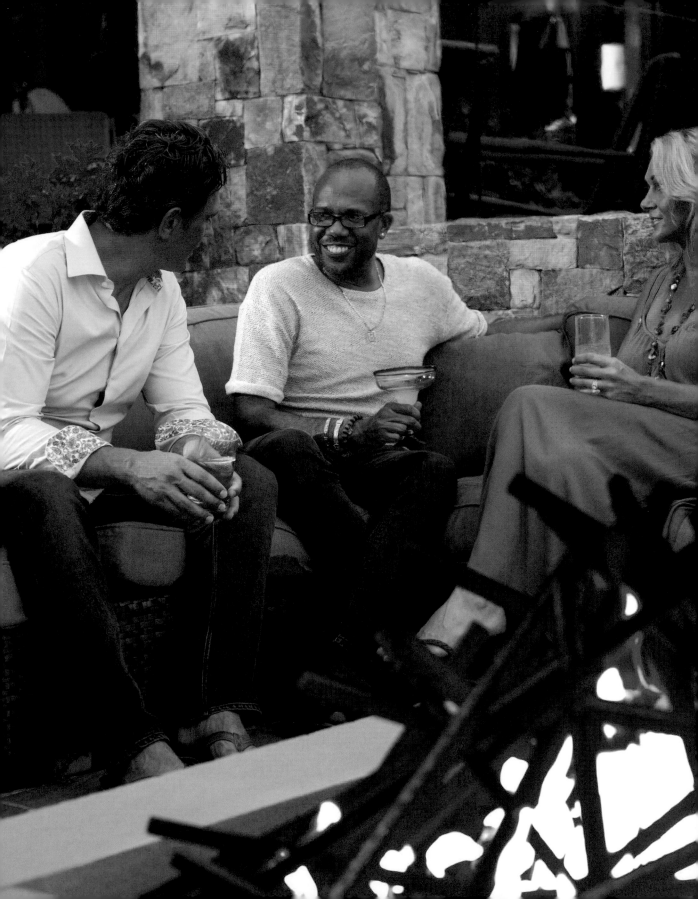

INFLAMMATION: DOUSING THE FLAME

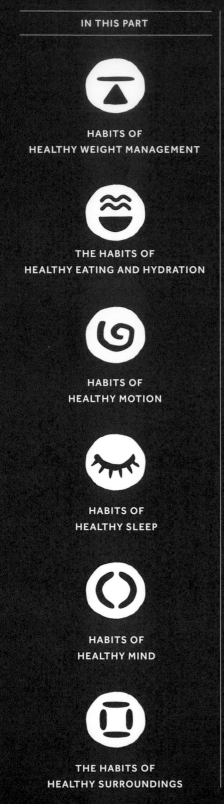

IN THIS PART

**HABITS OF
HEALTHY WEIGHT MANAGEMENT**

**THE HABITS OF
HEALTHY EATING AND HYDRATION**

**HABITS OF
HEALTHY MOTION**

**HABITS OF
HEALTHY SLEEP**

**HABITS OF
HEALTHY MIND**

**THE HABITS OF
HEALTHY SURROUNDINGS**

All six MacroHabits are involved in this part because unless the body is optimized, then the opportunity for your body to be attacked by your surroundings is a real threat that can easily become an all-out assault. The assault doesn't just come from the world around us, but from our inner world, especially if we have not provided it with the proper type and amount of nutrition, the right amount of movement and sleep, the benefit of balanced relationships, or attended to the healthy mind that can create internal calm and balance.

For most of us, inflammation probably conjures up images of a swollen sore throat that keeps us in bed all weekend gargling salt water or a red infected lump that swells around a cut. In cases like these, our immune system jumps into appropriate action by sending in white blood cells, bombarding the invading bacteria, and then we're back to normal in a few days.

The immune system—our own personal 24/7 on-call emergency service— has an incredible ability to seek out intruders such as bacteria, viruses, and parasites. In fact, it's the most complex system in the body. It not only defends us, but it remembers every battle it's ever fought so it can recognize repeated threats and avoid wasting time on harmless ones. Its purpose is to restore balance to an unbalanced body, and once it's done its job, it should settle down into its normal, vigilant state to await the next crisis.

Unfortunately, that's not always what happens. As medical science is beginning to discover, this benevolent protector has a darker side that can all too easily turn on its master, especially if we make the Habits of Disease our way of life.

When you eat donuts and coffee for breakfast, a fatty cheeseburger for lunch, and a bowl of ice cream before bed or when you carry extra fat around your middle, smoke cigarettes, and refuse to get off the couch, your immune system goes on alert. Instead of an all-out attack, it trickles inflammatory molecules into your blood in quantities so small they can only be detected through a special test. Unnoticed, these inflammatory biochemicals work their sinister effect against your blood vessels, joints, brain, and other critical systems. It may start with stiff, painful joints, or tired-looking skin, or something far more menacing, like cancer, a stroke, or Alzheimer's disease.

Our hostile environment stimulates our immune system every day through thousands of little exposures, and the resulting damage to our health and longevity can be staggering. In fact, we're only beginning to understand the magnitude of the effect that a chronically elevated immune system has on our body. What we do know is this: the continual production of inflammatory markers is aging our organs, and us, prematurely. In fact, it's quite likely that human longevity could stretch to 150 years or more, if only we could get our immune systems under control.

THE SILENT ENEMY

Most of us only pay attention to inflammation when it has become acute, but we now know that chronic, low-grade inflammation attacks our health and plays a central role in degenerative diseases and aging. Just look at the following chart to see the many ways a hyperactive immune system can affect your body. The negative effects, however, begin long before these disease states express themselves.

"*The negative effects of an overactive immune system aren't felt overnight. But over time, if we keep our immune system in action on bad habits such as eating unhealthy foods, avoiding exercise, neglecting our sleep, or handling stress poorly, then our bodies will begin to age and break down prematurely.*"

2.14

INFLAMMATION: DOUSING THE FLAME

Inflammation:
A Key Player in Heart Disease

Until just a few years ago, the medical community focused on cholesterol and triglycerides as the main culprits in heart disease. Now, thanks to a landmark study at the Harvard School of Public Health, we know that chronic inflammation—specifically the presence of C-reactive protein, an inflammatory marker—plays a major role in the development of heart disease.[1]

It begins when the immune system becomes over-stimulated. It could be something you breathe, eat, drink, see, feel, hear, or think, even from something as benign as sitting on the couch for too long. Carrying those extra pounds around your middle is a major contributor as well. Whether precipitated by the need to fight dangerous bacteria or as the result of a Big Gulp loaded with high-fructose corn syrup, the result is the same: inflammatory molecules begin circulating at high levels in your blood. They kill the enemy, but, at the same time, they have serious consequences on innocent bystanders, including your heart, blood vessels, brain, pancreas, kidneys, and other blood-rich organs, which begin a series of small conflicts against you.

The Silent Enemy: Conditions Caused by an Inflammatory State

CARDIOVASCULAR SYSTEM	• High cholesterol/triglycerides • High blood pressure • Atrial fibrillation	• Abdominal aortic aneurysm • Stroke • Sudden death
RESPIRATORY SYSTEM	• Light sleep • Nasal polyps	• Sinus infections
GASTRO-INTESTINAL SYSTEM	• Ulcerative colitis • Crohns disease • Obesity	• Inflammatory bowel disease
KIDNEYS	• Glomerulonephritis • Nephrotic syndrome • Nephritic syndrome	• Acute or chronic renal failure
IMMUNE SYSTEM	• Atopic dermatitis • Rheumatoid arthritis • Multiple sclerosis	• Psoriasis • Allergies
BRAIN	• Alzheimers • Mood disorders	• Depression • Schizophrenia
ENDOCRINE SYSTEM	• Non-alcoholic fatty liver disease	• Diabetes
EYES	• Macular degeneration	
OTHER	• Breast colon and prostate cancers	

Chronic, low-grade inflammation attacks our health and plays a central role in degenerative diseases and aging.

The good news is that you have an antidote to these insurgencies: the Habits of Health. The MacroHabits you have been learning and applying to your daily life will help protect you against inflammation. In this part, we are going to focus on additional habits that will optimize and guard you against each mini-mutiny and turn your immune system back into the protector it's meant to be. Let's start by looking at how your immune system operates: what is it that puts the bad guys in motion, and how do they cause so much trouble?

FREE RADICALS AND OXIDATIVE STRESS

In a controlled state, the oxygen in your body fuels health. When oxygen molecules are disrupted—forming what you've probably heard described as free radicals—they can kill cells, damage your DNA, and cause you to age prematurely.

Actually, in short-lived, local release, these oxygen radicals aren't harmful. Produced through a process called oxidative stress, they're actually used by the immune system to protect you by killing dangerous invaders, but if oxidative stress and inflammation are allowed to continue, a dangerous cycle is set in motion, with inflammation creating more oxidative stress. More oxidative stress fuels the inflammatory process. As you can see from the following illustration, the Habits of Disease have a profound effect on that cycle.

Habits of Disease that Cause Inflammation

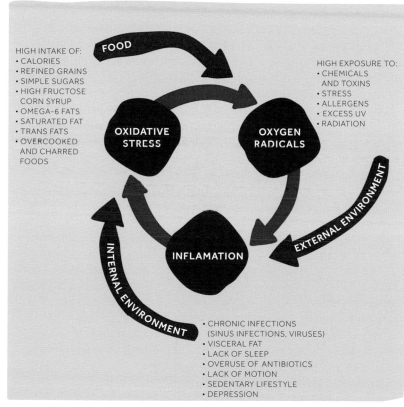

Inflammation is spurred by internal factors, external factors, and the type of food we eat. These Habits of Disease increase oxidative stress, causing our body to create oxygen radicals which, when left unchecked, produce chronic inflammation and cause further oxidative stress— a vicious cycle that slowly erodes our health and brings about disease.

> *Sitting is the most ignored health threat of our times. This lack of movement is activating our immune system and eroding our health, now killing more people in world than smoking![2]*

Eskimos have a similar prevalence of coronary artery disease as non-Eskimo populations, they have excessive mortality due to cerebrovascular strokes, their overall mortality is twice as high as that of non-Eskimo populations, and their life expectancy is approximately 10 years shorter than the Danish population.[3]

INFLAMMATION: DOUSING THE FLAME

Nix the Barbie!

Overcooking, and especially charring food on the grill, creates extremely dangerous compounds called advanced glycation end products (AGES) that are potent inflammatory agents and can actually increase your level of LDL—the bad cholesterol. Steam, bake, or boil your foods instead.

mHoH

Remove sources of harmful chemicals from your home by taking clothes out of dry-cleaning bags and avoiding harsh pesticides used on your lawn, which then get tracked inside.

Internal Environment

Exposing our bodies again and again to the Habits of Disease and environments that support them eventually chips away at our health. Like a boulder slowly eroding in a mountain stream, the effect doesn't happen overnight but eventually leaves us with a battered body, premature aging, and a shortened life. Our blood vessels and organs actually wear out, leaving us vulnerable to attack. You may have experienced a taste of this when you've been run down and more susceptible to infection. Your immune system just gets too fatigued to strike back.

To get rid of this dangerous inflammatory state, we need to create a microenvironment of health, both through the Habits of Health you've already learned and through some new ones you're about to discover.

Are You At Risk?

There's actually a way to measure your level of immune activation, using the C-reactive protein (CRP) test. Elevated CRP, which occurs when inflammation is present in the body, is highly predictive of cardiovascular disease. In fact, elevated CRP can boost your heart attack risk by 300%, even if your cholesterol levels are normal. This test can also predict your risk of other inflammatory diseases, such as arthritis and cancer.[4]

While anything under three mg/L is considered a normal CRP, our goal is to get you down to under one mg/L through healthy diet, exercise, healthy sleep and rest, and by looking closely at three important contributors to inflammation—the food we eat, our environment, and our stress level.

Food and Inflammation

Food provides us with critical nutrients that keep us healthy and help us grow, but many types of foods also contain toxins that harm or even poison our bodies.

The typical Western diet—known as the Standard American Diet (SAD)—is full of processed, high-glycemic carbohydrates and saturated animal fats, both of which are extremely inflammatory. In fact, many of the elements that make up these foods actually provide more toxins than nutrients. In the following chart you can see over half of the SAD diet is inflammatory. One of our chief enemies, and a major contributor to ill health, is processed food.

Pro-inflammatory Components in the American Diet (in Orange)

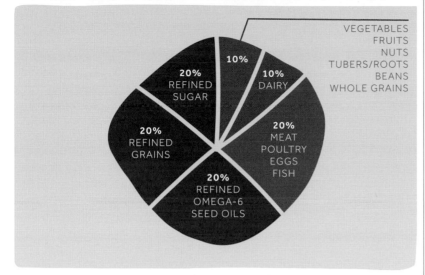

An astounding percentage of the average Western diet—over 70% —is now made up of processed foods.[5] The high level of chemicals in processed foods stimulates the immune system, which senses those chemicals as foreign intruders and attackers. And so it stands to reason that you can lower your state of inflammation by eating healthy, unprocessed whole foods. If, due to time constraints, you absolutely must eat processed foods, try to choose those with the fewest chemical ingredients. Here are some foods to look out for:

Carbohydrates
Processed, high-glycemic carbohydrates contribute to inflammation. But the good news is that the healthy, low-glycemic foods we've discussed in the parts on healthy eating for life can actually help reduce it. To help your body scavenge free radicals and quell inflammation, you should increase your consumption of the following:

- Low-glycemic foods
- Fruits and vegetables, especially those that are red, orange, or yellow
- Carotenoids (found in papaya, tangerine, yellow peppers, pumpkin, winter squash, sweet potato, carrots, apricot, cantaloupe)
- Vitamin C (found in citrus fruits, tomatoes, berries, peppers, sweet potato, broccoli, cauliflower, asparagus, dark green leafy vegetables)
- Quercetin (found in blueberries, blackberries, dark cherries, grapefruit, onions, apples)

Fats
The literature on this topic is very confusing, and most people struggle to understand which are the healthy fats and oils. The Standard

> *Ask your healthcare provider about testing your* CRP. *You should be tested at least every five years using a high-sensitivity C-reactive protein assay (hs-*CRP*), which can help determine your risk of heart disease and other inflammation-related conditions.*

2.14

Keep Inflammation in Check with These Handy Diet Tips

- Maintain a healthy weight by lowering your daily calorie consumption.
- Eat good fats (omega-3, monounsaturated fats).
- Avoid bad fats (trans-fats, saturated fats, animal fats, excess omega-6).
- Avoid overcooking and charring foods.
- Eat more fruits and vegetables, especially low-glycemic vegetables and antioxidant-rich colored vegetables.
- Eat more fiber through whole-grains.
- Avoid sugar, highly refined carbohydrates, and high-fructose corn syrup.
- Cook with anti-inflammatory herbs and spices.
- Incorporate modest amounts of antioxidant-rich supplements and foods such as red wine, dark chocolate, and green tea.

Fight Inflammation while You Eat!

According to research from the U.S. Department of Agriculture, eating antioxidant-rich foods can help ward off inflammation by blunting the oxidative stress produced by a meal high in carbohydrates, proteins, and fats. So when it comes to antioxidants, timing is everything!

American Diet (SAD) provides way too much of the wrong kinds of fat and oils. The SAD diet fats and oils promote the free radicals we discussed earlier, increasing our risk of chronic inflammatory disorders.

What we'll do is create clarity on what you can do to maximize your healthy fat intake and optimize your health and help you understand that fats can have amazing anti-inflammatory properties, as long as they're the right type of fats and in the right amounts.

There are four areas to guide you on how you optimize your daily fat ingestion:

First: you need to understand that fats and oils are extremely calorie-dense and it is important to eat them as part of a well-balanced diet. If you are eating too many calories, even good ones, and you are gaining weight that is stored as visceral adiposity, then you are in a pro-inflammatory state.

Second: polyunsaturated fats occur in two main types of fats—omega-3 and omega-6—both of which contain essential fatty acids. The term "essential" means our bodies cannot produce them naturally so they must be obtained from our diet. Both are considered polyunsaturated fats, but the way our body responds to them is different.

- Omega-3 fatty acids have an anti-inflammatory effect on the body. Two vital dietary omega-3 fatty acids are eicosapentaenoic acid (EPA) and docosahexaenoic acid (DHA), which reduce inflammation, cardiovascular disease, and even blood clotting. Omega-3s are abundant in cold water fish, like salmon and sardines, but can also be found in vegetarian sources such as whole flaxseed, chia seeds, hemp seeds, walnuts, and blue green algae.

- Omega-6 fatty acids also help to produce hormones, but they differ from those created by omega-3s. Omega-6 fatty acids tend to *increase* inflammation, cell proliferation, and blood clotting. Inflammation is caused by a type of omega-6 called eicosanoids. The more eicosanoids in your body, the more inflammation you risk experiencing, especially if you are not counteracting them with anti-inflammatory omega-3s.

Both types of omegas are needed for your body to function properly, but problems begin to occur when the system and the amount of each is off balance. Like everything else, balance brings harmony to our health. Because it seems easier for us to get omega-6s, you will need to make an effort to make sure and get your omega-3s.

The SAD diet tends to include too much omega-6. To keep inflammation in balance, it's important to maintain a ratio of no more than 4:1 (omega-6 to omega-3), though a 1:1 ratio is ideal!

Anti-Inflammatory Omega-3 and Inflammatory Omega-6 Fats

ANTI INFLAMMATORY OMEGA-3	
Oils	Flaxseed, canola, walnut, olive
Fish	Mackerel, sardines, herring salmon, bluefish, cod, scallops, tuna, lobster
Nuts/seeds	Flaxseed, walnuts, pecans
Greens/beans	Soybeans, tofu
Greens	Spinach, kale, collard greens
INFLAMMATORY OMEGA-6	
Oils	Corn, cottonseed, safflower, sesame, soybean
Margarine	
Ultra-processed foods or food with a long shelf life	

Omega-3 fats are an essential part of a healthy, anti-inflammatory diet. However, most Western diets are too high in omega-6. Be sure to keep your ratio of omega-6 to omega-3 less than 4:1 (a ratio of 1:1 is ideal).

Third: monosaturated fats are another very important type of healthy fat. They have proven health benefits that include reducing cholesterol, inflammation, and cardiovascular risk. Olive oil is perhaps the most important and useful of these fats, with its own unique antioxidant properties, including a large dose of oleocanthal—a powerful healthy anti-inflammatory compound that works like ibuprofen and similar over-the-counter medications to reduce inflammation and pain. Using cold-pressed extra virgin olive oil in your meals will give you a higher concentration of monounsaturated fat than any other edible oil.

You can also increase your consumption of monosaturated fats by eating more nuts, butters, and spreads that are made from raw nuts, avocados, olives, and high-quality oils. The following chart will give you a quick guide, but on the whole it's best to stick with monounsaturated and some polyunsaturated fats whenever possible.

Fourth: you should choose cooking oils with a high smoke point. The smoke point is partly determined by the type of oil. For example, walnut oil starts to smoke when it's at about 320°F, whereas grapeseed oil can be heated to 475°F before it begins to smoke. The refining process of the oil is another important factor when it comes to cooking. Removing the impurities from oil through the refining process will also increase its smoke point. For instance, extra virgin olive oil starts smoking at 325°F, but light or refined olive oil can be heated to 450°F or higher.

High-Heat Cooking

For frying, searing, grilling, stir-frying, or roasting, use oils with low polyunsaturated fats and a high smoke point, such as a light or refined olive oil, avocado oil, refined palm, or coconut oil.

" Refined vegetable oils and saturated fats are full of eicosanoids, without the anti-inflammatory, heart-healthy benefits of omega-3s. These are found in almost all ultra-processed food and should be reduced or eliminated from your diet. Avoid seed oils such as corn, sunflower, safflower, peanut, and soybean. "

2.14

INFLAMMATION: DOUSING THE FLAME

Which oils are best and which should you avoid?

A healthy, anti-inflammatory diet should include the following oils:

- **Olive:** Highest in oleocanthal, a powerful anti-inflammatory that works like ibuprofen to reduce pain and swelling
- **Flaxseed:** Rich in omega-3 and low in omega-6
- **Canola:** The least saturated oil, high in vitamin E
- **Coconut oil**

Use sparingly, if at all:

- Corn oil
- Sunflower oil
- Safflower oil
- Peanut oil
- Soybean oil

Steer clear of the following:

- **Trans-fats:** An extremely inflammatory fat
- **Fatty meats, especially overcooked or charred foods:** Can increase inflammation through the breakdown of protein and fats

Medium-Heat Cooking

For sautéing, stewing, baking, or braising use a light or refined olive oil, avocado oil, refined palm, or coconut oil. They all will work fine. But if you prefer extra flavor, choose a filtered olive oil.

Reuse of Cooking Oil

You should avoid reusing vegetable oils, as they rapidly become breeding grounds for hydrogenated byproducts and oxygen radicals. Even food that is cooked in trans-fat-free vegetable oil becomes saturated on repeat cooking.

Off-Heat Cooking

For salad dressings or drizzling over a dish, an unfiltered extra virgin olive oil, or unrefined or toasted nut oil will give you great flavor and maximum health benefits.

Anti-Inflammatory and Inflammatory Fats

ANTI-INFLAMMATORY		
MONO-UNSATURATED FATS		
• Olive oil • Almonds • Canola oil	• Avocado • Peanut oil	
POLY-UNSATURATED FATS		
• Vegetable oils (corn, soybean, safflower, cottonseed)	• Fish	
SATURATED FATS		
• Whole milk • Red meat • Butter	• Coconut oil (healthy in small amounts) • Cheese	
TRANS FATS		
• Partially hydrogenated vegetable oils • Most margarines • Baked goods	• Vegetable shortening • Commercially prepared French fries	

A healthy, anti-inflammatory diet should contain primarily monounsaturated and, to a lesser extent, polyunsaturated fats. Saturated fats and trans-fats are inflammatory and should be avoided.

Other Anti-Inflammatory Foods

Fighting inflammation doesn't mean depriving yourself. Here's a list of some specialty foods and spices with unique properties that can help you quell the fire of inflammation, including some favorites that you might enjoy adding to your diet:

- *Herbs:* many herbs are great for countering inflammation, including ginger, rosemary, turmeric (and its component, curcumin), oregano, cayenne, cloves, nutmeg, feverfew, and boswellia.

- **Teas:** teas contain catechins, a powerful anti-inflammatory and antioxidant. White tea contains the most, followed by green tea, and then black tea. Try to drink two to three cups per day to begin receiving the benefits.
- **Chocolate:** chocolate also contains catechins, and well as polyphenols, another antioxidant. Choose dark chocolate (at least 70% cacao), which contains 10 times the antioxidants found in milk chocolate.
- **Wine:** you've probably heard of the French paradox. Despite a diet high in saturated fats, the French have lower rates of heart disease than many other Western nations. Why? Because they enjoy wine in moderation. Moderate amounts of alcohol (one drink a day for women, one to two for men) lowers inflammation and the risk of heart disease and type 2 diabetes. Red wine in particular is a potent antioxidant and anti-inflammatory and has even been shown to extend life in animal studies.

For more information on red wine and longevity, visit HabitsofHealth.com.

YOUR ENVIRONMENT AND INFLAMMATION

Like the foods we eat, the world around us can affect our immune system. But by paying attention and making the necessary changes in the way we live, we can decrease our exposure to potential immune activators.

The Air You Breathe

We would all want to lower the amount of smog and pollution in the environment. But did you know that our greatest air pollution risk is actually inside our homes and offices?

The development of more energy-efficient houses and buildings, combined with a greater use of synthetics, has resulted in a new medical condition called sick building syndrome. Even brief exposure to volatile organic compounds such as radon, chloroform, and styrene can raise your CRP level. If that's the case, how do you know if you're affected? If you suffer from headaches, fatigue, or respiratory symptoms that are relieved when you're away from home or work—on vacation, for example—but that come back immediately on your return, you may want to get tested (or get a new job!). A simple CRP screen can help determine if you're being exposed to an inflammatory environment.

Other toxins include bacteria, molds, mites, and biological toxins in the air, including the very dangerous Stach toxic mold. Treatment begins by identifying the source of the toxins and removing them from your environment. Air filters may help, as well as increasing

> *Only buy first-press olive oil that have the highest levels of antioxidants and anti-inflammatory properties. Keep your bottle fresh, buying only what you will use in a month. Store it in the dark, and away from a hot stove.*

What is Canola Oil?

Is it a seed or nut? Actually it's derived from rapeseed oil (which originally had too much erucic acid and caused heart lesions in lab animals). Canadian researchers have bred strains of rapeseed with very low to inconsequential levels of erucic acid which are safe. Safe processing to make the oil healthier meant it was given a new name: Canola (Canada, Oil, Low, Acid). There are no studies to date that show it to be a problem, but it is new. We know, olive oil, coconut oil, and even butter have been used safely for many generations.

"

Want to learn some great anti-inflammatory recipes and find out more about the relationship between food and inflammation? Check out Anti-Inflammatory Foods for Health, by Barbara Rowe, MPH, RD, LD, CNSD, *and Lisa M. Davis,* PHD, PA-C, CNS, LDN *(Fair Winds Press, 2008).*

"

ventilation by opening windows and doors, especially in new buildings.

I highly recommend that you use a HEPA (high-efficiency particulate air) filter, either through a whole-house system or in individual rooms. Available on vacuum cleaners, HEPA filters are capable of filtering even tiny particles that are as small as one micron. These filters can be expensive, but every particle they filter out of the air you breathe would otherwise be inhaled into your lungs and make its way into your blood, leaving your overburdened immune system with the task of locating, identifying, and disposing of each and every particle.

Your Water Supply

Focusing on healthy hydration is one of our MacroHabits and a key building block of optimal health. One of the vital roles in anti-inflammation is to help your immune system—through lymphatics—flush out any toxins that build up and are sequestered by our immune system. Unfortunately unless you have a safe source of obtaining your water and fluids you could be adding to the inflammation. Your water may not be helping.

It's hard to look at the news these days without hearing about another contaminant found in our tap water. Painkillers, hormones, pesticides, household cleaners are all potent inflammatory agents and then there are the plasticizers, dioxin, and heavy metals that have been linked to autoimmune diseases. More and more people are turning to bottled and filtered water to avoid substances like these, but deciding which type is best can be confusing.

Bottled water comes from a variety of sources, usually indicated on the packaging. Artesian well water taps into an aquifer under the earth's surface, which helps protect the water from contamination. Mineral water comes from an underground source that contains natural minerals and trace elements. Spring water is sourced from underground springs that flow naturally to the earth's surface. Other bottled water sources include well water and even plain old municipal water that's been specially treated before bottling. Any of these sources can provide clean, safe water but just make sure that whichever brand you choose has been properly inspected.

Filtered water, available through a home filtration system, is a good option that's typically more cost-effective than bottled water. According to the Brita company, their widely available home filter system can produce water for 18 cents a gallon, compared to a dollar or more for an eight to 12-ounce bottled water. Home filtration systems generally attach to the faucet, filtering water as it comes through the tap. Systems like Brita and PUR also use containers that have the filter built right into them.

According to the Water Quality Association, consumers can feel confident about the quality of water provided by brand-name home filtration systems. However, it's important to maintain the filters according to the manufacturer's instructions in order to avoid build-up of bacteria and other contaminants. In addition, you should be aware that these systems do not eliminate volatile organic compounds. For the purest water available through a home system, choose a reverse osmosis (RO) system, though these tend to be more expensive.

Noise, Noise, Noise

Loud sounds from traffic, construction, and even high-volume music in your ear buds can over activate your immune system, as can noisy distractions when you're trying to concentrate. Soft, inexpensive foam earplugs are one solution. Even better, you can invest in a good pair of noise-cancelling headphones.

Sounds aren't all bad, though. Listening to or making music can actually be a therapeutic way to lower stress, reduce inflammation, and calm the immune system and release endorphins.

X-rays and Other Radiological Techniques

While the dose of radiation from X-rays is extremely low, it makes sense to avoid excess or unnecessary radiological diagnostic tests and to use a lead shield during dental X-rays and other tests that focus on specific areas of the body.

Excess Antibiotics

Unnecessary use of antibiotics can disturb intestinal flora, allowing opportunistic bacteria to invade and spur inflammation.

Multiple Sex Partners and Other High-Risk Behaviors

These increase your risk of contracting acute or chronic infections that cause inflammation.

Exercise

We've already discussed how a lack of activity can directly raise your inflammatory state. The flip side is that getting sufficient exercise is probably the single most effective way to lower your inflammatory state, counteract stress, and decrease your CRP level.

Get Out and About

One of the best ways to decrease stress is to spend time with people we like and who support our Habits of Health. Whether it's other new moms, dog lovers, fishing buddies, or siblings, just knowing you're not alone can go a long way toward helping you cope with stress. Remember, the Japanese have found an amazing way to unwind and enhance their immune system by using forest baths and walking amongst the evergreens.[6]

Go Natural

I'm convinced that we all need to get out in nature and get in touch with our 10,000-year-old design. We are now considered an indoor species with us spending almost all our time inside. If you've got kids, you should grab them and take them outside as well, as they are only outside eight minutes a day on average! Nothing is more important than leaving

Beware These Toxins in the Home!

While many of us already filter our water and air, other sources of toxins in the home may not be so obvious.

- **Your lawn:** Pesticides and herbicides contain toxic substances that can be absorbed through the skin. Don't walk barefoot on your lawn, and remove your shoes before going in. Better yet, manage your lawn organically.

- **Your closets:** Plastic covers and dry cleaning bags contain a dangerous substance called perchloroethylene, which has been shown to cause dizziness, confusion, inflammation, and even cancer. Keep it out of your house and off of your body by machine-washing clothes instead of dry cleaning, or by choosing a dry cleaner that uses less toxic substances such as carbon dioxide or wet dry-cleaning processes. To find a professional near you, check out www.nodryclean.com or www.findco2.com.

Beat Stress and Curb Inflammation with These Healthy Behaviors

- **Get a massage. Nothing works like human touch to promote feelings of wellbeing.**
- **Do some yoga. You'll learn to breathe deep, stretch unused muscles, and even find a little inner peace. For more information, see the section on stress reduction in Part 3.4, *Brain and Mind Longevity: Protecting and Enhancing Your Future*.**
- **Take a warm bath. Soothe your muscles and your mind by taking some time for yourself.**
- **Make your home cozy and inspiring. Turn on soft music, put up some beautiful art, plant a garden, create a spot for meditation, hang wind chimes, or build a waterfall or reflection pond.**

behind the madness of our high-tech world to spend some time simply absorbing all that connects us to each other and to nature.

Treat Your Body
Anything from a light massage to deep structural therapy can help you relax and restore balance to your musculoskeletal system when you're stressed, stiff, or just worn out. And it even helps lower CRP and inflammation!

We have now taken another step in approving our surroundings and addressing the risks to your health and wellbeing. Our next steps are to address how we can augment your healthy immune system and ensure that you have the optimal supplementation to fortify your body and become as healthy as you can at any age.

Laugh
Laughter has been shown to reduce stress, decrease CRP, and lower unhealthy hormone levels. Watch a funny movie, tell jokes, and find time to laugh with friends and family. Or next time you feel stressed, just try rustling up a great big smile. While it may feel forced at first, smiling by its very nature smiling reduces bad feelings.

Focus on the positive
It's easy to slip into a negative self-image. But why say something bad about yourself that you wouldn't even dream of saying about someone else? Turn that internal dialogue into a running commentary on all the reasons you have to be grateful.

Stop. Challenge. Choose.™
We all have to deal with day-to-day problems. Learning to focus on the outcome you want can help defuse a potentially stress-filled situation. Revisit Part 1.6, *You in Charge of Yourself: Setting Up for Success*, or the Habits of Health App for a refresher on this technique if you need more practice or instruction.

And no discussion of inflammation would be complete without addressing stress, one of the biggest contributors to a host of health complications. When our bodies are stressed—locked in fight or flight mode—we struggle to function at our best. Though much of the material we covered in this part and in previous parts can help you reduce stress—such as Stop. Challenge. Choose.™ or exercising more frequently. This is because stress is best addressed in the context of your mind.

If stress is a significant challenge for you today, you might benefit from jumping ahead to Part 3.4, *Brain and Mind Longevity: Protecting and Enhancing Your Future*, to learn more about the MacroHabit of a Healthy Mind. In the meantime, begin to extinguish the flame of inflammation as you grow and improve your Habits of Health, optimizing your life, one choice at a time.

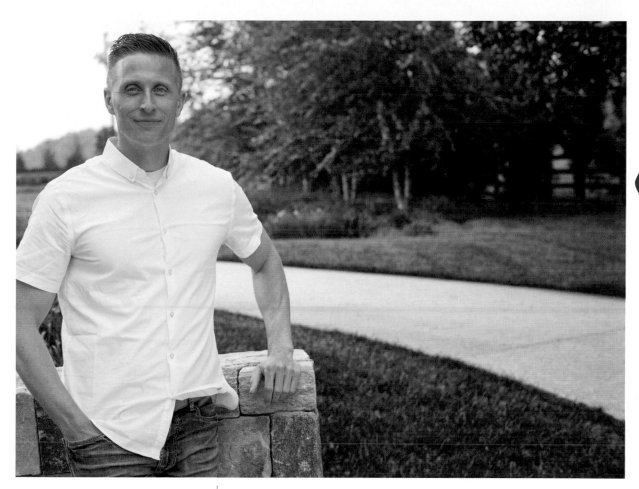

> **I had actually started to hate exercise because I was just doing it to lose or maintain the weight that I had put on.**

TRANSFORMATION: JARED SMITHSON

I've been an athlete my whole life and, although I was skinny, I wasn't healthy. I ate a lot of junk food, and I felt like I was lucky because I had good genetics. I just never gained any weight until I started a more sedentary life when I got out of college. But I really didn't know anything, despite being an athlete.

The biggest difference for me in the Habits of Health was the mindset. I had become good at shedding a few pounds here and there, and then it would go back up, but it was because I wasn't living what I learned to be an integrated life. I would piece little bits together here and there, but then we would go on a trip or I would have a week of work where I was traveling, and everything kind of unraveled.

The good, the bad, and all the experiences of life had led me to the habits that I had created. This world is really created by chain breakers, and I felt like this was my opportunity to become a chain breaker of what I had created in my own life. I started becoming a more conscious individual because of those Habits of Health that we focus on.

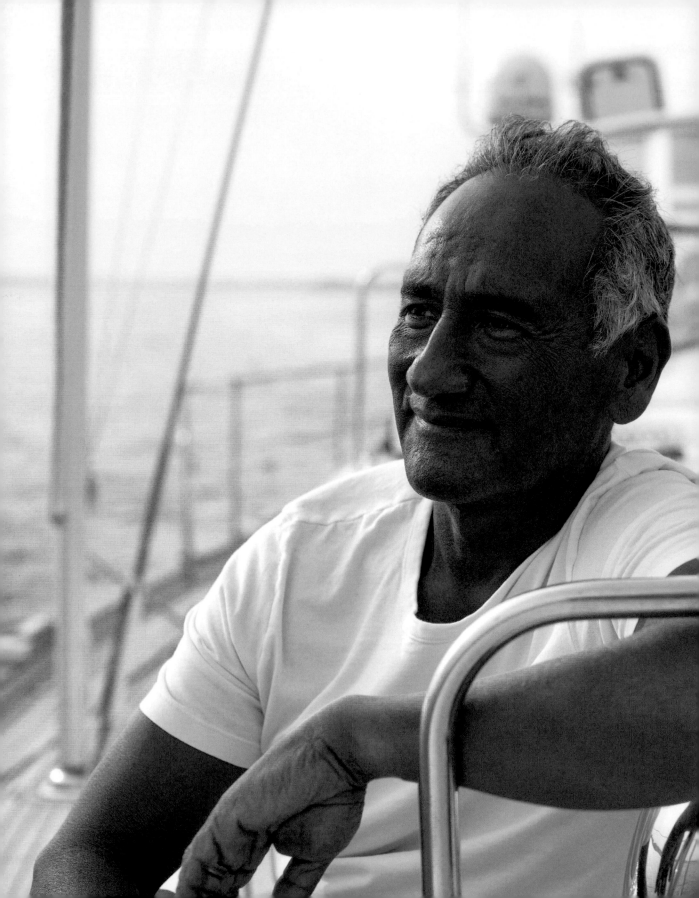

THE BEST YOU CAN BE: OPTIMIZING YOUR LIFE AT ANY AGE

As you continue on your journey to optimal health and wellbeing, there are a few more tools in our arsenal that can help optimize your current state and help keep you in the best possible condition at any age.
They could even extend your life.

Take a look at the following illustration, which shows the Optimal Health Journey. The red line represents the lifeline of those who remain passive to the daily insults and attacks of our obesigenic world. Their optimal health quickly becomes a state of non-sickness—they are overweight, have a poor diet, and are in a state of sarcopenia (flabby, weak muscles, insomnia, over-stressed, a higher state of inflammation) which decays to disease over time. Medications may bring about some limited improvement by decreasing the symptoms, but these folks never really regain their health.

Contrast this with the graduates of the Habits of Health (green line), who continue to enjoy optimal health for life. It's worth taking note of something interesting: in order for our graduate to reach and maintain optimal health, he or she must continue to adjust to the changing conditions of aging and their environment to remain in the optimal health zone.

The upshot? Optimal health isn't static. It looks different at age 20 than at age 80, and it requires vigilance and constant adjustment to the changes your body undergoes as you mature.

It's now a good time to look at your body's changing needs to help you learn how to adapt as you follow your path to better and more vibrant health.

Half of America is Now on Meds

For the first time in history, 55% of all insured Americans are taking prescription medications regularly for chronic health problems such as high blood pressure and cholesterol—problems often linked to heart disease, obesity, and diabetes. And on average, they take four different medications! The U.S. Office of Disease Prevention and Health Promotion has more on safe medicine use.

Source: Consumer Reports, news release, August 3, 2017

2.15

The Optimal Health Journey

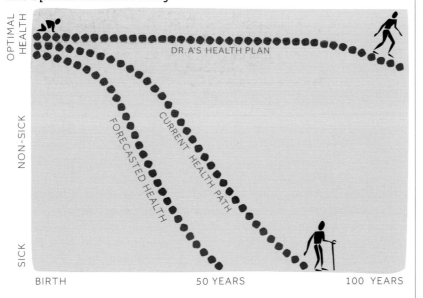

DR. A'S HEALTH PLAN

CURRENT HEALTH PATH

FORECASTED HEALTH

OPTIMAL HEALTH · NON-SICK · SICK

BIRTH · 50 YEARS · 100 YEARS

The red line represents the path that many people take—a premature decline into non-sickness and sickness. The green line represents the path of optimal health—a steady journey of vibrant living into your 100s. Staying in this state takes vigilance and the ability to adapt as you age and your body's needs change.

THE BEST YOU CAN BE: OPTIMIZING YOUR LIFE AT ANY AGE

Nutrients aren't like medications. While medications are foreign intruders that work temporarily in acute situations (often with side effects), nutrients are already present in our body. By supplementing them in just the right amount, you're simply helping your body reach its optimal efficiency. In fact, nutrients are the very fuel of optimal health!

When it comes to the new specialty of creating optimal health and wellbeing, nutrients, not medications, are key.

REACHING THE SUMMIT

Up to this point, we've utilized your body's inherent capacity to heal itself, accomplished by reaching a healthy weight, healthy eating and nutrition, increased daily movement, better sleep and energy habits, increasing your support, and creating healthy surroundings by removing the toxins from your internal and external environments.

Now we're going to augment these normal physiological processes with some valuable tools that can take you even further up the summit of optimal health—namely vitamins, minerals, and other critical nutrients for enhanced vitality.

It's important to reiterate the differences. Nutrients are very different from the medications that today's medical delivery system relies on to treat disease. Medications work rapidly and effectively in acute situations, but they're not naturally created by our own body. Most medications become problematic—first, because they interrupt normal body functions and, second, because they cause a large number of secondary side effects. Medications have their uses, but creating health isn't one of them.

Nutrients, on the other hand, are great facilitators. They may take a bit more time to create an effect but, since they're already present in the body, they're extremely safe. Nutrients can help you create a thriving, healthy life and augment the health of every cell and organ in your body. They're the very fuel of optimal health.

I'm actually a bit embarrassed to admit that my understanding of the significance of nutrients in health and disease treatment didn't come from my medical education. The nutritional focus in medical school and my postgraduate training was based on little more than replacing the nutrients that patients lost as a result of particular diseases, such as pernicious anemia, scurvy, or iron deficiency. The role of nutrients seemed to be little more than as replacement therapy.

It wasn't until years later, when I began to use nutritional intervention in critically ill patients, that I came to understand the pivotal function that nutrients play in creating health. I'm now convinced that in the not-too-distant future, the role of medications will be relegated to secondary status, treating cases that resist our primary tools of nutritional and behavioral intervention. When it comes to the new specialty of coaching and helping create optimal health and wellbeing, the use of nutritional intervention will play a role through a robust intake of fruits and vegetables, but also by spotting potential areas of vita-nutrient supplementation. While medications will have no role in the creation of truly optimal health.

NUTRIENT RESTORATION:
REVERSING THE EFFECTS OF A DEFICIENT DIET

Today's modern farming techniques have caused our foods to become nutrient deficient. That's a sad reality, not some crazy premise cooked up by vitamin manufacturers.

Inorganic fertilizers, susceptible crops laden with pesticides, over-farmed soils lacking iodine, zinc, and selenium all contribute to producing foods that are nutritionally inadequate. Combine that with vegetables treated with sulfites (to give the appearance of freshness), and you can see that the foods available in our markets have become inferior products.

There are also nutritionally degraded processed foods, which now make up over 70% of a typical Western diet, and the canning, cooking, and reheating leaves us with serious micronutrient deficiencies.[1] In addition, we rely heavily on refined grains, sugar, and barely enriched cereals that lack the normal complex array of vitamins, minerals, and other nutrients essential for optimal health. What it all adds up to is this—the food we're eating is seriously depleted and, as a result, so are we.

In fact, less than half of a typical modern diet—which is mostly fast foods and sodas filled with high-fructose corn syrup—has any nutritional value whatsoever. As a result, our bodies begin to crave more food, hoping that the next bite will provide the fuels and nutrients we need (which is a very different and worrying way of looking at cravings).

Making up for these deficiencies is critical if we are to reestablish our equilibrium and our health. The Habits of Health go a long way toward this but, to create optimal health, we need to look for supplements.

Nutrient Augmentation: Customizing to Create Optimal Health

Taking some extra nutrients to make up for a deficient diet is an important part of health maintenance but, in fact, nutrients can do much more by providing us with a premium fuel that can actually enhance cellular and organ function.

Scientist Linus Pauling coined the term "orthomolecular" to describe the process of providing optimal amounts of the substances already present in the body—a concept that's been embraced by a number of innovative physicians, including the legendary Dr. Robert Atkins, who pioneered the role of vitanutrients in health.

One particular group of nutrients we'll be paying close attention to are antioxidants. As we discussed in the previous section, antioxidants play a central role in health optimization by shielding us from the attacks of dangerous free radicals that can damage our cells. And that's in addition to the inflammation-beating diet tips you've already learned—consuming deep green and brightly colored vegetables, for example, as well as green tea, certain spices, and even red wine. We will now focus on fish oils, vitamins, and other supplements that

"Pesticides, preservatives, depleted soils, and processed foods all add up to a diet that's nutritionally inadequate. Today's typical diet simply can't build or sustain optimal health."

2.15

THE BEST YOU CAN BE:
OPTIMIZING YOUR LIFE AT ANY AGE

Do Supplements Work as Well as Whole Foods?

You've probably read that the best way to get the proper nutrients is through healthy whole foods. Well, that's absolutely right. Filling your plate with fresh fruits, vegetables, and unrefined grains that contain all the complexities of nature is the best way to create optimal health. And we do that by putting the right raw materials into our bodies: real, whole, local, fresh, unadulterated, unprocessed, and chemical, hormone, and antibiotic-free food.

Unfortunately, hectic schedules, high costs, and limited availability sometimes prevent us from having healthy foods at our fingertips. That's why the prudent, informed use of complete, complex supplements—especially antioxidants—is a smart idea. One of the reasons I like prepackaged portion-controlled meals is they make sure you get a wide range of necessary nutrients and are fortified with strong vitamin and mineral premixes, as well as providing an additional means of obtaining supplementation.

are chock full of antioxidants, which we can add to your arsenal to help optimize your current health.

RENEWING AND OPTIMIZING THROUGH NUTRIENTS: YOUR PERSONAL GUIDE

The guidelines that follow will help you add supplements to your daily diet in the ideal amounts to support optimal health. You'll also learn how to maximize your antioxidant production to avoid immune stimulation and prevent damage to skin and organs and learn the first steps of your lifelong anti-aging strategy.

Its important you check with your healthcare provider before adding any supplements, as some may interfere with medications.

Fish Oils

The omega-3 oils in fish provide numerous health benefits, although last year the benefits of their ability to reduce heart attack or stroke were removed because recent research could not substantiate such claims. They are still capable of boosting heart health by improving numerous heart disease risk factors, including lowering blood pressure, decreasing cancer risk (especially breast and colon cancers), and decreasing immune activation and autoimmune diseases.[2] In addition, the DHA in fish protects the brain and our retinas. A recent study confirmed that fish oil supplements combined with regular exercise help reduce body fat and improve cardiovascular and metabolic health.[3]

Proven Benefits of Omega-3 Fatty Acids

Omega-3 fatty acids have all sorts of powerful health benefits for your body and brain; indeed, few nutrients have been studied as thoroughly. Here are the incredible health benefits of omega-3 fatty acids that are supported by science.

Omega-3s in Heart Health

The benefits against risk factors include:

- Triglycerides: omega-3s can cause a major reduction in triglycerides, usually in the range of 15–30%.[4]
- Blood pressure: omega-3s may reduce blood pressure levels in people with high blood pressure.[5]
- HDL-cholesterol: omega-3s can raise HDL ("good") cholesterol levels.[6]
- Blood clots: omega-3s can keep blood platelets from clumping together. This helps prevent the formation of harmful blood clots.[7]
- Plaque: by keeping the arteries smooth and free from damage, omega-3s help prevent the plaque that can restrict and harden the arteries.[8]
- Inflammation: omega-3s reduce the production of some substances released during the inflammatory response.[9]

Interestingly, despite all these beneficial effects on heart disease risk factors, there is no convincing evidence that omega-3 supplements can prevent heart attacks or strokes. Indeed, many studies find they provide no benefits in this area.[10]

Omega-3s Reduce Inflammation

Inflammation is a silent killer. Omega-3 fatty acids can reduce the production of molecules and substances linked to inflammation, such as inflammatory eicosanoids and cytokines.[11] Studies have consistently shown a link between higher omega-3 intake and reduced inflammation. Omega-3 fatty acids can help fight several autoimmune diseases (PB1), including type 1 diabetes, rheumatoid arthritis, ulcerative colitis, Crohn's disease, and psoriasis.[12]

> **Conclusion:** *Omega-3s reduce chronic inflammation and can lower the risk of heart disease, cancer, arthritis, cognitive decline, autoimmune diseases, and various other diseases.*

Omega-3 Fatty Acids May Improve Sleep

As one of the MacroHabits of Health, sleep is a foundation of optimal health.

- Low levels of omega-3 fatty acids are associated with sleep problems in children and obstructive sleep apnea in adults.[13]
- Low levels of DHA have also been linked to lower levels of the hormone melatonin, which helps you fall asleep.[14]
- Studies in both children and adults have shown that supplementing with omega-3 increases the length and quality of sleep.[15]

> **Conclusion:** *Omega-3 fatty acids, especially DHA, may improve the length and quality of sleep in children and adults.*

Omega-3s Are Helpful in Depression and Anxiety

Depression, whose symptoms include sadness, lethargy and a general loss of interest in life, has become one of the most common mental disorders in the world, and its incidence is increasing along with anxiety (another very common disorder characterized by constant worry and nervousness).

- Studies have found that people who consume omega-3s regularly are less likely to be depressed.[16]
- People who have depression or anxiety who start taking omega-3 supplements, may experience decreased symptoms.[17] A study shows that of the three types of omega-3 fatty acids, EPA is the most effective for reducing depression, and it can be as helpful as Prozac.[18, 19]

DR. A SAYS...

> *"Despite the fact that multivitamins have been proven extremely effective for health, only two in five people actually take them."*

2.15

Antioxidants: Your Daily Dose of Protection

Antioxidants protect our cells from the damage caused by free radicals— the dangerous byproducts of a hyperactive immune system, brought on by today's Habits of Disease. Try to consume between 3,000 and 5,000 ORAC units (oxygen radical absorbance capacity) each day through a combination of healthy foods, such as green and colored vegetables, green tea, and supplements such as fish oil, vitamins C and E, carotenoids, zinc, selenium, and glutathione.

Do We Need Vitamins or Not?

"I agree that you don't need vitamins and that they are a waste of money, but *only* if you eat wild, fresh, whole, organic, local, non-genetically modified food grown in virgin mineral and nutrient-rich soils, and not transported across vast distances and stored for months before eaten. It is true *only* if you work and live outside, breathe only fresh unpolluted air, drink only pure, clean water, sleep nine hours a night, move your body every day, and are free from chronic stressors and exposures to environmental toxins.

Then you don't need vitamins.

But, of course, this describes absolutely no one on the planet! Therefore, in reality, we *all* need vitamins. To get the most out of your supplements, just make sure they're from a reliable source. For extra reassurance that you're getting full functionality, choose combined forms (such as B complex) rather than isolated versions."
Mark Hyman MD, leading nutritional interventionalist.[20]

Conclusion: Omega-3 supplements may help prevent and treat depression and anxiety. EPA may be the most effective at fighting depression.

Omega-3s May Help Prevent Cancer
Cancer is one of the leading causes of death in the Western world, and omega-3 fatty acids may reduce the risk of certain cancers.

- Studies have shown that people who consume the most omega-3s have up to a 55% lower risk of colon cancer.[21]
- Omega-3 consumption has been linked to a reduced risk of prostate cancer in men and breast cancer in women. However, not all studies agree on this.[22]

Conclusion: Omega-3 intake may decrease the risk of colon, prostate, and breast cancer.

Omega-3s May be Beneficial For:
- Brain development in pregnancy and infancy[23]
- Eye health[24]
- ADHD and reducing asthma in children[25, 26]
- Metabolic syndrome[27]
- Age-related mental decline, Alzheimer's disease, improving mental disorders[28, 29]
- Improving bone and joint health[30]
- Help with menstrual pain[31]
- Health of your skin[32]

Where Should You Get Your Omega-3?
Getting omega-3 from whole foods, such as eating fatty fish twice a week, is the best way to ensure optimal omega-3 intake. However, if you don't eat a lot of fatty fish, then you may want to consider taking an omega-3 supplement. For people who are lacking in omega-3, this is a cheap and highly effective way to improve your health. However, there are hundreds of different omega-3 supplements available. Not all of them have the same health benefits. Fish oil comes in both natural and processed forms. The processing can affect the form of the fatty acids. This is important because some forms are absorbed more effectively than others. Omega-3s come in several forms, most commonly as triglycerides. Some fish oils that are more processed may contain omega-3 ethyl esters, which aren't absorbed well.

Summary on Fish Oils
For most people, a regular fish oil supplement is probably sufficient. However, make sure the supplement actually contains what it says it does, and check out the EPA and DHA content. EPA and DHA (important for brain health) are best found in animal-based omega-3 products. Vegetarian options are available, but they usually only contain ALA. I recommend algal oil, which is an excellent source of quality omega-

3s and suitable for everyone, including vegans. It is best to take these supplements with a meal that contains fat, as fat increases the absorption of omega-3s.

Finally, keep in mind that omega-3s are perishable, just like fish, so do not buy a lot. If you buy the enteric coated type, which have been processed, occasionally open one to make sure the oil has not turned rancid. Omega-3s may be one of the most beneficial supplements you can take. Just make sure you buy it from a reputable source.

Note: While eating fish regularly is a good way to gain these benefits, there's a growing shortage of safe fish on the world market. That's why I've become a big advocate of supplementing your diet with one to three grams of pharmaceutical-grade fish oil daily. Be sure to choose oil that's been tested and does not contain heavy metals.

VITAMINS, MINERALS, AND AMINO ACIDS

The term "vitamin" refers to certain organic compounds that we need in tiny amounts as nutrients but that we can't synthesize in sufficient quantities by ourselves and, therefore, must obtain through our diet. This category doesn't include other essential nutrients, such as dietary minerals, essential fatty acids, essential amino acids, or the large number of other nutrients that promote health but are required less often.

Vitamins serve a number of functions, acting as hormones (as in vitamin D), antioxidants (vitamin E), growth regulators for tissue and cells (vitamin A), and precursors for enzymes involved in metabolism (vitamin B complex). Minerals and amino acids, like vitamins, also play a range of roles to help you achieve optimal health.

The good news is that following the Habits of Healthy Eating will help you to reach your daily recommended amounts of vitamins, minerals, and amino acids. In some cases, supplementation may still be necessary, but not always.

Because this topic is dense and because the research continues to evolve rapidly in terms of the precise amounts to supplement, I've provided more content on this section at HabitsofHealth.com. Go there for the most up-to-date insights!

FIBER

In the sections on eating healthy, we discussed the importance of fiber in lowering cholesterol and blood sugar, creating satiety (fullness), and improving intestinal health. But there's even more to this important nutrient—a high intake of fiber directly decreases the inflammatory state.

" *Fiber does so much! Along with being a great anti-inflammatory agent, it can lower cholesterol and blood sugar, improve intestinal health, and make you feel fuller.*[33–39] "

2.15

Açaí: The Super-Berry

Açaí (ah-sigh-ee), the high-energy berry of an Amazonian palm tree, is a veritable powerhouse of antioxidants, amino acids, and essential fatty acids. Available in many whole food and health stores, açaí has the vibrant flavor of chocolate and berries. While it can be taken in juice form, you're much better off consuming it as pulp to reap the full benefits of the following:[40]

- High levels of antioxidants (30 times the anthocyanins in red wine).[41]
- Monounsaturated (healthy) fats, dietary fiber, and phytosterols for cardiovascular and digestive health. Açaí's fatty acid content resembles that of olive oil and is rich in monounsaturated oleic acid—an important partner to omega-3 fish oils in promoting cellular health and longevity.[42]
- Essential amino acid complex and valuable trace minerals for muscle contraction and regeneration.

Much of today's increase in heart disease, diabetes, degenerative diseases, and cancers can be attributed to the development and profusion of refined grains and sugar.[43] Adding fiber to your diet can immediately improve your intestinal flora by giving beneficial bacteria, such as lactobacilli and bifidobacterium, abundant food. These healthy intestinal dwellers flourish on the fiber that we can't digest, enabling them to overcrowd and wipe out dangerous bacteria.

Fiber also slows down the absorption of glucose, which helps control blood sugar and allows more time for the process of offloading cholesterol. And, by preventing toxins from entering the bloodstream, fiber takes the burden away from the immune system, making it a powerful tool for optimal health.

Let's take another look at the two types of fiber:

- Soluble fiber slows the breakdown of complex carbohydrates and helps reduce blood sugar. It dissolves in water, forming a gel-like mass that binds cholesterol in the stool. If you eat enough, it can actually help lower blood cholesterol. Good sources of soluble fiber include vegetables, legumes, fruits, and grains such as rye, barley, and oats.
- Insoluble fiber does not dissolve in water and is not absorbed or digested by the body and because it's filling, it reduces hunger. It also helps keep your gastrointestinal tract clean and aids in regular bowel movements by pulling water into the colon. Good sources of insoluble fiber include brown rice, whole-wheat breads, cereals, seeds, fruit skins, vegetables and, my favorite food, legumes!

The foods listed above average around three grams of fiber per cup. Men need at least 38 g of fiber per day, and women at least 25 g. As a general rule, you should try to eat 20 g of fiber per thousand calories. While this should be doable under the Habits of Health, which encourages you to eat significant amounts of vegetables and fruits, it doesn't hurt to supplement! The following fiber supplements are sugar-free:

- Methylcellulose (Citrucel®)
- Guar gum (Benefiber®)
- Psyllium husks (Konsyl®)
- Pectin

PROBIOTICS

On occasion, we may find ourselves forced into a period of unhealthy eating or extra stress, or need an antibiotic for acute infection. These stressors can wreak havoc on our intestinal flora and cause gastrointestinal distress in the form of gas, cramping, bloating, and diarrhea. Some people may find that their existing sinus, ear, and respiratory problems or food allergies are exacerbated as well.

At times like these, the addition of friendly bacteria in the form of probiotics can help you re-establish a healthy intestinal tract and recover optimal health. Probiotics can also help reduce CRP and immune hyperactivity, and assist in the manufacture of such nutrients as biotin, folic acid, and vitamin K.

To supplement, look for a high-quality brand with at least four million bacteria per dose, including the following:

- Acidophilus to help augment the immune system and inhibit growth of candida and E. coli
- Bifidobacterium, our most abundant and important bacteria, which lowers cholesterol, digests lactose, and helps with the manufacture of B vitamins
- Bulgaricus, a powerful immunity enhancer

Probiotics are enhanced by the addition of FOS (fructooligosaccharide), a sugar that's not absorbed by the body. As a prebiotic, FOS has been shown to help lower sugar and cholesterol and alleviate constipation and diarrhea.[44]

It's been said by some researchers that up to 90% of all diseases can be traced back to the gut and health of the microbiome. Believe it or not, your microbiome is home to trillions of microbes: diverse organisms that help govern nearly every function of the human body in some way. The importance of our gut microbiome cannot be overstated: poor gut health can contribute to leaky gut syndrome, autoimmune diseases, and disorders like arthritis, dementia, heart disease, and cancer.[45] Our health, fertility, and longevity are also highly reliant on the balance of critters living within our guts. Throughout our lives, we help shape our own microbiomes and they also adapt to changes in our environment. For example, the foods you eat, how you sleep, the amount of bacteria you're exposed to on a daily basis, and the level of stress you live with all help establish the state of your gut flora. Probiotics and prebiotics play a vital role in its health. Probiotic foods contain good bacteria that populate your gut and fight off bad bacterial strains. Try to include probiotic foods like yogurt, kombucha, kvass, kefir, or cultured veggies in your diet daily or supplement as described above.

Phytonutrients

Phytonutrients are produced by plants to protect them from infection, disease, and oxidation. They give plants their vibrant colors and have been shown to help protect humans as well. Here are some phytonutrients you should know about.

- Polyphenols are powerful antioxidants that have anti-cancer properties. They're found in extra virgin olive oil, dark chocolate, fruit skins, green and white tea, and red wine.

"

Many of these powerful antioxidants can be enjoyed in the form of tea, dark chocolate, and red wine.

"

2.15

Prebiotics and Probiotics: Different Animals

Probiotics aren't the same thing as prebiotics. While probiotics add helpful bacteria to your digestive system, prebiotics contain non-digestible food ingredients that selectively stimulate the growth and activity of beneficial micro-organisms that are already in your colon. When probiotics and prebiotics are mixed together, they form yet another type of substance—a synbiotic.

THE BEST YOU CAN BE: OPTIMIZING YOUR LIFE AT ANY AGE

What is Your Microbiome?

Each of us has an internal complex ecosystem of bacteria located within our bodies that we call the microbiome. The microbiome is defined as a "community of microbes". The majority of the bacterial species that make up our microbiome live in our digestive systems and can reach levels of 10–100 trillion symbiotic microbial cells. The word "microbiome" tells you a lot about how it works and the importance of its roles, since "micro" means small and "biome" means a habitat of living things.

Place a roll of dental floss or preformed sticks in a small dish or container by your tooth brush. Decide to floss at least one tooth after brushing and you will probably end up doing them all.

- Resveratrol is a potent antioxidant that can help us live longer.[46] It's found in the skins and stems of grapes, and in higher concentrations in red wine. You can supplement with around 50–200 mg per day, or just open up a good cabernet and have a daily glass.
- Genistein, an isoflavone found in soy, can provide both antioxidant and anti-inflammatory protection with a resulting decrease in immune activation.
- Curcumin is a spice derived from the turmeric root, which is used commonly in curry dishes. It's an anti-inflammatory that can also help autoimmune diseases as well. Use the powder in cooking or take 250 mgs per day, divided into three doses every eight hours.

MEDICATIONS

Aspirin

Aspirin (acetylsalicylic acid) is the only medication I include with nutrients. It has a wonderful ability to block the immune system's production of cytokines and CRP. In small doses, it is a weapon against immune hyperactivity. It's well known for its antiplatelet, or anti-clotting, effect, which makes it an important ally for anyone at risk for cardiovascular disease due to family history or Habits of Disease such as smoking, excess abdominal fat, high LDL, low HDL, inactivity, and high triglycerides. It's also helpful for those at risk due to diabetes or aging. Additionally, recent studies show that aspirin affects colon cancer and polyp formation by preventing the ability of cancers to create a blood supply for growth.

I consider aspirin a safe and inexpensive weapon in the health arsenal. I take the recommended dose of 81 mg in the morning, with a glass of warm water to help it dissolve and minimize gastric irritation. To achieve the right dose, use the 81 mg low dose but avoid formulated, enteric-coated low-dose aspirin because there are some studies that say absorption is affected. There are some new studies that question whether aspirin is beneficial in healthy individuals and worth the small risk of increased bleeding. Plus a brand new study says that a low dose is not effective in people who are overweight or obese.

Because of the uncertainty, please do not start any aspirin protocol without first consulting with your healthcare provider.[47]

WHERE DO YOU GO FROM HERE?

We've just covered a lot of ground! Obviously, if you took each and every one of these recommendations for supplementation, you'd have no time or money left for anything else. So our goal is to identify areas where you have specific deficiencies or special needs and to focus on adjusting your current intake to reach an optimum level. I'll also highlight some key areas where nutrition augmentation can help you reach and maintain optimal health.

One simple way to pinpoint areas of deficiency is to take a look at your current health by going to your healthcare provider and having them evaluate any abnormal lab, paying particular attention to your lipid evaluation, nutritional evaluation, current diseases and medications, and family history of disease. Another way to get more information is to ask your healthcare provider for a hs-CRP test (high-sensitivity C-reactive protein), which can help determine your risk of heart disease and other inflammation-related conditions.

Once you've identified your areas of deficiency and current health challenges, you'll be able to create an individualized, targeted plan that not only brings you into better balance, but actually augments your health for optimal living. To do that, we'll first look at some general guidelines from the U.S. government and then at some more specific recommendations of my own that you can use to guide your choices.

U.S. GOVERNMENT RECOMMENDATIONS

U.S. Government recommendations are used on commercial food and nutritional products to give consumers a general idea of the amount of daily nutrients they should obtain and the amount that each product provides. But bear in mind that these are general guidelines only and not tailored to your specific needs. Let's take a look at some of these recommendations.

First, you'll need to learn a few terms. RDI (reference daily intake) calculates the recommended amount of vitamins and minerals. DRV (daily reference value) calculates the recommended amount of energy producing nutrients (fat, carbohydrates, protein, and fiber). For the purposes of food and product labels, the U.S. Government calculates DRV as a percentage of a 2,000 calorie diet. This means that your own recommended amount may be higher or lower, depending on the number of calories you eat in a day. Here are the percentages the U.S. Government uses to calculate their DRV, versus the percentages we've set as our goals for healthy weight maintenance and optimal health.

U.S. Government RDI (Recommended Daily Intake)

FOOD GROUP	U.S. GOVERNMENT RECOMMENDATION	OUR GOAL (% DAILY CALORIE INTAKE)
FAT	30% OF CALORIES	LESS THAN 25%
SATURATED FAT	10% OF CALORIES	LESS THAN 5%
CARBOHYDRATE	60% OF CALORIES	45–60%
PROTEIN	10% OF CALORIES	15–25%
FIBER	11.5g PER 1,000 CALORIES	11.5g PER 1,000 CALORIES

FOOD COMPONENT	DRV
FAT	65 GRAMS (g)
SATURATED FAT	FATTY ACIDS 20g
CHOLESTEROL	300 MILLIGRAMS (mg)
TOTAL CARBOHYDRATE	300g
FIBER	25g
SODIUM	2,400g
POTASSIUM	3,500mg
PROTEIN (ADULT	50g

These are the amounts of nutrients that the U.S. Government recommends you obtain daily, based on a diet of 2,000 calories per day.

U.S. Government DRV (Daily Reference Values) for Energy-Producing Nutrients (Fat, Carbohydrates, Protein, and Fiber)

NEW LABEL   ORIGINAL LABEL

These are the amounts of vitamins and minerals that the U.S. government recommends you obtain daily.

U.S. Government RDI (Recommended Daily Intake) for Vitamins and Minerals

FOOD COMPONENT	AMOUNT
VITAMIN A	5,000 INTERNATIONAL UNITS (IU)
VITAMIN C	60 MILLIGRAMS (mg)
THIAMIN	1.5mg
RIBOFLAVIN	1.7mg
NIACIN	20mg
CALCIUM	1.0g
IRON	18mg
VITAMIN D	400 IU
VITAMIN E	30IU
VITAMIN B6	2.0mg
FOLIC ACID	0.4mg
VITAMIN B12	6 micrograms (mcg)
PHOSPHOROUS	1.0g
IODINE	150mcg
MAGNESIUM	400 mg
ZINC	15mg
COPPER	2mg
BIOTIN	0.3mg
PANTOTHENIC ACID	10mg

These are the amounts of vitamins and minerals that the U.S. government recommends you obtain daily.

DR. A'S SUPPLEMENT GUIDELINES

Your Optimal Health Guidelines

Now let's take a look at some guidelines that are based on you, rather than just focusing on a model calculated around deficiencies.

Note: Before starting any new supplement protocols meet with your healthcare provider to make sure none of your medicines or conditions will be affected by a nutritional intervention.

Step 1: Add Fish Oil

Make one of the following a part of your daily routine:
- 4 oz of fatty fish three times a week (e.g., salmon, mackerel, sardines)
- 3–6 walnuts a day
- One to three grams of omega derived from a cold-water arctic fish, with EPA and DHA, taken 30 minutes before meals (sprinkle flaxseed on your breakfast as well). Long-chain omega-3 fatty acids are EPA (eicosapentaenoic acid) and DHA (docosahexaenoic acid). These are plentiful in fish and shellfish. Short-chain omega-3 fatty acids are

" *The U.S. government recommendations that are published on food labels only go so far. Because they're just general guidelines, they're not tailored to your specific needs.* "

2.15

The various terms used in U.S. Government nutritional guidelines can be confusing. Here's a quick synopsis:

- RDA (Recommended Dietary Allowance): A set of estimated nutrient allowances established by the National Academy of Sciences. It is updated periodically to reflect current scientific knowledge.
- DRV (Daily Reference Value): A set of dietary references that applies to fat, saturated fat, cholesterol, carbohydrate, protein, fiber, sodium, and potassium.
- RDI (Reference Daily Intake): A set of dietary references for essential vitamins and minerals and, in selected groups, protein. It replaces the term U.S. RDA (Recommended Dietary Allowance).
- DV (Daily Value): A relatively new term that attempts to simplify the guidelines by combining both DRV and RDI.

alpha-linolenic acid (ALA). These are found in plants, such as flaxseed.

Step 2: Take a Daily Multivitamin

If you're not already taking a multivitamin, start today with a one-a-day multivitamin specifically designed for your sex and age. Make sure it's a high-quality bioavailable vitamin, not one from a wax matrix (some companies use a petroleum-based process that interferes with proper vitamin and mineral absorption).

Step 3: Add B Complex Vitamins

The B complex vitamins work as a team. Unless you have specific needs, it's usually best to take them in the form of a high-potency B complex formula. If these aren't included in your one-a-day multivitamin, add them as needed to reach the following daily doses.

VITAMIN	FULL NAME	AMOUNT PER DAY
B1	THIAMINE	25mg
B2	RIBOFLAVIN	25mg
B3*	NIACIN	0mg
B5	PANTOTHENIC	100–300mg
B6	PYRIDOXINE	4–50mg
B12**	CYANOCOBALAMIN	100-400mg
	BIOTIN	100–300mg
FOLATE	FOLIC ACID	400mg

If you're at high risk for heart disease, talk to your healthcare provider about increasing this amount.
*** 100 mcg/day until age 40, 200 mcg/day from age 40 to 60, and 400 mcg/day after age 60. Take only in combination with other B vitamins, not on its own.*

Step 4: Augment with Other Key Vitamins

Add any necessary vitamins and minerals that aren't part of your multivitamin and B complex.

Other Key Vitamins

VITAMIN	AMOUNT PER DAY
A*	5,000 IU
C**	1,000mg
D	400–1,000 IU
E (MIXED TOCOPHEROLS)*	100–400 IU
K	20–100MCG

Get your vitamin A from food.
*** These two powerful antioxidants can compete with the anti-inflammatory effects of statin drugs. If you take statins, check with*

your healthcare provider and decrease vitamin C to 200mg/day and vitamin E to 100 IU/day.

Step 5: Add Antioxidant Power

To enhance vitamin C antioxidant capacity, combine it with one or both of the following:

- *Quercetin:* found in apples, onions, broccoli, and tea; includes citrus compounds. Take 500 mg per day on an empty stomach.
- *Pycnogenol:* part of a group of powerful antioxidants called proanthocyanidins. Take 50–300 mg per day as pycnogenol or grape seed extract.

For further antioxidant support, try these:

- *Lutein:* obtain from kale, collard greens, spinach, and other green leafy vegetables, or take 40 mcg per day.
- *Lycopenes:* found in high levels in cooked tomatoes. Eat half a cup tomato sauce per week (500 mcg) or take 10–20 mg per day as a supplement.

Step 6: Add Key Minerals

Take the following daily dose of these important minerals:

- *Calcium:* check with your healthcare provider for more on cardiovascular risk research before starting. Women after menopause should take 1,200 mg, men at risk for osteoporosis should take 1,000 mg.
- *Magnesium:* supplement with 200–400 mg or take a warm Epsom salts bath.
- *Selenium:* take 200 mcg as sodium selenite, selenomethionine or, if you're not prone to yeast infections, yeast-derived selenium, or eat two Brazil nuts. Take with vitamin E for enhanced effectiveness.
- *Zinc:* Take 15–25 mg of zinc per day. If you can't taste it on your tongue, increase the dose until you do. A note of caution is that zinc competes with other minerals, especially copper, manganese, and iron. Don't exceed 200 mg per day.

Step 7: Take an Anti-inflammatory Package

Inflammation is an area that often goes unnoticed by both patients and healthcare providers, but as you've discovered throughout Phase III, extinguishing the inflammatory flame is a major part of our core strategic plan to optimize your health.

As we discussed in the last part, an hs-CRP (high-sensitivity C-reactive protein) test is a good way to determine your current level of inflammation. Here are some guidelines that might be helpful but please discuss with your healthcare provider and follow their guidelines once you know the results of your test.

2.15

THE BEST YOU CAN BE: OPTIMIZING YOUR LIFE AT ANY AGE

> *Red fruits and vegetables like tomatoes and watermelon are full of lycopenes— an important antioxidant that may help protect against cardiovascular disease and certain types of cancer. Cooking tomatoes actually increases their lycopene content.*

- **If your hs-CRP is over three,** you may want to consider adopting an aggressive plan to lower it. Begin by reviewing the information in Part 2.14, *Inflammation: Dowsing the Flame*, and applying all possible techniques to reduce your immune activators. In addition to the Habits of Health, you may want to consider starting the following: at least two grams a day of vitamin C; 800 IU of mixed vitamin E; a mega B complex; three grams of fish oil; 1,000 units of vitamin D; chromium, magnesium, selenium, and zinc supplements; and increase your fiber to more than 40 g per day.
- **If your hs-CRP is between one and three,** evaluate your risk factors and, in addition to applying the Habits of Health, you may want to consider taking a multivitamin and fish oil.
- **If your hs-CRP is less than one,** your immune system is in great shape! While this is a fine goal, you can actually do even better. In fact, our ultimate goal over time is to lower your hs-CRP to less than 0.5—a great marker which optimizes your chances for long-term health!

Step 8: Bonus Round

Ask your healthcare provider about these other key nutrients that can help you reach and maintain optimal health.

- **Alpha lipoic acid:** Take 100–300 mg per day. (Diabetics should note that this may lower your need for medications.)
- **Coenzyme Q10:** Yes, it's expensive, but by using a hydro-soluble form, you can cut the dose to 100–200 mg per day.
- **Chromium:** Found in brewer's yeast, eggs, chicken, apples, bananas, and spinach, or supplement with 200–600 mcg per day. (May cause mild insomnia. Diabetics should watch blood sugar closely with their healthcare provider, as levels will drop.)
- **Aspirin:** Take 81 mg per day in the morning with warm liquid. Check with your healthcare provider before beginning aspirin therapy.
- **Probiotics:** Take a dose that provides four billion lactobacillus per day, including acidophilus, bulgaricus, and bifido.

You now have a great outline of the nutritional support you need, not only to correct any deficiencies that have resulted from our modern lifestyle, but to flourish and thrive at your best today and for many years to come. Add this to the anti-inflammatory practices you learned in the last part, and you're nearly ready to take on the world!

But first, we're going to spend the next section taking a closer look deep inside where the seeds of health are planted. This is not the physical you that we've been optimizing through healthy foods and supplements, but the emotional you, whose ability to deal with stress and find happiness and fulfillment is a key component of the journey to optimal health.

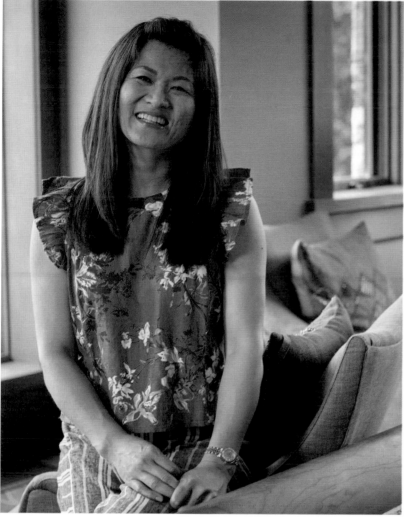

TRANSFORMATION:
MOLLY KIM

A couple months ago, I started Dr. A's program through a friend. She looked great, so I asked her about it, and she said she was a coach.

This program really helped me to control my appetite. As an Asian, we eat lot of rice, but I know that eating a lot of rice over the years just made me feel very sluggish and tired. Dr. A taught me that rice can turn into fat, and it's making me really not who I really want to be. I want to live an active life now, and with the Habits of Health, I am much more active. I'm enjoying more activities and, after work, I want to be able to enjoy more time with my children. This is really teaching me to do the things that I'm able to do.

I've been only in this program a couple of months, but already I've been surrounded by such a supportive group of friends. I feel so encouraged, and I feel like I can do this.

With the new habits I've learned, I'm very excited to continue this journey. I look forward to spending more time with my children and family and doing more with life.

> "
> *I want to live an active life now, and with the Habits of Health, I am much more active. I'm enjoying more activities and, after work, I want to be able to enjoy more time with my children.*
> "

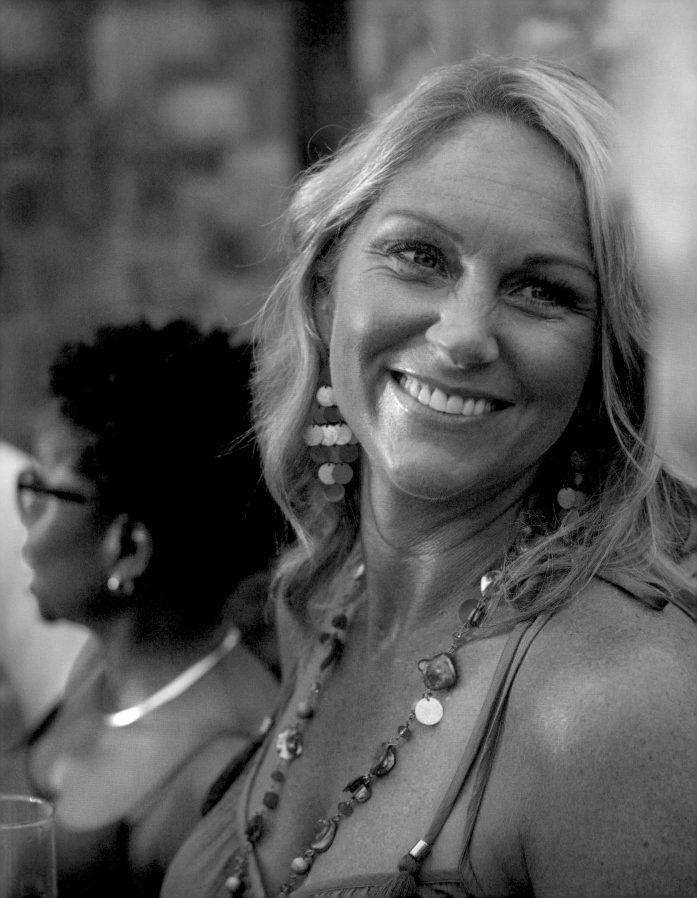

CREATING OPTIMAL WELLBEING: ALIGNING HABITS WITH WHAT MATTERS MOST

You haul yourself out of bed, drink a cup of coffee, rush to the car, get to work, turn on your computer, answer your emails, grab a quick lunch, struggle to focus all afternoon, drive to the dry cleaners, stop at the grocery store, go home, fix dinner, watch a little TV, and hit the bed to rest a few hours before getting up and doing it all again.

And then it's the weekend. You get home late Friday night, do chores on Saturday, sleep in on Sunday morning out of pure exhaustion, maybe spend some time at your place of worship, watch some afternoon TV and just about the time 60 Minutes, or your favorite series comes on, you get a sinking feeling in your gut because you know that in less than 12 hours you're going to launch yourself into another chaotic, energy-draining week of work. Sound familiar?

Recall the story I've told again and again about our ancestors living 10,000 years ago under the stars in tribal communities. Think about their days of gathering food, resting when the sun is highest, and sharing stories around a campfire.

Now contrast that picture with today's overworked, overstressed, overweight, flabby, and sleepless society. We're the first generation ever to actually rank the quality of our lives lower than that of our parents.

How did this happen? Well, here I go again with my familiar refrain. It comes down to our love affair with technology. We've become used to measuring success by our possessions, our house, our car, our income, and our status. As a result, our preoccupation with having the most best "stuff" has taken us away from what really matters. So, let's try and answer that question first.

Do you know what really matters to you? Sadly, many of us don't have any idea. We look to the Internet, the latest TV commercials, or our neighbor's driveway, as if someone else can answer that question for us.

And if we do try, what answer do we come up with? For many, it's financial security, or the resources to be able to buy whatever they desire. But if you dig a little deeper and ask why they want those things, their answer is more fundamental. They believe that those things will make them feel better, happier, or more secure.

I have an important message for you. First of all, money and material goods won't make you happy if you're unhappy to begin with. Second, in our lives, there's no such thing as security.

I want to help you create not only optimal health but also optimal wellbeing for yourself and for the people who matter to you. As a physician and lifestyle professional, I've found that if an individual does not have purpose in their life, helping them create long-term health is an uphill battle. Conversely, aligning your mind with your heart's desire is a powerful force that can do much to support a lifetime of health.

The truth is that the modern world is a complicated, unsettling, and sometimes threatening place. Thanks to technology, we're more aware than ever of tragedies, political unrest, economic challenges, and climate change all around the globe. The chaos of modern life affects us all and our friends, families, and our neighbors may face challenges they want us to help them fix.

All of this means that if we're not in control of our intent, we can easily get caught in a vortex that feeds on stress and frustration— the vicious cycle of buying more things on credit, needing more vacations, working more hours in the hopes of a promotion. We search desperately for relief, hoping that the sleekest car, the most sophisticated possessions, or a new position will make us feel better, reduce our stress, or bring more meaning to our existence.

But there's a way to get back in touch with what's really important and a way to regain a sense of direction and create the life you really want, whatever that may be. You've worked hard to learn and install new systems for healthy eating, movement, and sleep. Now I'm going to teach

"

Despite our material wealth, our generation ranks the quality of our lives lower than our parents' for the first time in history.

"

2.16

As a physician and life coach, I've found that if someone is lacking a true sense of purpose and direction in their life, creating health is an uphill battle.

you a system to help build your life around what really matters to you.

Even if you're already happy on the whole, these techniques will teach you new ways to reduce stress and make your day-to-day life even more enjoyable. And if you feel you've lost touch with your guiding purpose, the lessons you learn will be just what the doctor ordered.

IF YOU COULD LIVE YOUR LIFE OVER...

In the end, what really matters? That's what Richard Leider, author of *The Power of Purpose*, wanted to know. He spent over 20 years interviewing people in the final years of their lives, asking them "If you could live your life over again, what would you change?"

Three universal truths emerged:

- They would have paid more attention to the big picture. They spent so much time being busy that life just seemed to pass them by.
- They would have taken more risks, found work that was more meaningful to them, and had the courage to be better friends, parents, sons, and daughters.
- They would have left a legacy and made more of a difference.

Waiting until the sunset years of life to make these discoveries is just about the most tragic realization I can imagine. Connecting what really matters to the fabric of everyday life should be one of our highest priorities.

The fact is, if you're living for your vacations, you're not going to enjoy a long, optimally healthy life. In fact, finding out what really matters and acting on it can make all the difference in the world. It has for me.

MY OWN JOURNEY TO A LIFE OF PURPOSE

When I was very young, I lived with my mother and grandparents in a crowded apartment in an asphalt jungle. My father was in the military, assigned overseas, my mother worked for an airline, and my grandfather was a beat cop.

One weekend, as a special treat, my grandmother drove me down to Annapolis, Maryland, to see the Naval Academy. I loved to read books about boats and the sea, but at that point my experience with water had been limited to playing in a gushing fire hydrant on a hot summer day.

I fell in love with Annapolis, a historic town surrounded by water and full of all kinds of boats. All the way home, I told my grandmother that someday I would be a ship's captain and live on the water in that wonderful place. I was five years old at the time, and no one in my family had even been to college, yet my grandmother helped me set up a piggy bank and I started saving my pennies.

Years passed. As a military brat, I traveled all over the world, including faraway places like Spain and Japan. And eventually I went to college, followed by medical school, and then started my medical residency.

Upon finishing my fellowship in the newly emerging specialty of critical care from the nation's top program, I began my practice in landlocked Ohio. I became director of critical care and soon found the love of my life—my wife, Lori. We were married and built a beautiful house on a creek which, just to give me my water fix, included a 500-gallon saltwater aquarium. A few years later, we were blessed with our first daughter, Savannah, and three years later Erica came into our lives. And we had an amazing life.

That could have been the end of story, but it's actually only the beginning. For the first 15 years, I was fully immersed in taking care of my patients, working 100 hours a week and loving life. Somewhere along the way, however, stress started creeping in. Jumping out of bed in the morning, eager to start the day, gave way to hassles with HMOs, belligerent healthcare providers, and overworked, stressed-out nurses. I started gaining weight, my sleep deteriorated, and I just wasn't having fun. To top it off, I was growing more and more frustrated with the little I could do to help people recover from lifestyle-induced diseases. All I could see was patients getting sicker. I wasn't dealing well with the stress and was starting to resent having to spend time away from my family.

I left my practice behind. Lori and I gave it all up, gathered a few belongings, sold everything else, and with our one and three-year-old daughters in tow—and amid heavy protests from our friends, family, and colleagues—we moved across the country.

Our goal was to redirect our efforts to help people create health and in the process rediscover our own health. In the beginning, we made no money and were forced to live on credit cards in a small rented house, with no one to rely on but ourselves. But then a curious thing happened. Despite the fact that we'd left the trappings of success in our rearview mirror, I started having fun again. My stress level went down considerably, and I began to thoroughly enjoy this simpler, less material life that left me with time to go for rides with my wife and my girls. I even shed those extra pounds and started exercising.

Seven years later, I had an incredible, thriving life. We were financially sound, and I had time to attend every one of my children's parent-teacher conferences, even in the middle of the day (of course, I was usually the only father there). I was living on the water with a boat at the end of my dock, less than a half mile from where this story began 50 years earlier, in Annapolis, Maryland.

"

In order to create and maintain optimal health, you need to organize your life around what matters most to you.

"

2.16

CREATING OPTIMAL WELLBEING: ALIGNING HABITS WITH WHAT MATTERS MOST

Organizing our life around the pursuit of what's most important to us appears to convey a type of immunity, an enhanced tolerance of whatever life dishes out.

The Next Chapter…

In the last 10 years since I wrote that piece for the first edition, the story has become even better. I have used the principles of the Habits of Health to further my health and wellbeing, and although I am 10 years older I can do more things and have better physical, mental, and overall optimal wellbeing.

I am now heli-skiing in British Columbia, dropping out of helicopter at 10,000 feet into billowing powder in mountains so remote we are the only ones there. Last summer, I sailed across the Atlantic in my boat last year to Bermuda to watch the America's Cup series so close to the race course.

Most importantly, my understanding of how the mind works and how I can use that personally and professionally to optimize my relationships with my family, my colleagues, my friends, and myself has taken my level of fulfillment to a growth level that I cannot even describe.

Note: Recently, completely unexpectedly, I lost my soul mate and wife, Lori. Although it is a tremendous loss, having the foundations that we will discuss in this part have allowed me to continue to live fully with clear purpose. The support and guidance during this tough adjustment period has enabled me to be fully present for my daughters, with a strong determination to help them build an amazing future. I am still totally on purpose, I just wish I had my best friend by my side.

With all this in mind, I am going to spend this section talking to you about how you can really grow and develop your mind so you can experience truly becoming the dominant force in your life and thriving for the rest of your days.

We'll discuss the importance of knowing what is most important to make sure your daily life is aligned with what you want for your future.

THE QUEST FOR FULFILLMENT

If having the things that modern life provides doesn't complete us, what does? The one ingredient that seems to be missing for most of us is fulfillment—a dimension that's critical to our happiness and our health.

Psychiatrist and author Viktor E. Frankl, who wrote his seminal *Man's Search for Meaning* based on observations he made while being held in World War II concentration camps, discusses fulfillment as a separate yet essential component of our lives—one that's determined by internal rather than external measures. Does your life have purpose? Is it going in the right direction? Do you feel complete?

Success is great, and no doubt financial freedom beats being destitute, but the bottom line is that your status and your material things do not define you. As Nietzsche put it, "He who has a why to live can bear almost any how."

Our modern lives are not as complicated or unsettling as they may seem, and they are certainly nothing like the horrific experiences that Frankl and his fellow prisoners suffered. If we can discover what really matters to us and find a way to bring our needs for both success and fulfillment into alignment, we can elevate ourselves to lives full of order and purpose. As an immediate benefit, when our minds and hearts are in alignment this way, our daily joy increases and our stress begins to vanish. The hassles of everyday life become more tolerable and that, in itself, has a direct, positive influence on your immune system and your health.

It starts by looking at the level of fulfillment and sense of purpose in your life as it stands today.

FULLFILLMENT AND SUCCESS

Are you happy? Are you doing what you really want? Are you financially successful? Can you do the things you want and have the things you want?

These are all important questions. In this section, we are going to put into perspective for you what it means to organize your life around what matters most. There are six types of life aspirations and three of these are extrinsic aspirations—the stuff that the American Dream is made of, the ones that define us, and the ones that society says we need. It is whispered in our ear at an early age: Success.

Success

Most people define their lives around success. This is the extrinsic measures of things we want: the nice car, beautiful house, great position at work, and rich stock portfolio. It's what we are told we need to be happy. These things are all external measures that we can divide into three main categories:

1. **Attractiveness:** How appealing am I compared to others?
2. **Fame:** How important and well known am I?
3. **Wealth:** How rich am I?

The interesting thing about each of these external measures is if you are using these judge to how successful and happy you are, it won't work.

> *"Hang on a moment," you say "you are telling me that if I have a model's looks and body, a movie star's fame, and have enough money to do what I want, I won't be happy?"*

mHoH

Enjoy the sunset with your family, unplugging and turning off electronics so that you can be fully present.

Well, you might be happy for a while. Money brings power and material possessions. Fame opens doors and may lead to showers of gifts. A beautiful image provides for glamorous dates, marketing opportunities and lots of attention. But it is never going to be enough if you are using these extrinsic motivators to judge your happiness and whether you're fulfilling your reason for living.

The models that measure their lives on their attractiveness have plastic surgery, continually diet, and live an extremely unhealthy world that isolates them from a real life. Later in life, as their beauty fades, if they have nothing else that brings them joy, their lives will not be a have a happy ending.

The actors that live for their fame often have flawed lives with many marriages, substance abuse, and loneliness. When they're no longer getting the lead roles and the limelight, life for them can be miserable and frustrating. And the very wealthy are often less healthy, stressed by the magnitude of their responsibility, and constantly trying to make more money in the elusive search for happiness that never seems to come despite their growing wealth.

Of course, there are actors and models that are thriving. Lots of them. But I will bet that this is because they also are extremely fulfilled and are doing what they want to do and loving it. They are continually getting better at it and they are using money, not as a goal but rather as a means to have greater experiences, to create amazing experiences with family and friends, and to eliminate the stress that a lack of finances creates.

Those reasons are actually about fulfillment, which is determined by our intrinsic motivation. They are the three aspirations that come from our inner purpose. Unlike the extrinsic aspirations which never seem to be enough and always lead to wanting more, the intrinsic aspirations work because they provide their own rewards.

Now let's switch and talk about the three intrinsic measures that create wellbeing and the enduring joy of fulfillment.

Fulfillment

Fulfillment is the sense that my life matters—I have meaning and purpose, my days are filled with something I love to do, and I have a strong sense of pride. I am doing what I am doing because it is my choice and I enjoy sharing with others. I have a strong sense of purpose, and I am connected in a meaningful way to others. These reasons give meaning to life, and show that what is important to me is guiding me to a sense of satisfaction and joy.

The three aspirations and intrinsic goals we want are:

1. Having satisfying personal relationships
2. Growing as individuals
3. Making contributions to the community

Unlike extrinsic aspirations, the intrinsic ones are satisfying in their own right. They create significant personal satisfaction whether or not they lead to other ends.

The most interesting part is that research shows that in individuals where the aspiration for money, fame, or beauty was much higher than the intrinsic aspiration, the individual was much more likely to exhibit poorer mental health. In comparison, strong aspirations for any of the intrinsic goals (meaningful relationships, personal growth, and community contribution) were positively associated with wellbeing.

People who wholeheartedly desired to contribute to their community had more vitality and higher feelings of connection. Those that covet and organize their behaviors more around internal strivings are more content than those that focus on external strivings and, as a result, display a much higher level of psychological health.

Those that are healthiest focus on the intrinsic measures, although they also enjoy the benefits of having financial success and the ability to live comfortably. Wealth, fame, and beauty do not disproportionately occupy their consciousness like those that seem to obsess and have less mental stability.

A strong emphasis on extrinsic strivings throws a light on what you have, but it lacks a solid grounding because material things are not lasting and in contrast to living your purpose and looking toward what you want to become. This lack of feeling deeply satisfied leads people to seek more superficial goals and creates a false self.

Maslow defined a human need—either physiological or psychological—as something that must be satisfied in order for a human to remain healthy.

Let's take a look at where you are currently and how we can make any necessary adjustments to help you create optimal health and wellbeing.

Fulfillment and Success Continuums: Where are You Right Now?

Take a look at the following illustration showing the failure-success continuum. Where would you say you are on this continuum (1–10)?

Remember, success is defined primarily by external factors, like financial status, your place in the community, and your job. Are you comfortable with your current house, car, and professional position? What level of achievement would you say you enjoy now, compared to where you'd like to be?

Failure-Success Continuum

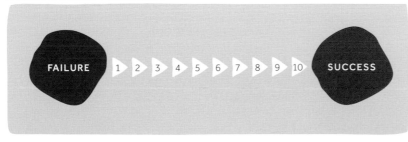

> The intrinsic needs to become better, to do what is most important to us, and relate it with others are fundamental to our wellbeing.
>
> In contrast, the wants or desires for money, fame, or beauty are not basic psychological needs and certainly will not create wellbeing.

2.16

At the end of life, when asked what they'd do differently, no one wishes for a bigger house or a better car. It's the things that make us feel fulfilled that matter in the long run.

How successful would you say you are right now in terms of external, more material factors such as finances, your job, and your standing in the community?

Fulfillment-Depression: Where are You on a Scale of One to 10?

Now, let's look at the Fulfillment-Depression Continuum and determine where you would place yourself on this axis.

Fulfillment-Depression Continuumn

FULFILLMENT

10
9
8
7
6
5
4
3
2
1

DEPRESSION

Figuring out where you are on this continuum—happy and fulfilled, purposeless and depressed, or (like most of us) somewhere in between— is the first step in creating a life of purpose. Where are you on a scale of one to 10?

Now let's put these two parameters together to see how the internal (fulfillment-depression) and external (failure-success) determinants balance out on the Wellbeing Chart. Looking at your current reality in two dimensions allows you to see if what you're doing with your life is in alignment with what matters most to you. Which quadrant would you say you're in right now?

Wellbeing Chart: What Quadrant Are You Currently In?

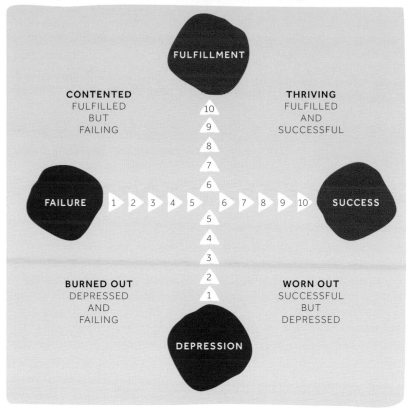

Which quadrant are you in now? By putting both axes together, we can get a more objective picture of our current state of wellbeing and see more clearly whether the way we're living now is aligned with what matters to us most.

Comparing your success track to your degree of fulfillment can be an enlightening exercise. Think back to the elderly subjects in Leider's interviews. When asked what they'd do differently, they all responded with wishes from the fulfillment-depression axis—less focus on the daily grind, more meaningful work and relationships, making a difference. Not one of those people said they wish they'd had a better car, a bigger house, or more money.

What it comes down to is balance in creating a comfortable life arranged around the things that matter most to you—whatever it is that puts you in that upper-right quadrant that signifies abundance.

Once you do, you'll find that when your life is guided by what really matters, the very way you respond to daily life changes. The inconveniences, the complications, the changes, the difficult relationships—when you're immersed in creating the things that are important to you, it suddenly all seems so much more tolerable. Whether you're working toward a new occupation, hobby, or relationship, having a purpose frees your mind from sweating the

"

A Habit of Health: Having the flexibility to recognize when change needs to happen and to adjust accordingly

"

small stuff. You're too busy going after what really matters!

Even if over time things change and what you thought mattered turns out to be something else entirely, what's important is having the flexibility to recognize these changes and adjust accordingly. In fact, it's a fundamental Habit of Health. Without that flexibility, stress will return, and in time you'll be back on your old path to non-sickness and disease. That's why being able to identify and reassess your position on the wellbeing chart is so important. It was for me.

Using the Wellbeing Chart to Illustrate How Life and Wellbeing Evolves

Fresh from my fellowship in critical care, I felt ready to take on the world. In my quest to become the best physician I could be, I threw myself into my work, even staying up all night in the operating room or the intensive care unit on many occasions. I was single and driven by the satisfaction my work gave me, so that even at the bedside of a patient whose life hung in the balance, I felt little stress. In fact, the toughest cases only fueled my passion. My finances, my position as chief of the department, and my level of fulfillment all contributed to great health (with a little fatigue at times, perhaps), and my life was thriving.

Fast-forward 15 years. Stressed, with no time to see my family, and experiencing a change in philosophy stemming from my growing desire to help others create health rather than merely react to disease, I had sunk into the "worn out" quadrant of the wellbeing chart. My physical and mental health were putting me on the path to the very diseases I was treating.

Fortunately, I did something about it. Leaving my practice, taking those risks, seemed scary at times, but I knew I had to align myself with what was important. And I also knew that what was important wasn't the big house or the respected position and, instead, it was my family and my desire to help create health. Changing my life immediately put me way back up on the fulfillment scale. Now that I had decided and was going after my newfound purpose, I was unstoppable. Despite many setbacks and a serious slide backward on the success continuum as I lived on credit cards and we went almost two years without income, Lori and I dived into this vision of helping people create health.

Over time, refusing to give up, we started making traction and yet, during that period, the intense fulfillment satisfied a need that keep us going. By 2008, we were back up in the thriving quadrant, and the last 10 years have been a continual journey of becoming a higher version of myself. Today, I am smack dab in the middle of the abundancy quadrant. The last 10 years have been amazing. As a family we have traveled all over the world including an amazing trip to the Galapagos and hang with incredible wildlife. Last summer we sailed from our house across the ocean to Bermuda for the America's Cup. I started heli-skiing in British Columbia, which I could not have done 10 years ago. Lori and I were honored last year for positivly affecting over a million live which moved us both so deeply. And although our family suffered a major loss with Lori's unexpected passing earlier this year, we have become even closer as a family. And my purpose and resolve to help others create optimal health and wellbeing has never been stronger. I feel so fulfilled and grateful to have helped so many people change their lives and become the dominant force in their own lives. We can help you as well thrive in your life. Let's spend some time and rewrite your story as well. You can be too.

My Wellbeing Chart from 1986 to 2008 shows you an example how our wellbeing changes overall time. Make sure you make one for yourself once you review and understand my example.

My Wellbeing Chart from 1986 to 2008

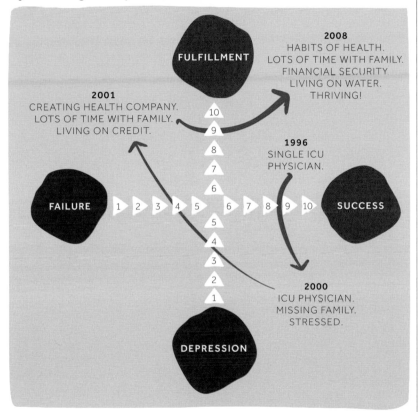

In my own journey, I've gone from being successful and fulfilled, to depressed, to happy but broke, to where I am now—thriving!

Make one of these charts for yourself. Sketch it in your journal or follow the detailed guide in *Your LifeBook*. However you do it, taking the time to reflect and to map out where you are relative to where you'd like to be can lay the foundation for a transformational catalyst in your life.

"If you find you want a lot of external things, ask yourself why. Make sure that the reason is truly aligned with your fundamental aspirations and not just a short-term effort to feel successful at the cost of your long-term goals.

REWRITE YOUR STORY

So many people have written the story of how their life is, and they follow that script like a playbook. Unless that story is currently leading you to an amazing life of optimal health and wellbeing, we need to start writing a new story.

You can either be the victim or you can become the dominant force in your life. *Your LifeBook* is designed to guide you over the next 12 months to create a very different story, one in which we build your new set of habits that leads you up the trail to optimal health and wellbeing. This year of transformation will allow you to truly organize and live your life the way you want.

What I have seen so many times is that as someone really works on their inside and aligning their goals with what matters most, they will grow and excel. I have seen them flourish in their occupations or leave them to find something brand new that aligns their heart and their head so that they are fully involved, satisfied, and no longer settling for less.

If you have not yet taken out *Your LifeBook,* let's do that now and start the first part of your new story. Before we close and move on to our focus on living longer, list some things you can do right now to shift the alignment in your life. I like to think of it as breaking the habit of being yourself!

FINDING WHAT REALLY MATTERS: SOME FINAL TIPS

Most of us are familiar with the idea of reaching and setting goals for external things. However, it's important to ask yourself why you want what you do, until you can honestly answer that it directly satisfies a dynamic urge based on your most fundamental aspirations.

Here's an example: Sam has a very intense job. According to his wellbeing chart, he is in the wornout quadrant. He's successful, but he works so many hours that he is frustrated and misses spending time with his children. Sam's boss has a Porsche that he's thinking of trading in, and Sam knows that if he takes on an extra account and works weekends, he can afford to buy it. If I were Sam, I would ask myself why I want that particular car. If it's for status, he might want to think twice. Having a Porsche might bring him some happiness while he's driving it (trust me, it will) and move him a couple of points forward on the success line, but the long-term effect—less time with the kids—will bring his already poor fulfillment score even lower (after all, they can't even fit in that two-seater!).

Knowing what's really going to fulfill us can be hard to figure out, especially for those of us who've been driven by today's success-at-all-costs mentality. I recommend you read *Your Life as Art* by Robert Fritz for a more detailed explanation of how to build the life you want, but, for now, I'd like to give you a few concrete ideas for enjoying some areas of life that are too often neglected in our drive for success:

- **Follow your passion:** in an unforgettable scene from the movie *American Beauty*, the main character asks his wife what happened to the passion in their lives. "When did you become so... joyless?" he asks.

- **Find something or someone to be passionate about:** You want something that has you jumping out of the bed in the morning, and love is one of nature's greatest healers. If you had it before, you can get it back! It can be restored, rediscovered, renewed. Take a word of wisdom from the elders in Richard Leider's interviews: If you're struggling in a relationship, be courageous enough to reach out and call a truce. Let your loved ones know how much you care, then sit down and rediscover each other. If your paths have diverged so far that they can't realign, you need to accept that too, and move on to find your true love.

- **Rekindle your romance in large or small ways, perhaps by leaving love notes:** on a past visit to the Ronald Reagan Museum, I found myself fascinated by the handwritten notes the former president would leave for his wife, Nancy, before departing on Air Force One. Even as he led the free world, he made time to pay attention to the person who was most important to him. Remember, kindness and love can bridge any chasm.

Here are some other ideas:

- **Take up a new hobby:** find a craft, sport, or adventure that you've always wanted to do, and do it.
- **Enjoy the arts:** learn an instrument, act with a local theater company, or take up dancing.
- **Explore nature:** reconnect with nature and breathing fresh air on your daily walks, while strolling on the beach or in the woods, or just by spending time in your backyard can do wonders for your stress level.
- **Get in touch with your spiritual side:** if matters of the spirit are important to you, join a church, synagogue, or other place of worship or spiritual growth.
- **Spend time with others:** join a special interest group in an area that appeals to you, whether you're an advocate for peace, an environmentalist, an animal lover, or a political junkie.

And since most of us have to work, here's a final guideline: Do what you love or love what you do. It really is that simple. This may require you to quit your job, go to school, enter a new line of work, or invent what it is you want to do, or it may simply mean finding new ways to bring meaning to what you're doing right now. Whatever you do, it should bring you passion, spur your interest, and tap into your talents.

"Living a fulfilling life not only satisfies us emotionally, it also has the power to make us more physically vibrant. In fact, without fulfillment, we can't achieve optimal health."

2.16

Get out and live to the fullest every day, and your body will respond with glee.

Becoming the dominant force in your life is a big opportunity for your wellbeing, and I hope that this section becomes the spark that ignites an entirely new beginning for you. There is a lot of work for us to do in this area, so don't forget to open *Your LifeBook* and work through the exercises and material there to continue building your momentum into action. One of the key areas you will want to work on is your emotional management. There is a great Element in *Your LifeBook* that will challenge you to step up and truly change the habits of being you. It will examine your emotions and how you navigate your day including how you interact around others. It can be a real eye opener to put you on track to providing a different perspective. If you are ready to shake it up and start playing at the deep end of the pool, break out *Your LifeBook* and jump into Element 23, *Master Your Thoughts and Emotions*.

In the next part, now that you know how to be optimally healthy, we will start exploring ways to live longer in that healthier state.

But first, I will leave you with a quote from author James A. Michener, who wrote so powerfully and movingly about far-off lands like Tahiti and Hawaii:

"The master in the art of living makes little distinction between his work and his play, his labor and his leisure, his mind and his body, his information and his recreation, his love and his religion. He hardly knows which is which. He simply pursues his vision of excellence at whatever he does, leaving others to decide whether he is working or playing. To him he's always doing both!"

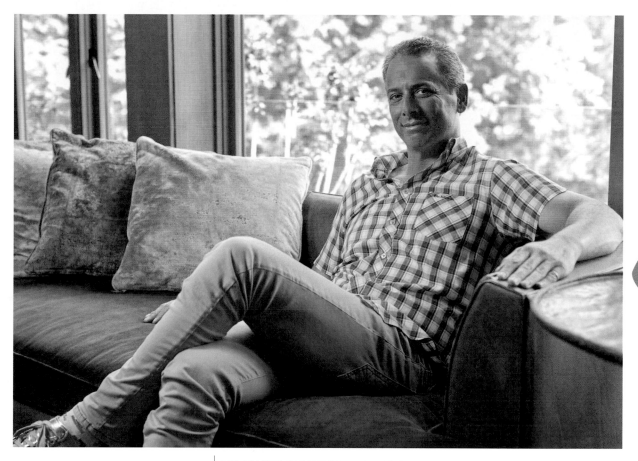

> **"** *I needed a program that had structure because I was a workaholic and I didn't have any free time to get to the gym.* **"**

TRANSFORMATION: JC DOORNICK

In May 2007, I found myself on a beach in North Carolina on a beautiful sunny day as a health professional. I was swimming with my shirt on, and that was a pivotal day for me because I recognized I was incongruent as a health professional. I was a workaholic, always just slaving away at the business of the health industry. I felt a calling that day to get my health straight.

As a health professional, I had no free time to do the right thing. I knew that I needed to eat more frequently, get nutrition, and get my calories straight, but I could not execute it. I love Dr.

A's program because it made it goof proof and it took care of the nutrition, which was important to me even with an extremely busy schedule.

I lost 55 lbs.* My energy was better, my sleep improved. I had a little bit of mental clarity and, at that moment, I started to really engage in the program and recognize that I wasn't on a diet. I was actually building these little microHabits that I kind of always knew I needed to have, like drinking water and getting better sleep and exercise.

*Average weight loss on the Optimal Weight 5 & 1 Plan® is 12 lbs.

LONGEVITY
AND
BEYOND

In Part Two, Your Journey to Optimal Health, we thoroughly unpacked all six MacroHabits of Health. Mirroring the story of the mason jar, we spent the entire second part of your journey carefully exploring and placing each of these foundational bedrocks on your path for your long-term success. If we fail to address each of these keystones and prevent them from becoming an integral contributor to your optimal health and wellbeing, your journey will remain vulnerable and lower your ability to withstand the negative effects of our modern world.

In each of the sections in Part Two, you progressed along the path to optimal health and wellbeing assisted by the primary and secondary habits—represented visually as pebbles—which are derived from the six MacroHabits.

These daily actions surround, reinforce, and actually arise from the foundational rocks that make it all possible. You will continue to install these daily new behaviors by using your App, Your LifeBook, and surrounding support system. And to make them easier to consistently install, these habits can be further broken down into the microHabits of Health (represented by the sand)—extremely small positive actions that are so small and easy to complete we can always do them.

We spent Part One teaching you why, how, and what is needed to build a new transformational life at your own pace in order to begin building the surrounding structures that will support this new world.

This Habits of Health based infrastructure is specifically designed to be digested in bite-size pieces to both support and balance each other. They are also interdependent.

As an example, you addressed your weight management MacroHabit in the beginning of Part Two by learning, applying, and progressing through a series of advancing phases that taught you the knowledge, skills, and techniques you need to take control of your eating, moving, and behaviors for lasting health.

Each phase on your journey has followed the next in a logical fashion, based on one unifying principle: using energy management—the relationship between the energy you consume, the quality of that energy, and the energy you use and create—as a catalyst for health. As you continue to work on optimizing your health you can begin to explore in the innovative leading edge things you can do to create Ultrahealth™ and potentially live a longer healthier life.

In this part, we will continue to enhance your physical health and fitness. We will also explore the development of your mind and brain and the many options you have available because of all the work you have done to date.

Do thoughts of living a long life conjure up images of lonely nursing home patients slumped in their chairs, or a confused relative who calls you by the name of the cat she had 20 years ago? Or maybe thinking about old age makes you mutter to yourself, "I can't drive at night; I have pain in my knee, hip and back; and the last time I even thought about sex is a distant memory."

Hopefully not, because those scenarios describe living in a state of less-than-optimal health—in other words, just surviving—and that's not what we're talking about. Rather, what I want to know is this: if you could live longer in a thriving state of wellbeing while maintaining your optimal health, would you make that choice?

PHASE IV: THRIVING LONGER: THE PRINCIPLES, PRACTICE, AND FUTURE OF LONGEVITY

Now if you are ready, this is the final piece in the optimal health puzzle: staying as healthy as you can for as long as you can. We will begin to fine-tune your mastery and skills so you can enjoy lasting optimal health and wellbeing potentially longer as you continue to become a higher version of yourself. My take on longevity is that it only makes sense when you have both long life and thriving health. And, in fact, the best way to do that is to keep doing the things I've already taught you. Practice the Habits of Health forever. They're your guarantee that you're giving your body the best possible chance to live out your genetic programming which, based on our current understanding of the aging process, means you could live 100 years or more.

THE THREE ERAS OF MEDICINE

Modern medicine has been a bit slow to enter what some call the third era—the revolution of health. But it's done a great job during the first two eras at eliminating most of the diseases that prevented us from living to 100.

The first era, from the beginning of medicine to the middle of the twentieth century, focused on battling infectious disease and improving infant mortality through the advent of vaccines and antibiotics, better sanitation, and an emphasis on hygiene. Once deadly killers such as cholera, typhoid, and polio were eliminated, around the 1950s, we entered the *second era of medicine.* This era involved wrestling with chronic diseases, especially heart disease and, as a result, people are now living longer than ever.

Today, although medicine remains focused on degenerative diseases such as diabetes and cancer, the time has arrived to shift our emphasis to the *third era*. This groundbreaking movement involves more than just keeping blood pressure, cholesterol, and body mass index out of the disease danger zone. It requires a synergistic partnership between patients and healthcare professionals to optimize health and wellbeing. The good news is that more physicians and other medical personnel than ever before are joining this revolution, helping to move our medical model forward from one of reaction and repair to a new school of thought focused on creating health. So if you're looking for a partner in optimal health and longevity, these third era physicians are the ones you should seek. Many of them, like myself, have joined the American College of Lifestyle Medicine, which is a progressive organization of innovative physicians.

Now that medicine has removed the X-factor for longevity by eliminating so many of the diseases that could kill you, you have the advantage. And with the habits you learn in this book, you're well equipped to thrive in medicine's third era.

" *Some of us in the medical profession are shifting our emphasis to what's called the third era of medicine— a new model that's focused on creating health, not just reacting to disease.* "

LONGEVITY AND BEYOND

481

"

Longevity practices such as calorie restriction— modifying your diet by reducing the amount of high-glycemic carbohydrates and saturated fats, along with calories— require only a small adjustment for those of us who've already adopted the Habits of Health.

"

OUR LONGEVITY PLAN

To set the stage for your healthy life extension plan, let's revisit our trusty companion, the energy management diagram. You can see that in Phase IV, the longevity phase, your balance of energy in and energy out stays coupled, as it has since we established equilibrium at the end of Phase II. This coupling helps you control your health and is fundamental to extending your new healthy life.

Energy Management in Phase IV: Longevity

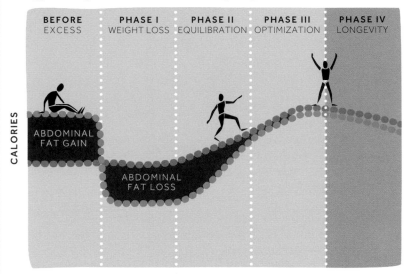

Longevity. Your plan for healthy longevity in Phase IV includes a decrease in calorie intake (blue line), with a resulting decrease in calorie expenditure (beige line). Your body mass index will also shrink and you will become leaner, so you calorie expenditure will also be lower which, at least theoretically, slows the aging process.

And what's the overriding principle of that longevity? It's simple— eat less! It's all about reducing your calorie intake and eating healthier food. Sound familiar? It should, because you're already doing it as part of the Habits of Health. We're just going to tweak your energy plan a bit to put you on our thriving life extension plan. At the same time, we are altering your body composition so you have less fat and leaner muscle. Your body mass index will also shrink and you will become leaner, so your calorie expenditure will also be lower which, at least theoretically, slows the aging process.

Here's how it works: now that you've reached your optimal health and have reduced your body fat and increased your lean muscle, your body will follow your lead and slow down its rate of cellular aging if you simply reduce your calories by a small amount. This principle— the foundation of almost all current longevity work—is called calorie restriction (CR). A more apt term would be dietary restriction, because what we're really talking about is restricting our intake of high-glycemic carbohydrates and saturated animal fat, along with total calories. Now, to some people, that may sound punitive, but that's because the vast majority of those individuals are still in the "before" stage. The chasm between the way they eat now and the way research tells us you need to eat for longevity is huge.

For you, though, it's just the next phase of our plan and, when you're ready for it, you'll find that living longer is something you really can do. Now that the Habits of Health are part of your daily life, the adjustments you need to make in order to live longer and healthier are well within your reach. In fact, the very principles and practice of longevity are embedded in the Habits of Health. It's the only scientifically validated, safe method of life extension, and it's on the very cutting edge of the practice of longevity.

But I'm getting ahead of myself. What's important to know right off the bat is that our longevity plan simply takes the daily choices you're making right now for optimal health and wellbeing and refines them a bit. Like the changes you've already made, these are doable, easy baby steps that you can learn and use for the rest of your life and hopefully that's a good long time to come!

In the next five sections of Part Three, *Longevity*, we'll explore the principles, practice, and future of longevity, including where science might take us next. But we'll keep our discussion grounded in simple actions you can apply right now as you take control of your future by applying the Habits of Health.

- Part 3.1, *The Principles of Longevity: The Secret of Life Extension*, reviews the principles of longevity, including what the most current scientific research tells us about how we can prolong our lives.
- Part 3.2, *The Habits of Longevity: Living Longer in Ultrahealth™*, teaches you the expectations of longevity and outlines our plan to utilize the Habits of Health to create the Habits of Longevity, in order to support a longer, healthier life as a result of optimal health.
- Part 3.3, *Ultimate Energy Control: Extending Your Health through Dietary Optimization and Movement*, describes how dietary optimization and enhanced movement can create ultimate energy control to extend your health.
- Part 3.4, *Brain and Mind Longevity: Protecting and Enhancing Your Future*, discusses important ways to create brain longevity, an important factor in protecting and enhancing your future.
- Part 3.5, *Reaching a State of Ultrahealth™: Living the Future of Wellbeing*, describes what it is like to be Ultrahealthy and looks into the future of the science of longevity.

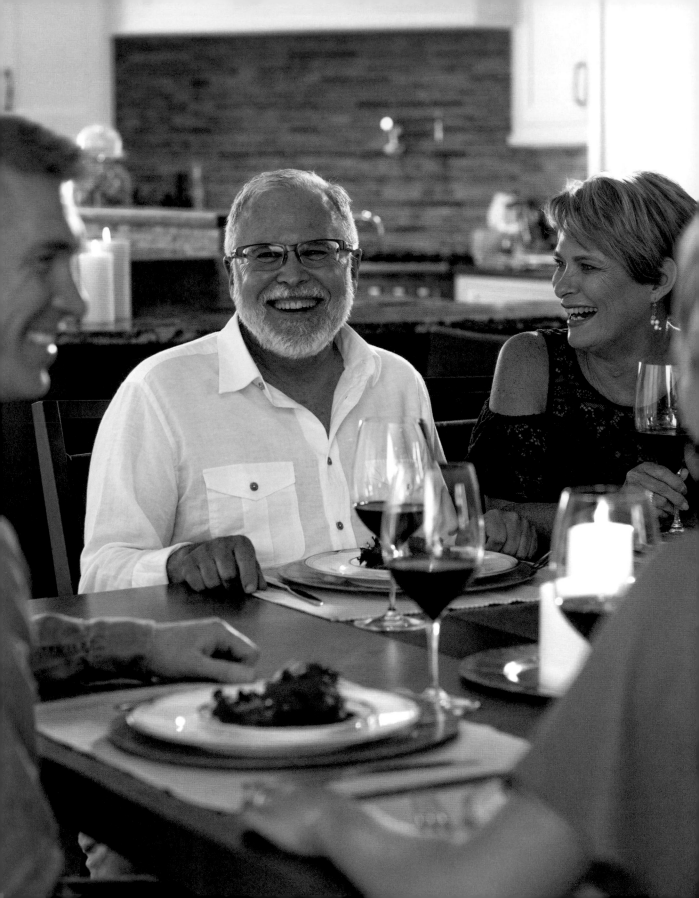

PART 3.1

THE PRINCIPLES OF LONGEVITY: THE SECRET OF LIFE EXTENSION

The image on the right was the first slide of a lecture I once gave to the International Anti-Aging Society. It said almost everything I wanted to say. If you look at all the people who've reached 100 years of age, not one of them is obese.

Why is that the case? Aging is a cellular process that happens in every one of us. How long we live is directly related to how well we take care of ourselves and our cells. The good news is that aging is reversible. Immediate changes can affect your life expectancy in as little as three months. If you start the Habits of Health today, it will take just three years for you to enjoy the same health you would have if you had been practicing them your whole life.

If that's the case, and if you begin your longevity practices right now, just how long can you expect to live?

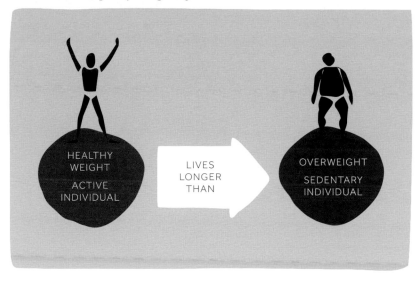

> *The good news is if you have made it to 65 years of age, your lifespan predictively goes up: A man reaching age 65 today can expect to live, on average, until 84.3. A woman turning 65 today can expect to live, on average, until 86.6.*[3]

THE SECRET OF LIFE EXTENSION

Early science perpetuated a fallacy that our life span is predetermined. Well, if we're talking about genetics, we can say with certainty your genes are important and have some influence on how long you're going to live, but studies of identical twins raised in different environments and exposed to different lifestyles, have demonstrated that genetics determines only about 20–30% of health and longevity. Lifestyle and daily behaviors make up the rest to be the dominant factor.[1]

Let's look at this another way. You buy a Porsche (as cars go, it's a genetic purebred) but you don't change the oil or have it serviced regularly. Without proper, routine maintenance, there's every chance it could be outlasted by a plain old Ford Escort; however good its start in life.

What's My Expiration Date?

According to insurance actuarial tables, today's average life expectancy for women is around 80, and for men it's around 75.

Now, that's just the average, meaning that half the population makes it to that age, but by applying the Habits of Health you've already learned, along with the ones I'll be teaching you over the next few sections, you have the capability to extend your life by as much as 35% beyond the average.[2] Studies show an extension of seven years just by maintaining a normal weight, not smoking, and drinking alcohol at moderate levels. Our focus on emotional management, stress reduction, and healthy sleeping can all potentially help us live longer.

What's frustrating is that most of us are born in optimal health. Our modern environment moves us away from it and down the

The oldest documented person in recent history is Jeanne Louise Calment, who lived her whole life in Arles, France, and died in 1997 at age 122. Jean-Marie Robine, a public health researcher and one of the authors of a book about Mrs. Calment commented:

"I think she was someone who, constitutionally and biologically speaking, was immune to stress," he said in a telephone interview. "She once said, 'If you can't do anything about it, don't worry about it.'"

path to non-sickness. It's a tragedy that children as young as five are already suffering the effects of inactivity and high-fat, high-glycemic diets. By the time we reach our thirties, our rate of aging accelerates, and if we don't control our daily choices, it actually begins to double about every eight years. Before long, we're in poorer health, which leads to disease, which leads to death in our mid- to late-seventies. Like a poorly maintained Porsche, we start in perfect condition, and then we just go and rust right through!

But here's the trick: it doesn't have to be that way. You can actually disconnect your biological aging from your chronological age and live longer simply by making the decision today to change your path. By adopting the strategies and choices of the Habits of Health, you can achieve better health almost immediately, slowing the aging process and thriving for many more years to come. The lifestyle changes and improvement in your overall wellbeing are the only real ways (based on the outcome of research studies with many thousands of people)that you can potentially prolong your life.

Of course, there are no guarantees as to how long you'll live (especially if you are a bad driver), but the potential is there if you are willing to do the work and stay safe.

We'll have to wait a few years before we know if what we're doing today has produced a whole generation of healthy 100-year-olds. My educated guess is that it will, and here's some of the science to support it.

LONGEVITY RESEARCH: THE CUTTING EDGE OF MEDICINE

Why do we age? We're here to sustain the species, driven by our ability to pass along genetic material. Once we reproduce and then leave our reproductive usefulness, we're on our own, so it becomes important for each of us to understand how to keep our machinery going for ourselves, as individuals. For that we need to look at tiny structures within our cells called telomeres and mitochondria.

Your chromosomes—organized structures inside your cells that contain your genetic information—are like blueprints that tell your body what you look like and determine how your cells function. Every time our cells reproduce, these chromosomes duplicate themselves. On the end of each chromosome is a telomere, which protects the genetic information that's inside (like tape placed on the end of a rope to stop it from fraying). Each time a cell divides, the telomeres get slightly shorter, until eventually the cell can no longer duplicate.

There's more to learn before we can be absolutely certain, but what we can say is that if you eliminate emotional and oxidative stress and create a rich environment of antioxidant protection, your cells won't need to divide as frequently and will be better able to repair themselves, slowing the shortening of your telomeres.[4]

THE BEST POSSIBLE TIME TO BE ALIVE

Why live longer? Well, because there's never been a more exciting time to be alive. You can communicate with loved ones anywhere in the world at a moment's notice. You can run your business right from the beach and have strawberries in the dead of winter. Travel has become safer, whether you're flying in the latest passenger jet or driving your own car. And medical technology has virtually eliminated most random threats to our survival.

And there's more to come. Ray Kurzweil, a futurist who's made in-depth analyses of the history of technology, believes that our technological growth today is no less than exponential. During the twenty-first century, he says, we'll experience not 100 years of progress, but closer to 20,000. So I want to be here for as long as possible to see what comes next.

Now it's up to you to do your part—to take control of your health and your life; to harness technology and put it in its proper place as your servant, not your master. All these things are within your grasp and available to help you maximize your healthy time on this earth; my longevity plan will show you how.

In the end, we all have a choice. To paraphrase Morgan Freeman's character in *The Shawshank Redemption*, you need to get busy living or you'll get busy dying.

> *The latest scientific research into pathways to longevity confirm what the Habits of Health have been saying all along— exercise, a healthy diet, low body fat, quality sleep, stress reduction, and proper nutritional support all contribute to a long and thriving life!*

THE PRINCIPLES OF LONGEVITY:
THE SECRET OF LIFE EXTENSION

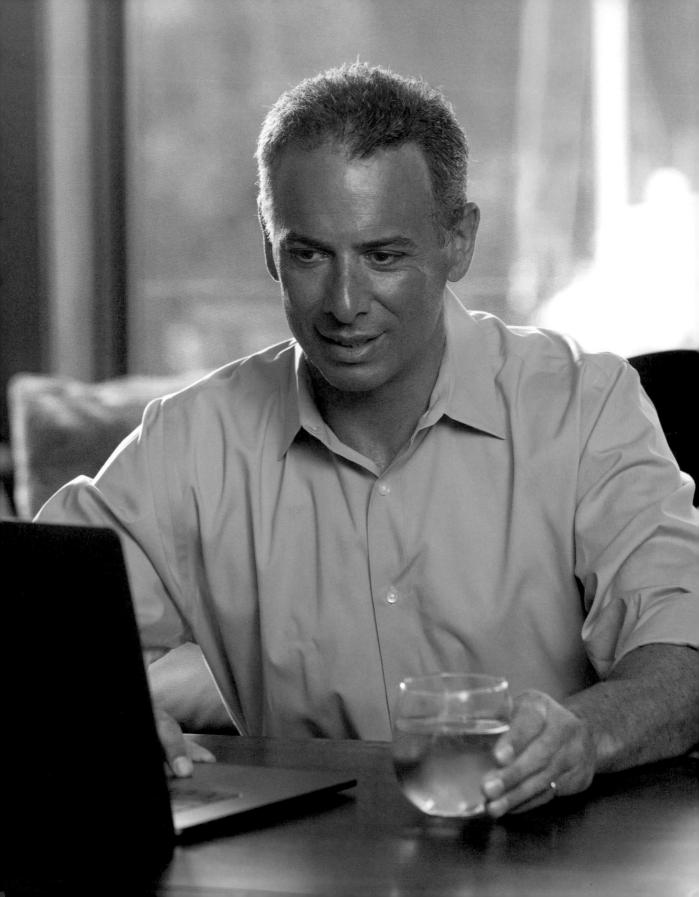

PART 3.2

THE HABITS OF LONGEVITY: LIVING LONGER IN ULTRAHEALTH™

We're now going to design a plan to help you live longer in optimal health and wellbeing, based on current scientific research, observation, and experience. No matter what shape you're in right now, these Habits of Longevity will slow your aging process. In as little as three months, you'll see measurable changes that directly affect your life expectancy and in three years your body will have repaired itself to such an extent that, in physiological terms, it will be as if you've practiced these habits your whole life.

Our strategy is, first, to make sure you're using all the original Habits of Health that can help slow biological aging. And that you are continuing to explore all six MacroHabit categories and continue to master them and progressively install them in higher versions for the rest of your life. We know that these ensure a longer life. Second, we'll reach out to the very edge of safe science and add new advancements that show the most promise and which form the Habits of Longevity.

At the core of these habits is a practice I call dietary optimization (DO), which uses a combination of nutrients and fuel in just the right amounts to maximize health and longevity. Dietary optimization is based on the science of nutritional intervention and includes current research on calorie restriction. While we know that calorie restriction can extend the life span of long-lived mammals, like rhesus monkeys, its ability to extend our own lives is less clear, even though the research is encouraging.[1]

There are factors that we know for certain will have an effect on our health. We know that obesity impairs the functioning of most of our organ systems, paving the way to non-sickness, disease, and premature death. In fact, if the 67% of our people who are overweight[2] (and that includes 18% of children) don't get down to a healthy weight, our society's life expectancy will progressively drop. I predicted 10 years ago it would start dropping in the not too distant future. That prediction has become true as our life expectancies have actually dropped in the last two years. It may be partially driven by opioid overdose but that is part of emotional mismanagement that is a major habit of disease. We will discuss this in detail in Element 23, *Master Your Thoughts and Emotions*, in *Your LifeBook*.[3]

We know that by making the decision to adopt and practice the Habits of Health you can improve your risk factors for cardiovascular disease and a whole host of other conditions that rob you of vitality and health. And we know that as you reach a healthier weight and adopt a healthier lifestyle, you're more likely to live a longer, healthier life.

MAXIMUM LIFE SPAN: LIVING TO OUR POTENTIAL

So realistically, just how much can you extend your life? The answer to that question depends on two governing principles that determine longevity.

The first principle is the limitation of your current design, known as the principle of primary aging. In other words, what is the predicted maximum life span of humans—the longest we can possibly live before our parts simply wear out?

Primary aging is very different from life expectancy (a term that refers to the age at which 50% of the population has died). Life expectancy today is 75 years for men and 80 years for women. But as I mentioned as a result of lifestyle and emotional mismanagement the

"Increasing our maximum life span is a bit like breaking the four-minute mile. People once said the human body couldn't tolerate such intense demands. But they were proved wrong, and today hundreds of runners have managed to push themselves beyond what was believed to be the limit of human capability."

Want a Longer Life?
Give Your Brain a Boost!

Your brain may not be the first thing you think of when you consider the benefits of diet and exercise. But these essential Habits of Health have an enormous impact on this most critical organ. Just consider the following:

- Habits of Disease, such as poor diet, lack of exercise, and too much stress, cause a buildup of beta-amyloid, a key component in Alzheimer's.
- Inflammation and the resulting atherosclerosis can cause brain function to deteriorate by altering the blood flow to the brain.
- Neurotrophins, a substance vital to memory, have been shown to increase through exercise, calorie restriction, and the use of certain spices such as curcumin. They also decrease with stress and inflammation. (for more information, see Part 3.4, *Brain and Mind Longevity, Protecting and Enhancing Your Future*).
- Decreasing diastolic blood pressure to below 90 can make a dramatic difference in the onset of brain aging.

last two years American's life expectancy has been decreasing for the first time in two decades our lifespan.[4] Before this recent decline, life expectancy had risen dramatically since the early 20th century thanks to improved sanitation, medical technology, vaccines, and antibiotics, but many scientists believe that our shelf life—our maximum life span—could actually be as high as 150 years.

It's like the four-minute mile. Some people said it couldn't be done and came up with all sorts of reasons why the human body simply wouldn't tolerate such intense demands. Then, in 1954, Roger Bannister proved them wrong. Since then, our expectations have changed, and several hundred people have run a mile in three minutes 49 seconds or less.

You might recall we talked about Jeanne Louise Calment, who was 122 years old at the time of her death. She holds the record for human maximum life span, but I predict that within a few years, science will be able to extend the life of a healthy individual—one who's mastered the Habits of Health Lifestyle—to closer to 150 years.

And to think that most of us only live half that time.

Expectancy vs. Predicted Maximum Life Span

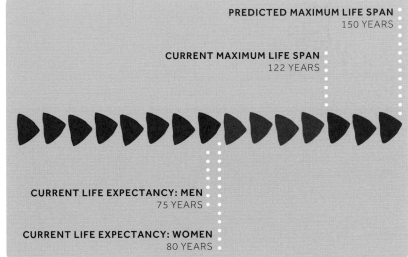

Today's human life expectancy is around 75 years for men and 80 years for women. The longest any human has actually lived (actual maximum life span) is 122 years. But many scientists believe that humans could live as long as 150 years (predicted maximum life span).

RESTORING YOUR BRAIN THROUGH THE HABITS OF LONGEVITY

Why is there such a discrepancy between the life span of most humans and Jeanne Louise Calment?

For the answer we need to look at the second governing principle— the principle of secondary aging. This is the process by which the Habits of Disease produce an insidious deterioration of our organ structure and function, resulting in degenerative disease and cellular aging. This process has begun to accelerate so rapidly that, without drastic intervention and lifestyle change, we will soon counter the medical advances of the twentieth century and see our life expectancy as a society shrink. This is why we are seeing some people's lifespan decreasing, when it would improve if they were living the Habits of Health.

Secondary aging affects all our organ systems, but one that's of particular concern is the brain. While genetics certainly play an important role in memory loss and Alzheimer's, an unhealthy lifestyle and environment make these conditions much more likely to occur. Fortunately, the Habits of Longevity can actually reverse decreases in vital brain chemicals.

Why so much discussion on brain aging? Well, if you make it past 100, we want to make sure you have a fully functioning CPU! That's why in Part 3.4, *Brain and Mind Longevity, Protecting and Enhancing Your Future,* as we look at brain longevity, we'll spend time focusing on specific strategies you can use to keep your brain humming. When we combine the work you are doing to improve your emotional management (Element 23, *Master Your Thoughts and Emotions,* in *Your LifeBook*), you are also setting your brain and mind up for optimization.

Of course, there are no guarantees, but by making the decision to adopt the Habits of Health, you've made the first step. The next step is to ingrain your new healthy habits for 12–24 months to ensure that you can maintain and stabilize your new lifestyle. It may not take you that long, but it's vital that you're comfortable and have solidified your new optimal health lifestyle before taking that next step. This is where *Your LifeBook* helps you write your new story.

3.2

> *Habits of Disease cause our cells to age and our organs deteriorate— including our brain. The Habits of Health help to reverse that process.*

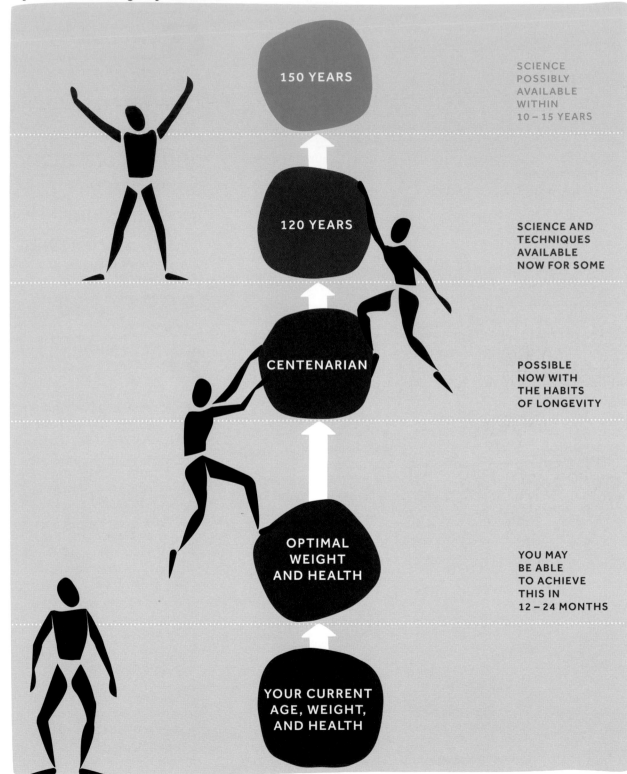

150 YEARS

SCIENCE
POSSIBLY
AVAILABLE
WITHIN
10 – 15 YEARS

120 YEARS

SCIENCE AND
TECHNIQUES
AVAILABLE
NOW FOR SOME

CENTENARIAN

POSSIBLE
NOW WITH
THE HABITS
OF LONGEVITY

OPTIMAL
WEIGHT
AND HEALTH

YOU MAY
BE ABLE
TO ACHIEVE
THIS IN
12 – 24 MONTHS

YOUR CURRENT
AGE, WEIGHT,
AND HEALTH

Adopting the Habits of Health is the first step. After 12–24 months, when you've reached optimal health and have added the Habits of Longevity, you may realistically be able to reach 100 years. And as science and technology advances, longer life spans become increasingly possible.

Once you're ready, have added in the Habits of Longevity, can maintain your optimal weight and health, and can continue to refine your approach by mastering all six MacroHabits, there are no guarantees but you could very well live to see the scientific advances that put a 150-year life span within our grasp.

DR. A'S LONGEVITY PLAN

Here's my plan for a longer life, broken down into simple steps that you can start taking today. These steps include a number of basic actions and behaviors that will reduce your likelihood of falling prey to preventable diseases, accidents and the ravages of an unhealthy lifestyle. They culminate in optimal health, but that's not the end of my longevity plan. In fact, these steps are really a prelude for a lifestyle that can take you even further, to cutting-edge techniques that many scientists and medical researchers believe can extend your life well into a second century. We call it Ultrahealth™.

THE HABITS OF HEALTH

Step 1: Right Now
- Eliminate tobacco.
- Eliminate all recreational drugs.
- Wear a passenger restraint system any time you're in a car, and purchase a vehicle with front and side airbags as soon as possible.
- Drive the speed limit (I don't want you dying at age 100 because you're showing off!)
- Limit your intake of alcoholic beverages to fewer than two drinks a day, and never drink while driving or operating machinery. For more information on red wine and longevity, see HabitsofHealth.com.
- Avoid situations that put you at risk of contracting a sexually transmitted disease (such as having multiple partners).
- Avoid sunburn at all costs.
- Don't exercise on roads used by motor vehicles.

Step 2: Create a Healthy Environment
- Eliminate toxic foods, cleaning supplies, and other poisons such as radon.
- Ensure that your water is clean.

Your Cancer-Screening Guide for Lifelong Health

- **Breast:** self examine monthly; healthcare provider exam once or twice a year; first mammogram at age 40, then yearly after 40.
- **Cervical:** first pap smear at age 21 or within three years of sexual activity.
- **Colon:** first colonoscopy at age 50, then every 10 years; hemoccult test every five years.
- **Prostate:** digital exam and PSA pros and cons considered with counsel from your physician.
- **Skin:** self-exam regularly for unusual or quick-growing lesions.

Oral Health and Inflammation: Pathways to Disease

Gum recession and medication-induced dry mouth—two common complaints related to aging—set us up for cavities and gum disease by creating an environment where bacteria can flourish. As plaque infects the tissues around the teeth, the gums become swollen and red and slowly begin to pull away, resulting in loose teeth and bad breath. But that's not all. This process also sets up an inflammatory state that can lead to heart disease and diabetes.

The cure? Follow my guidelines for dental health, which are important to follow as we age and especially for diabetics, who are at particular risk for progressive gum disease.[5]

Dental health is often neglected (until it's too late!) but it's an important part of optimal health and longevity. After all, you want to be able to continue to enjoy healthy fresh foods into your 100s!

- Ensure that your air is clean.
- Check your smoke detectors to make sure they're working.
- Cover or fence swimming pools.
- Eliminate potential hazards that could cause falls.
- Lock all doors when you're home.
- Lock up firearms.

Step 3: Get a Yearly Check-Up

If you didn't see your healthcare provider before you began your weight-loss and movement program, do so now. You're in the process of a whole-body makeover, and it's important to make sure your blood, heart, and general physical health are all in order. Tell your healthcare provider you're taking part in a program that includes healthy diet, regular movement, better sleep, and stress reduction see what they say! After they recover from fainting, have them check the following:

- Record your weight, waist measurement, height, blood pressure, heart rate, and body mass index so you can track your progress. (When you've reached a state of Ultrahealth™, go back for another check-up so you can watch them faint again!)
- See if you should lower any of your medications as you lose weight.
- Review the full list of medications you're currently putting in your body. Drug interactions can cause serious side effects, erode our health, and increase the likelihood of falls, motor vehicle accidents, and even cellular aging. And because records aren't always complete—not to mention the fact that many of us have multiple healthcare providers—it's really your responsibility to talk with your primary care physician about lowering or eliminating medications. Remember, prescription medications are one of the top five causes of death.
- Ask for a full lipid profile to assess your cardio-metabolic risk and a hs-CRP test to assess your current inflammatory state (to ensure you're staying in control of your immune system; it's also a good idea to continue with follow-up tests for life). If you're 50 or older, a baseline echocardiogram and stress test are in order as well.
- Have appropriate cancer screenings (see the sidebar on the previous page, Your Cancer-Screening Guide for Lifelong Health).
- Make sure you're up to date on your immunizations, including:
  – Pneumovax if you're over 50 (repeat at 65)
  – Tetanus (every ten years)
  – Whooping cough (once for adults)
  – Influenza (yearly)
- Get a baseline TSH to assess thyroid function if you're over 35.
- Have a mineral density scan if you're perimenopausal. Repeat every five years.
- Test sensory systems, including eyes, hearing, and balance. Repeat yearly.

Step 4: Go to Your Dentist

It may surprise you to know that dental health is critical for optimal health and longevity. Keeping your own teeth and maintaining excellent gum and oral health minimizes inflammation and is an important part of our plan.

As a whole, baby boomers, the nation's first fluoride generation, enjoy extraordinary oral health. But this may come to a halt as boomers enter their retirement years and come face to face with gum disease. In fact, if recent trends continue, three out of four boomers will develop gum disease as they age.

Why is that the case? As we get older, we're more prone to certain conditions that put our teeth and gums at peril, including hormonal changes, medical conditions such as diabetes, receding gums that leave roots exposed and vulnerable, and medication-induced dry mouth, which can cause bacteria to proliferate. In addition, the elderly are more likely to have poor dental hygiene and make fewer visits to the dentist.

What can you do about it? For starters:
- Brush at least twice a day with fluoride toothpaste.
- Floss daily.
- Get a yearly check-up from your dentist.
- Have your teeth cleaned twice a year.
- Don't use tobacco products, including cigarettes, chewing tobacco, snuff, pipes, and cigars.
- Drink alcohol in moderation, if at all.
- Use a lip balm that contains sunscreen.
- Avoid lipsticks that don't contain sunscreen (recent research has shown that the pigment in lipstick can actually intensify UV damage).
- Combat dry mouth and keep your oral cavity moist by taking sips of water or chewing sugar-free gum.

Step 5: Reach and Maintain Your Healthy Weight

Reaching a healthy weight not only lowers your risk for disease but actually lengthens your life by several years. If you haven't yet begun the healthy meal plan introduced in Phase I, there's no better time.[6]

Step 6: Incorporate the Habits of Health

From learning to eat right, reaching a healthy weight, incorporating movement into your daily schedule, to making better sleep a priority, and learning to reduce stress and manage your world through a healthy mind, the Habits of Health take you on a complete journey from surviving to thriving.

Step 7: Obtain Optimal Health

No matter what your age, optimizing your health is a fundamental principle of living longer. Not only is it necessary, it makes sense. After all, if you're going to have a longer life, why not be able to fully enjoy everything this big adventure has to offer?

> *Genetics—the cards you're dealt in terms of longevity—actually play a much smaller role in determining life span than your lifestyle. And fortunately, lifestyle is a factor you can control.*

3.2

1. Apply the Habits of Health lifestyle.
2. Reach and maintain optimal health.
3. Add Ultrahealth™ practices—an additional level of vigilance that focuses on increasing your resilience to aging and disease.

Now, if you stop right here at this step and focus on being at the height of health for your whole life, you may live longer. But there's even more you can do. Remember, just as there are no shortcuts to health, there are no shortcuts to longevity. It takes discipline. And just as you made a fundamental choice to be healthy, you can make a fundamental choice to be Ultrahealthy, and take your place among an exciting new generation—the New Centenarians.

ULTRAHEALTH™: THE FINAL STEP

A Practical Approach to Living Longer

The Ultrahealth™ system you're about to discover uses principles drawn from the cutting edge of scientific research. Once you've reached a state of optimal health by adopting the Habits of Health, you can use it to go to the next level and attain your maximum life span.

Let's look at the components that determine just who achieves this ultimate state. Basically, your maximum life span is determined by these three factors, in the following proportion (and we explored this in depth in the previous section):

- Genetic programming (20%–30%)
- Position on the health continuum (70%–80%)
- Luck (< 0.1%)

YOUR POSITION ON THE HEALTH CONTINUUM

Adopting a lifestyle that supports optimal health is by far the biggest factor in longevity. That means that the Habits of Health—which are all about moving forward on the health continuum—are a great way to position yourself for a long and healthy life.

In fact, I believe you can potentially add 10–20 years to your life just by adopting the optimal health lifestyle I've been teaching you. If you're a woman, that means extending your life from 80 years to potentially 100, or from 75–95 if you're a man—simply by living the Habits of Health.[7]

What I propose now is a state of health that pushes you to be the very best you can be, a state in which your body operates at optimal efficiency. A state of living a robust and thriving life, eating only the freshest, nutrient-rich foods, lean and strong, with terrific stamina—kind of like our prehistoric ancestors 10,000 years ago (just without the risk of saber-toothed tigers).

It's a state called Ultrahealth™, and it's really an augmentation of the Habits of Health lifestyle through dietary optimization, intensified weekly workouts, and a focus on brain health. And it has the potential to add another 10–20 years to your life beyond the extra years that optimal health can give you.[8] That potential is becoming a reality in the research as they have used these techniques on monkeys and they are living much longer. Whether this will translate to humans is too soon to know. But what I do know is that the strategies we use in Ultrahealth™ will keep you healthier.

Ultrahealth™ by the Numbers

The ultimate state of health— one that can take you well into your second century of life— is an entirely new standard for health optimization. Here are the key parameters we're aiming for:

- Systolic blood pressure: 110–95 or less
- Diastolic blood pressure: 75–60 or less
- Body mass index: 24.9–20, (21–23 is ideal; no less than 20)
- Body fat: 10% for men; 17–23% for women
- HDI (good cholesterol): 50–70 mg/dl
- Fasting blood sugar: 75 mg / dl
- hs-CRP: 0.5

Life Span Continuum

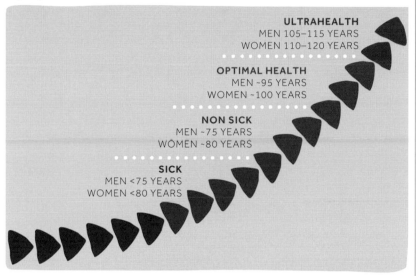

ULTRAHEALTH
MEN 105–115 YEARS
WOMEN 110–120 YEARS

OPTIMAL HEALTH
MEN ~95 YEARS
WOMEN ~100 YEARS

NON SICK
MEN ~75 YEARS
WOMEN ~80 YEARS

SICK
MEN <75 YEARS
WOMEN <80 YEARS

By moving from a state of sickness, to non-sickness, to optimal health, and finally to Ultrahealth™, you can add more than 50% to your life span and live well into your second century.

Ultrahealth™ Arrow

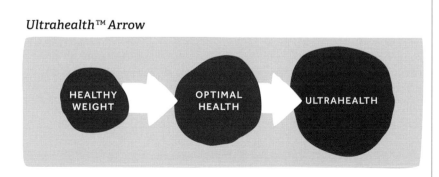

HEALTHY WEIGHT → OPTIMAL HEALTH → ULTRAHEALTH

THE ULTRAHEALTH™ PLAN: EXTEND AND THRIVE

Up to this point, you've learned a practical system to integrate all of ways medical science has to help us stay healthy and protect against disease. Now, the Ultrahealth™ plan will take all that and add yet another level of daily choices. Think of it as your postdoctorate degree in health optimization.

This state of Ultrahealth™ is obtained by making the decision to play full-out with all you have—to organize your life and your daily choices around what's best for your physical, mental, and social wellbeing.

Now before we go on, let me emphasize: if you haven't learned the Habits of Health and applied them to your daily life, and if you haven't reached a healthy weight and aren't currently living an active lifestyle, you aren't going to be able to apply the Ultrahealth™ program to your life.

Why? Well, it will simply be too hard for you. It would be like trying to perform jumps on a double black diamond ski run when you haven't even learned how to snowplow on the bunny slopes. And second, it won't work. If you're still eating a tub of ice cream at bedtime, your high-sugar, high-fat intake is creating an inflammatory state that totally negates the Ultrahealth™ activation of cellular protection and longevity signaling.

If you've already reached and are maintaining optimal health, however, Ultrahealth™ really won't seem like much of a stretch for you. Let's break it down and see why. The Ultrahealth™ plan has three major areas of focus:

- Dietary optimization (DO)
- Movement enhancement
- Brain-health optimization

In the next sections, I'll show you specific strategies to enhance your energy management and optimize your brainpower, starting by focusing on adjusting your dietary intake to improve your body's functioning, reinvigorate you on a cellular level, and set you up with the lowest possible risk for disease as you continue your extended journey through life.

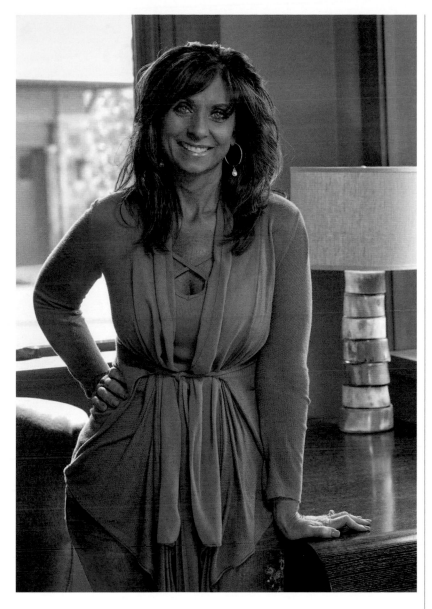

TRANSFORMATION: NANCY STRAUS

It was April of 2012. I was obese, losing my health, and not doing well at all. I was the "Diet Queen", always looking for the latest fad and gimmick. I could lose weight, but I always gained it back and more. At one point I had lost 70 lbs and gained that all back.

I reached out, got some help, and lost 54 lbs.* That's never happened before, as I always gained my weight back. It is such a blessing to have learned how to change my life through the Habits of Health, and I'm also paying it forward by helping others. This is a journey; it's ongoing.

My relationship with food and learning how to deal with emotions instead of using my food as my natural coping mechanism was probably the biggest change. Learning how to eat properly, the right balance, eating every three hours, that's huge. The way I shop at a grocery store is completely different. I'm sure the cereal aisle really misses me, but I don't miss it. Learning these skills is brand new to me, but that has been really life changing for me.

> ❝
> *I was the "Diet Queen", always looking for the latest fad and gimmick.*
> ❞

*Average weight loss on the Optimal Weight 5 & 1 Plan® is 12 lbs.

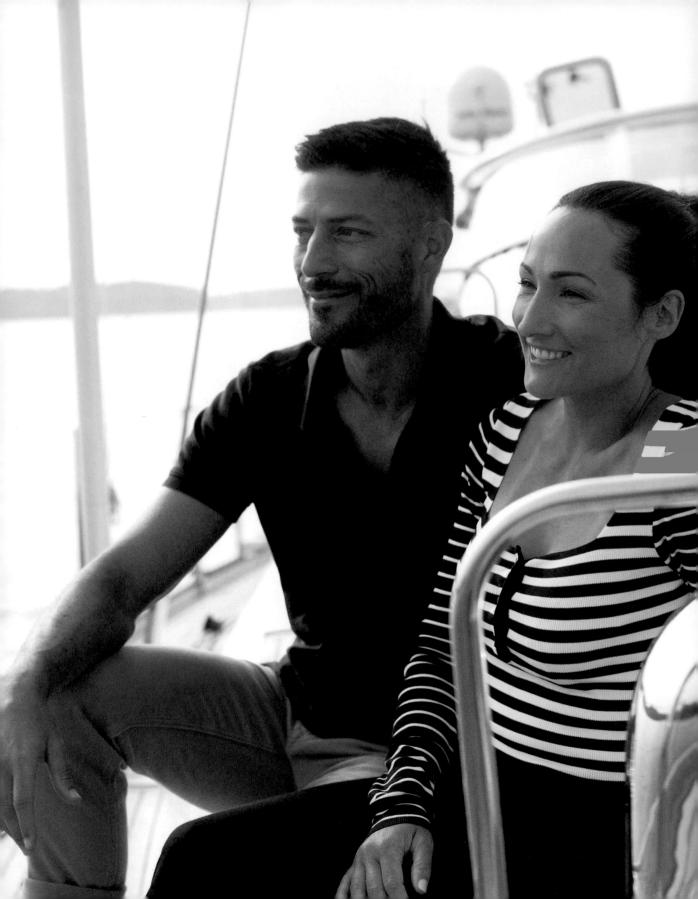

ULTIMATE ENERGY CONTROL: EXTENDING YOUR HEALTH THROUGH DIETARY OPTIMIZATION AND MOVEMENT

Now that you've learned more about the theory behind life extension and can envision just what's possible, you can begin creating a longer, healthier life for yourself through the three-part Ultrahealth™ program. It's a program that builds directly on the habits you've already adopted in your journey to optimal health and wellbeing. We're just going to add in some dietary optimization techniques, intensify your movement plan a bit, and teach you some brain-enhancing practices to keep you protected for life. Think of these as advanced applications of your MacroHabits of Health as we continue your journey to optimal health and wellbeing.

In Phase III, you reached a balance between energy in and energy out as part of your optimization plan for optimal health and wellbeing. For your longevity plan, we're going to tweak that slightly by reducing your daily caloric intake by 15%. That's because it's been scientifically proven that underfeeding with nutrient-dense foods is more conducive to health and longevity than overfeeding with nutrient-poor, energy-dense food.

But altering your energy consumption is just one part of our plan. We're also going to focus on eliminating all processed foods so that your diet consists of the freshest foods possible.

EATING FOR ULTRAHEALTH™: ADJUSTING YOUR DAILY INTAKE

First let's calculate your Ultrahealth™ daily energy intake. Now that we are advancing your understanding of caloric management we are going to use the more sophisticated way of calculating your total energy expenditure which is explained in detail at HabitsofHealth.com. We will use an example of a 46-year-old woman who has just finished *Your LifeBook* and her first year as a Habits of Health graduate and has decided to become ultrahealthy. Let's show you how to calculate her TEE:

- 46-year-old female
- five foot, nine inches (69 inches)
- Utilizing the EAT walking and two-day-a-week weight-training programs
- Body mass index of 24
- 162 lbs (down from 206 lbs)

We'll plug those numbers into the formula for calculating total energy expenditure (TEE), from the appendix:

TEE = BMR + PAL + TEF

Let's break that formula down to see how many calories she's currently burning in a day:

BMR (Basal Metabolic Rate)

BMR = $10 \times$ (WEIGHT IN POUNDS $\times 0.455$) $+ 6.25 \times$ (HEIGHT IN INCHES $\times 2.54$) $- 5 \times$ (AGE) $- 161$
BMR = $10 \times$ (164 $\times 0.455$) $+ 6.25 \times$ (69 $\times 2.54$) $- 5 \times$ (46) $- 161$
BMR = 1,450 CALORIES PER DAY

Be sure to consult your healthcare provider before you begin the Ultrahealth™ program.

When Can I Start the Ultrahealth™ Longevity Program?

Before starting the Ultrahealth™ program, I recommend that you reach optimal health and maintain a stable weight and reach normal lab results (lipid profile, hs-CRP, electrolytes, liver and kidney function, metabolic parameter including blood sugar, and thyroid function if you're over 35) for at least six months, preferably a year. You should also discuss your plan with your healthcare provider and, if they agree that it's safe for you to take part, follow up with visits based on their recommendations. (I would suggest a visit every three months for the first year and yearly visits after that.)

Warning: Do not allow your BMI (body mass index) to fall lower than 20. Monitor your progress closely with your physician. Any history of eating disorders, immune suppression, or other wasting disorders is an absolute contraindication to this program.

Activity Factor:

Multiply your TEE by:
- 1.2 (for light exercise)
- 1.5 (for moderate exercise)
- 1.7 (for heavy exercise)

PAL (physical activity level)

This is the difference between your baseline BMR and your BMR modified for activity (BMR × Activity Factor). To determine your modified BMR, which is called your EPAL, take the BMR from above and multiply it by the Activity Factor in the sidebar:

This modified BMR is called your EPAL.

EPAL =	BMR	X	ACTIVITY FACTOR
EPAL =	1,450 CALORIES	X	1.5 (ACTIVE)
EPAL =	2,175 CALORIES PER DAY		

As you can see, her BMR has increased as a result of her activity levels.

TEF (thermic effect of food)

TEF =	EPAL	X	0.1 (10% OF EPAL)
EPAL =	2,175	X	0.1
EPAL =	217 CALORIES		

TEE (Total Energy Requirement)

So, by taking the 2,175 calories we calculated by adding in her EPAL, and then adding the 217 calories she uses to process her food (her TEF), we come up with a total energy requirement of 2,392 calories per day—her TEE.

TEF =	EPAL	+	TEF
TEE =	2,175	+	217
TEE =	2,392		

Currently, this patient is consuming and expending approximately 2,400 calories per day through her new active lifestyle and has remained at a stable BMI (body mass index) of 24 for the past two years. Her blood chemistry is normal, including her glucose and hs-CRP; her lipid profile is within normal range.

Her thyroid function has never been better, her blood pressure is down to 125/80, and her body fat is 26%—all within normal limits. She is enjoying an optimally healthy, energy-filled life and has made the decision to take the next step—to achieve Ultrahealth™ and seize its potential to extend her new thriving life.

To take that step, she'll need to figure out her adjusted Ultrahealth™ calorie intake. To do so, she'll start with her optimal health TEE of 2,392 calories per day and use this formula:

NEW ENERGY INTAKE =	TEE	x	0.85
NEW ENERGY INTAKE =	2,400	x	0.85
EPAL =	2,040 CALORIES PER DAY		

So let's sum up. This woman's dietary optimization will include a decrease in daily calories to 2,040 calories. She'll accomplish this by eliminating all ultra-processed food and by choosing foods in the dark green section of the food charts. That way, she can be sure she's eating only nutrient-filled, low-glycemic carbohydrates, lean protein, and healthy fats. Here's how her daily eating plan will look:

- 2,040 kcal/day
- No ultra-processed foods
- Lowest-glycemic carbohydrates
- Increased soy intake (based on Okinawan longevity studies; see Part 3.1, *The Principles of Longevity: The Secret of Life Extension*)
- Healthy fats, especially olive oil, fish oils, walnuts, and flaxseed
- Every-three-hour eating schedule

Here's a snapshot of a typical daily meal plan for someone consuming about that number of calories under the Ultrahealth™ program.

Sample Ultrahealth™ Daily Meal Plan

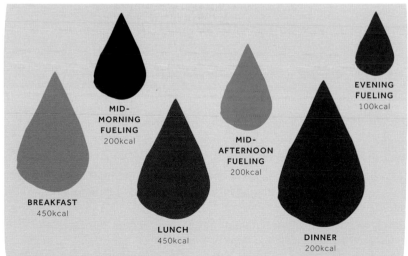

EVENING FUELING
100kcal

MID-MORNING FUELING
200kcal

MID-AFTERNOON FUELING
200kcal

BREAKFAST
450kcal

LUNCH
450kcal

DINNER
200kcal

With the Ultrahealth™ meal plan, you'll decrease your energy intake slightly from your optimal health level, but you'll still fuel every three hours. Here's an example of how a day's meals might look if you're taking in about 2,000 calories a day.

As you can see, while the calorie level of most of your daily fuelings has increased, you should keep your evening fueling at 100 calories

> *Start out slowly by incorporating these enhancements into the EAT resistance routines outlined in Part 2.12, Dr. A's Habits of Healthy Motion Part 2: EAT System.*

Low-intensity interval

Around 50–60% of your maximum heart rate (MHR), or a rate of perceived exertion (RPE) of around five to six.

High-intensity interval

Around 75–90% of your maximum heart rate (MHR), or a rate of perceived exertion (RPE) of around seven to nine.

Caution: Consult your healthcare provider before you begin any exercise program or increase the intensity of your workouts in order to ensure that your blood pressure, lung function, and musculoskeletal systems can handle the increased challenge.

For more information on MHR and the RPE scale, see Part 2.12, Dr. A's Habits of Healthy Motion Part 2: EAT System.

and, if you need to adjust your schedule to eat fewer calories, you steal those from your evening meal or decrease your mid-morning and mid-afternoon to 100 calories.

Note that while the Ultrahealth™ plan involves reduced caloric intake, it still requires you to fuel every three hours. To make this doable, I recommend you take another look at the fueling strategies in the healthy eating parts. It's worth noting that OPTAVIA®, as a pioneer and leader in restrictive-calorie meal plans, provides an excellent method to help you implement a regimen of dietary restriction. Scientifically formulated portion-controlled meals are particularly effective in delivering a nutrient-rich, low-calorie diet that also provides plenty of health-supporting soy!

Of course, in addition to eating a full range of nutrient-dense foods, you'll want to make sure you're getting the full range of supplementation outlined in Part 2.15, *The Best You Can Be: Optimizing Your Life at Any Age*. We'll augment that list in the next part by adding supplements that enhance your brain capacity and function for lasting health.

Exercise Enhancement: The Other Half of the Equation

Of course, it's not just your energy input that will change under the Ultrahealth™ system. You'll also be increasing your energy expenditure by 15% twice a week, on top of your current EAT walking and resistance program. Not only will you use more calories, you'll also receive increased cardiovascular benefits from these more intense workouts.

Here's the formula you'll use to calculate this increased energy expenditure:

ADDITIONAL ENERGY EXPENDITURE TWICE A WEEK = OPTIMAL HEALTH TEE × 0.15	
ADDITIONAL ENERGY EXPENDITURE TWICE A WEEK = 2,400 × 0.15	
ADDITIONAL ENERGY EXPENDITURE TWICE A WEEK = 360 CALORIES	

For our sample patient: 2,400 kcal × 0.15 = 360 kcal. That's the number of calories she'll be burning twice a week on top of her already robust EAT walking and resistance program. This can be accomplished either by adding intensity to the two weekly EAT Resistance Program workouts or by switching two of your weekly EAT Walking Program walks for two 20-minute interval-training sessions (plus 10-minute cool down), depending on your age, ability, and schedule.

In order to assure that your EAT Ultrahealth™ movements are on the cutting edge of exercise physiology, Greg Freitag, a top exercise physiologist at Johns Hopkins and an expert in the science of exercise help design this program. Together, we've designed an enhancement program that's sustainable, provides just the right intensity, and is minimally intrusive to your busy schedule. These additional movements complete our EAT System, enhancing your energy expenditure and cardiovascular fitness to help support maximum functional longevity.

Intensifying Your Workouts: Options for Enhancement

I've developed several options for increasing your energy output. First, let's look at some ways to boost your current resistance workouts. Second, we'll explore once again high intensity interval training, an option you can use to enhance the intensity of two of your 30-minute walks per week.

Six Options to Boost Your EAT Resistance Workouts

1. Increase repetitions: instead of performing five repetitions of each exercise, perform six to eight, while maintaining the 8-4-8 pattern (contraction-holding-relaxation) as well as your speed.

2. Increase resistance: increase the weight or resistance you use in each exercise by 10–15%, while maintaining the 8-4-8 pattern and your speed. You can accomplish this by using resistance bands and heavier dumbbells. Make sure your exercise ball is fully inflated to ensure the greatest balance challenge to your core. You'll also want to increase your own focus and effort of contraction.

3. Increase sets or rotations: complete three rotations instead of just two. This will increase your EAT resistance workout time by about one-third, or 10 minutes.

4. Decrease recovery time: decrease the amount of time you rest between exercises from 20 seconds to 10 seconds. Not only will this increase the demand on your muscle fibers, it will enable you to maintain an elevated heart rate throughout your resistance workout.

5. Increase your speed: increase the speed of each repetition from 8-4-8 (contraction-holding-relaxation) to 4-2-4. You'll generate more force per repetition, which means you should also increase the resistance or amount of weight by 15–25%.

6. Maintain muscular contraction: pay closer attention to keeping the contraction in your muscles, not your bones. It's common to "lock out" your joints during an exercise by straightening your elbows in a push-up or your knees in a squat, for example. But this transfers the weight onto your bone structure and away from working muscles, and is not recommended. By avoiding "locking out," you increase tension and maintain a high level of intensity throughout your repetitions.

Intensifying Your EAT Walking Workouts Through Interval Training

High Intensity Interval Training is a time-efficient way to train your aerobic (cardiovascular) and anaerobic (muscle) energy-burning systems. It's called interval training because it consists of short periods, or intervals, of high-intensity cardiovascular activity

"

If the weather's hot, exercise early or late in the day and remember to drink extra water to stay hydrated. Cut back or stop exercising completely if you feel dizzy, nauseous, light headed, or get a headache. And, of course, remember to wear sunscreen when exercising outdoors!

"

- NEAT
- EAT Walking
- EAT Resistance
- EAT enhancement (twice per week, replaces EAT walking or resistance training for that day)

followed by short periods of lower-intensity cardiovascular activity. By alternating high- and low-intensity intervals, you intensify the metabolic challenge to your muscles, increasing the amount of calories burned in each 20-minute session and that can help prevent injury by keeping exercise time shorter and saving muscles from overuse. In Element 18 of *Your LifeBook*, *Exercise is Your Gift to Yourself,* there are some great exercises for HIIT its called: High Intensity Interval Training (HIIT) at Home.

Just as we provided sample exercise routines for the early portions of your EAT journey at HabitsofHealth.com, we created Ultrahealth™ versions of EAT exercise routines as well. You are welcome to adjust them according to your preferences and needs, but the framework of the program is available to you online at HabitsofHealth.com.

Together, these increased activities provide a robust movement plan that builds optimal cardiovascular, musculoskeletal, and brain health. Combined with the nutrient-dense, calorie-reduced fuelings you'll be getting through dietary optimization, you'll have the tools you need to create an Ultrahealth™ state and stay in top physical shape into your seventies and eighties.

In fact, there's no reason you can't continue this high level of fitness even into your nineties. Just look at Jack LaLanne, my all-time optimal health hero. He lived to 96 years of age and was among the first to realize the importance of extreme fitness and proper nutrition. He lived in a state of Ultrahealth™ and was working with a group of innovative healthcare professionals to create a supervised program of EAT-type activities specially designed to help senior citizens get fit and stay fit. To find out more about it, visit www.HabitsofHealth.com.

Maintaining optimal health and fitness for as long as possible is key to supporting the most critical Ultrahealth™ determinant of all— your brain. By protecting and enhancing the health and wellbeing of your brain and following the Habits of Longevity, you have a real shot at reaching that three-digit life span.

Let's turn our focus to the inner workings of your mind and get you on your way to ultimate health!

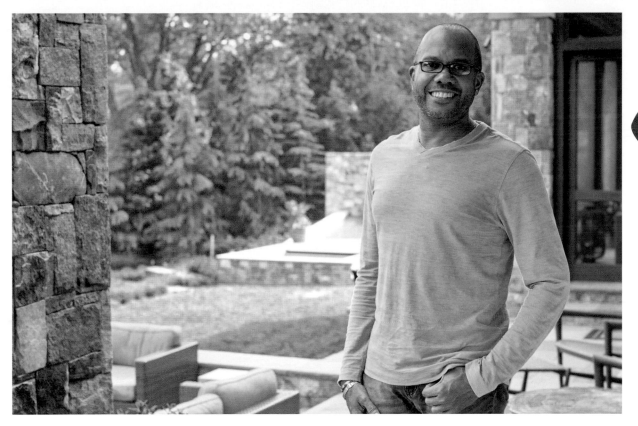

TRANSFORMATION: MARCUS CAILLET

> "
> I needed to gain
> control of my
> destiny and
> my health,
> so I thought
> why not take a
> chance and try?
> "

I started my journey with Dr. A because my mom told me I looked a little chubby and I needed to lose some weight. I was on blood pressure and cholesterol medicine. I needed to gain control of my destiny and my health, so I thought why not take a chance and try? In six weeks, I was 34 lbs* down, and my whole life changed.

Before I started, I put everything else before myself. Then I started realizing what was important to me: getting up in the morning, fueling my body with what I needed to go throughout the day, realizing that some days you just have to work on your mind and just relax, meditate, whatever it is that you like to do to give yourself that energy.

I definitely believe that your health is your wealth. For me it's one day at a time moving to what is important. I tell people that I've maintained my weight, and it happened by choice, not by chance. It's those choices that I continue to make on a day-to-day basis that enable to me to be where I am, feel the energy, and be in that great space.

*Average weight loss on the Optimal Weight 5 & 1 Plan® is 12 lbs. Clients are in weight loss, on average, for 12 weeks.

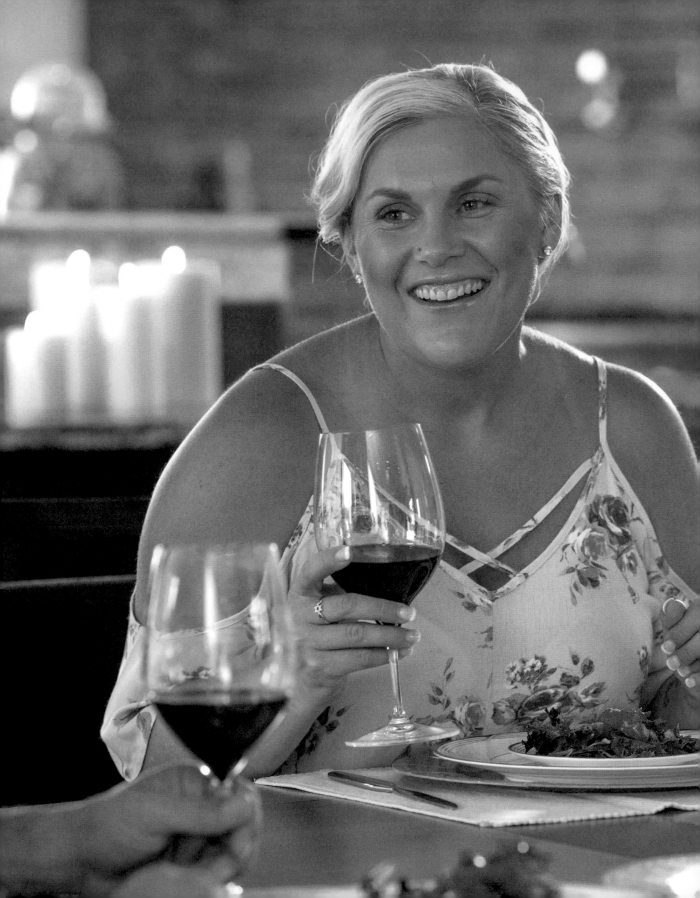

BRAIN AND MIND LONGEVITY: PROTECTING AND ENHANCING YOUR FUTURE

The brain and the mind are the source of all health and the master controller of aging. Its most fundamental function is to control the movement of the body. Without it, we would quickly go down the path to disease and death. In fact, the brain is one of the first organs to suffer if our daily movement is impeded. And, if we don't protect our master controller, we may lose our memory and our ability to think—at which point it really wouldn't make sense to extend our life anyway.

I've singled the brain out for special attention not only because of its central role in health and longevity, but also because it's become particularly vulnerable to injury in our rapidly advancing, technologically driven society. Our Western lifestyle, with a diet high in animal fats and high-glycemic carbohydrates, a lack of exercise, and excessive stress is pounding away at our brains as well as our hearts. Fortunately, reaching optimal health and wellbeing through the Habits of Health eliminates most of these negative factors.

Our goal in this part is to become laser-focused on the specific habits that will protect and enhance your brain and enable it to continue directing you toward a state of ever-increasing health. Our strategy concentrates on three major areas essential for brain health and longevity:

- Brain exercise (including physical exercise).
- Stress reduction.
- Brain food (we will address Brain Food (Nutritional Enhancement) in Element 26, *Ultrahealth™: Living Longer Full Out*, in *Your LifeBook*).

Let's give your brain a workout and some active rest!

THE SCIENCE OF THINKING

As science reveals the secrets of the three-pound CPU on top of your shoulders, we're discovering the brain's amazing resilience to changing conditions—what neuroscientists call "plasticity". Your brain will provide optimal levels of cognition and memory as long as you maintain it under the following conditions:

- Use it.
- Keep enough blood flowing to provide the oxygen it needs to flourish.
- Feed it enough of the right nutrients.

The brain cells we're going to be focusing on are neurons—the thinking cells that create and support memory. You have about 100 billion of them, yet they make up only 10% of your total brain cells. The remaining 90% are composed of support cells that provide housekeeping functions for the neurons. Neurons have several important components:

- *Axons*: long extensions that work like a TV cable to send messages out to other neurons and, through the spinal cord, to muscle cells
- *Dendrites*: antenna-like extensions that serve as receivers to pull information into the neuron and of course the brain
- *Synapses*: making neuron-to-neuron connections (there are up to 10,000 per neuron).

"

Studies show again and again that even moderate exercise like walking can improve brain health dramatically. And best of all, it's never too late to start.

"

Nomads and Neanderthals: Survival of the Fittest (Brains, That Is!)

10,000 years ago, our ancestors were nomadic. New environments and survival skills meant that their brains were constantly stimulated. Neanderthals, on the other hand, stayed close to their original territories and caves. As a result, they may have lacked the flexibility and innovation needed to survive.

"

Exercise to ward off strokes! According to recent research, older people who walked as little as 20 minutes a day reduced their risk of a stroke by 57%.[1]

"

Can Mental Activity Stave Off Alzheimer's?

Older adults who stay mentally active may be at lower risk for developing Alzheimer's disease, says recent (albeit limited) research. This includes reading, playing cards and other games, working crossword puzzles, going to museums, and even watching television or listening to the radio. Although this "use it or lose it" approach hasn't been proved, no harm can come from putting your brain to work on a regular basis.[2]

Through these components, each neuron acts as its own separate computer. Based on 100 billion neurons with 10,000 synapses each, that's a total of 100 trillion connections!

This amazing neural network transmits at 10 different levels of intensity, each capable of 200 calculations per second. In fact, the number of different brain states your neural network is capable of creating is greater than the total number of atoms in the universe. Think about that for a moment. (Aha! You just did a brain exercise!)

Memory and learning are dependent on changes in synapses. With each change that occurs, the size and health of the two—or 10,000—neurons involved actually increase, making it easier to communicate. This phenomenon is called long-term potentiation (LTP), and it explains why connections wither if you stop using them, just like muscles do from lack of exercise. And that fact leads us to our first area of enhancement.

BRAIN EXERCISE

Scientists at Brown University found that when rats were trained to accomplish a new motor skill, their brains changed over the course of the training. The synapses of the brain cells that were used actually grew. Just like doing curls increases the size of your biceps, doing mental exercises repairs damaged pathways and creates new ones, building memory and keeping your brain healthy.

So just what types of exercise can we do to increase our brain health and longevity?

Use It or Lose It: Mental Exercise for Brain Health

Our brains need a workout as much as our bodies do! But it doesn't need to be complicated. In fact, creating brain fitness can be as simple as reading, writing, doing crossword puzzles, hanging out talking to friends, going to meetings, learning how to play a musical instrument, playing video games, or spending the evening dancing.

Anytime you perform an activity that's different from your usual activity, you're creating new neural pathways. Here's an example to try: next time you're at your computer, try moving the mouse with your opposite hand. It will probably feel as awkward as the first time you tried to tie your shoelaces! At the beginning, as your brain builds new pathways, it can be hard to use precise movements, and you'll probably perform tasks more slowly but if you stick with it, you will improve.

Create new neural pathways by using your opposite hand to perform other daily activities, such as brushing your hair and teeth, grooming the dog, sending text messages, or dialing a phone number. You could even try changing the ear you use to talk on the phone.

Work on changing your sensory reality while doing daily chores. Eat dinner without talking, using only visual cues, or close your eyes while washing your hair and getting dressed. Challenge your brain to learn new and novel tasks, especially things you've never done before. Try playing chess or advanced card games, or take up tai chi, yoga, or sculpting. Travel to new places and explore new environments or, if you can't get away, just drive home following a different route.

The good news is that whatever our age, our brains can continue to grow and renew. In fact, according to renowned brain researcher Dr. Marian Diamond, senior citizens have even more highly developed neuronal networks than younger people, meaning they're even more responsive to intellectual enrichment. At birth, our neurons are just little spheres, sending out tiny preliminary branches of dendrites. But, as we grow, our neurons continue to reach out and gather information, communicating and creating a network of interconnectivity.

PUMP IT UP: PHYSICAL EXERCISE FOR BRAIN HEALTH

Statistics actually support the saying "What's good for the heart is good for the head." Adults who exercise at least three times a week have a 30–40% lower risk of developing dementia later in life than those who don't exercise. So why is exercise important for the brain? There are three factors:[3]

- It provides a healthy brain environment.
- It stimulates nerve growth factor (NGF).
- It reduces stress.

Let's look at these benefits one by one.

A Healthy Brain Environment
Exercise increases blood flow to the brain, delivering nutrients and oxygen and flushing out waste and necrotic debris such as beta-amyloid—toxic protein fragments that can jam up transmissions in the hippocampus (your memory command center). Exercise even helps prevent beta-amyloid from being produced in the first place.

Exercise can also increase neurotransmitters, such as norepinephrine and dopamine, and makes beneficial CoQ10 more easily available. It also boosts neuropeptides, such as endorphins, and decreases damaging cortisol. It stabilizes blood sugar and can relieve depression just as effectively as medication. And it plays a key role in lowering blood pressure, which improves cognition, slows Alzheimer's, and is an important determinant of long-term brain health.

And the great thing is, you don't even need to be an elite triathlete to enjoy this wealth of benefits. It turns out that plain old walking is especially good for the brain as it increases blood circulation, but it's not so strenuous as to cause your legs to take up the extra oxygen and glucose like other types of exercise can. And, according to a

Exercise your brain regularly with books of brain-teasers or other mental exercises. Here are some great choices:

- *Mensa Mind Teasers*, puzzles, games, and apps by Philip J. Carter and Kenneth A Russell (Sterling Publishing, 2017)
- *Sharpbrains*: Online resource 2018
- *Lumosity Online* daily trainer 2018
- *Get Your Brain in the Fast Lane*, by Michel Noir and Bernard Croisile (Mcgraw-Hill, 2006)

If we exercise our brains and increase these connections through continual stimulation, we can protect ourselves from memory loss and maintain our cognitive ability. After all, studies show that better-educated people have less risk of Alzheimer's, and that engaging in manual activities that require thought and action can increase and speed up cognition. So go play Bingo, engage in do-it-yourself projects, paint, participate in sports, or grow a garden! Just remember to vary your intellectual activities on a regular basis to keep stretching your brain.

Cognitive Training for Your Brain

One important study tracked 5,000 people between the ages of 20–90. When participants began experiencing mental decline, they were given a series of one-hour activities designed to improve inductive reasoning and spatial orientation. The results? Over half of the subjects improved significantly, showing that mental enrichment can increase intelligence at any age. In other words, if you haven't been using your brain, fire up the mental treadmill and watch your thinking power bounce back![4] Here are some mental practices you can follow to boost your brain's learning capacity:

- Practice the art of focusing— think about what you're doing ("I'm putting my keys on the table").
- Finding something you want to learn how to do and build some new circuitry by actually doing it!
- Mentally repeat information you've just learned to ensure it transfers to your long-term memory. Attaching emotion to an event can help you remember it as well.
- Think about what you're trying to learn. ("So why exactly is high-glycemic food bad for me?")
- Mentally summarize what you've just learned.
- Organize information into categories. Try classifying your grocery list, for example, use acronyms or create associations between things to tie information together and ground it in your memory.
- Use all of the exercises we created for improving you emotional management in Element 23 of *Your LifeBook*, *Master Your Thoughts and Emotions*.

recent study, walking is even more effective than weight training in preserving and enhancing brain health.

In fact, studies repeatedly show that this type of moderate exercise produces dramatic results. Here are findings from some of those studies:[5]

- Sedentary individuals were twice as likely to get Alzheimer's as those who exercised three times a week.[6]
- People 85 and older who remained active were spared significant heart disease and enjoyed 80% better memory functions than their inactive peers.[7]
- Seniors who walked regularly showed significant improvement over sedentary older people as they had better learning abilities, concentration, and abstract reasoning.[8]
- Woman walkers in their 70s experienced much less cognitive decline than their sedentary peers, and with each additional mile they further decreased the decline by 13%.[9]
- Exercisers exhibited much less decline in frontal and prefrontal regions of the brain, preserving executive function, such as planning, organization, and mental multitasking.
- Moderate exercise has been shown to improve brain cell survival in neurodegenerative disease.[10]
- Running boosts brain cells in the hippocampus—the area of the brain responsible for memory.

As you can see, it's never too late to start. In fact, exercising to boost your brain is more important than ever as we age. Older people who have heart disease and high blood pressure suffer cognitive decline because the blood flow to their brain is decreased. After all, the brain uses about 25% of our blood supply and exercise plays a critical role in increasing the strength of the entire circulatory system.

Nerve Growth Factor (NGF)

Nerve growth factor (NGF) and brain-derived neurotrophic factor (BDNF)—two powerful substances produced in the brain—are stimulated by exercise and suppressed by stress and high levels of saturated fats and refined sugars.

Why are these substances so important? NGF and BDNF repair and rescue damaged neurons, increase production of neurotransmitters and protect the neurons from oxygen stress radicals. They can help improve intelligence and are guardians that bathe, protect, and heal our precious neurons.

All we have to do to help them out is to go take a brisk walk! In fact, walking is just what the doctor ordered to clear your head.

Stress Reduction

Most of us rarely experience true relaxation (outside of vacation, that is). Yet, this state—being relaxed, creative, intuitive, vibrant, intelligent—should be our brain's normal default state. It's how we're supposed to be.

When we're stressed, our brain can't function optimally, and when stress becomes chronic, it can decrease brain health and accelerate cellular aging. In fact, reducing the amount of stress in our life is so critical to brain health that I've devoted the whole next section of this part to mental techniques that can help you relax and become more stress-free. This will allow you to take control of your life and choose the outcome that supports your long-term goal of a healthy brain and a healthy mind.

We have been talking since Part 1.1, *It's Not Your Fault That You're Struggling*, about how 10,000 years ago we were protected by our own flight-or-fight response to risk and how much of its ancient utility is no longer serving us in our modern life. Let's look deeper into the human stress response which served our ancestors so well. For them, stress was almost always induced by physical danger, and those dangers demanded a physical response. When they came face-to-face with a predator and their brains shot out norepinephrine, epinephrine, and cortisol, they used those chemicals to evade danger and stay alive.

But today, that stress response can turn on us. In the course of our modern, chaotic lives, our stress response may be activated several times a day. But unlike in ancient times, it's almost always in response to mental threats that don't elicit a physical response—like running or fighting. Instead, we internalize the stress, bathing our brain and heart with damaging substances that create systemic inflammation.

And here's something interesting, because the initial stress response gives us a jolt of energy and self-confidence, we can actually become addicted to it. The result? Chronic stress and a decline in brain function. Over time, ongoing stress reduces the neurotransmitters in the frontal lobe of our neocortex, where most of our abstract thinking occurs, and shunts norepinephrine away from the limbic system, which controls emotions. That can lead to anxiety, poor work performance, depression, and feelings of helplessness and lack of meaning.

Now how can we prevent those excess stress chemicals from just sitting there inside us causing all that damage? Exercise, of course! Exercise is a wonderfully effective way to dispose of these stress chemicals in just the way your body was designed to. All kinds of exercises are effective for this, but activities that mimic aggression such as kicks, lifts, or thrusts are especially therapeutic, as is physical labor like digging or whacking weeds. Not only will you burn off the stress you're feeling at the moment, you'll also create resistance to future stress and help your brain (and your garden) grow.

DR. A SAYS...

" *Want to learn more? For a great introduction to meditative techniques, you might enjoy reading "Notes to Myself", by Hugh Prather.* "

3.4

High Blood Pressure and Brain Risk

Having diastolic blood pressure of 90 or above for 20 years raises your risk of dementia to five times that of someone whose diastolic blood pressure is under 90.[11]

Counter the stress response with the relaxation response—a meditation-based technique to calm body and brain.

Stress Reduction: The Relaxation Response

Now that you've seen how exercise can help reverse the ill effects of stress, let's add to your arsenal with some specific techniques to help you respond to stress whenever it occurs, so you can take your brain back into its normal, default state of relaxation.

To do that, I'm going to teach you to develop a Habit of Health that's just the opposite of the stress response, called the relaxation response. Originally developed by Dr. Herbert Benson at Harvard, the relaxation response is based on meditation. But it just takes the parts that are connected with mental relaxation, enabling anyone to use this wonderful mechanism to reduce stress and improve brain health.

What we're going to do in essence is teach your neocortex—the part of your brain responsible for higher thought—to tell the emotional areas of your brain to relax. This stimulates the release of brain chemicals that change the body's state from one of stress to one of relaxation. It puts the brakes on our normal ways of thinking, slowing us down so that we actually begin to experience short pauses in which we have no thoughts at all. Our body's autonomic functions, such as heart rate and breathing, naturally begin to slow down and we feel calm. Stress chemicals recede and our brain gets a much needed rest.

It's a remarkable process, and there are a number of books available that can teach you the proper techniques in depth. We have many resources at the HabitsofHealth.com on relaxation, mediation and, of course, *Your Lifebook* is full of breathing exercises and ways to relax as well. But, for now, I'd like to show you some very basic methods that anyone can use to reach this relaxed and healthy stress-free state.

A Simple Relaxation Meditation

The goal here is to clear your mind of all thoughts—to turn off the mental merry-go-round that's feeding your brain and body with tension and creating a negative mental state.

Step 1: Set aside 10 to 20 minutes. Good choices might be in the morning, during your Model Morning, before breakfast or just before your evening meal, or during your Twilight Hour.

Step 2: Find a cozy spot—a quiet, serene place where you can be alone with your thoughts without interruption. Make sure to turn off any electronic communication devices. Silence is the overriding principle.

Step 3: Sit up straight on the floor, in a comfortable, relaxed position with your legs crossed. (Alternatively, you may sit in a chair with your feet flat, if sitting on the floor is difficult or uncomfortable for you.) Place your hands together in your lap, with your right hand resting in your left, palms up. Begin taking slow breaths using the abdominal breathing technique described throughout the system and on the HabitsofHealth.com.

Step 4: Close your eyes and let any tension release. Imagine that stress is seeping out of every pore in your skin. Starting with your feet, relax your muscles all the way to the top of your head.

A Habit of Health: Keep your brain in shape with daily exercise.

Step 5: Now let's turn off the internal dialogue in your brain and stop the thought process. Slowly repeat a word or phrase that you find calming, such as "love", "quiet", "peace", or a spiritual word that creates a serene state. Don't let other thoughts such as memories or events enter your brain. Just keep repeating that one word or phrase (your mantra) silently. This will help keep distracting thoughts at bay.

If thoughts come to you—which will happen until you perfect the technique and it becomes a Habit of Health—just repeat the word "relax", take a deep breath, and let the thought go as you exhale. Then return to your mantra.

Step 6: Once you've continued your internal chant for the length of time you've selected (long enough to reach a state of relaxation and calm), sit quietly for a minute or two. As you come back to your normal state, merge with the calmness of the meditative state and take one last deep inhalation. Hold your breath for about 15 seconds, exhale, and relax.

You've just created a new state of composure and control.

Progressive Relaxation for Body and Mind

Here's a great way to reset your body-mind connection. This is my favorite mind-body relaxation technique because it makes you more aware of the tension level in each part of your body and teaches you to shift your brain's directive from tension to relaxation using very precise control. As you relax your muscles, you'll enable background tension to dissipate as well.

Step 1: Find a quiet, comfortable place to lie down.

Step 2: Close your eyes and let all the tension melt from your body. Begin focusing on the toes of your left foot. Sense the level of tension, and then slowly relax every fiber in those toes, allowing the tension to flow out of you until it's completely gone. Now shift your attention from your toes to your foot, and repeat. Continue in the following progression:

- Left toes > left foot > left calf > left thigh > left hip
- Right toes > right foot > right calf > right thigh > right hip buttocks > belly > lower back > chest
- Left fingers > left hand > left forearm > left upper arm > left shoulder
- Right fingers > right hand > right forearm > right upper arm > right shoulder upper back > neck > face > scalp

Finally, let the last bit of tension escape from the top of your head.

Step 3: Spend a few minutes absorbing this new state of relaxation. As you go about your day, notice if tension begins to creep into certain areas. If it does, stop what you're doing as soon as possible and relax

" *A study of 1,350 patients with severe cardiac disease found that those with no support system were three times more likely to die as a result of their illness.*[12] "

Boost Your Brain... with Curry?

What do exercise, falling in love, reducing calories, and eating Indian food have in common? They all boost your level of BDNF (brain-derived neurotrophic factor), a powerful protector of cognitive intelligence. Curcumin, a spice from the turmeric plant, which has been shown to increase BDNF, is an important ingredient in curry and many spicy types of mustards. So dig in for a better brain!

More Stress Reducers

Try these techniques to create relaxation and lower internal stress.

- Deep breathing: Whenever you have a few moments and need to relax, revisit the deep breathing techniques we covered in *Your LifeBook* in Element 04, *Building a Healthy Mindset*, within the Conscious Breathing Skill section. Remember, these are especially useful during the challenge portion of Stop.Challenge. Choose.™, and it is the mental exercise you have been using throughout our time together to help you regain control and inhibit stress.
- Prayer: This healing stress reducer is especially beneficial for those who are experiencing severe situational stress as a result of illness or the loss of a family member or friend.
- Yoga.

For a complete mind-body practice, explore these ancient exercises that combine movement, breathing, posture, mantra, meditation, and even special healing finger positions.

those areas using an abbreviated version of the technique above. This will help prevent areas of tension from becoming stress reinforcers and stave off musculoskeletal dysfunction.

Get Help!

Remember, you can't hope to enjoy optimal health and extend life without addressing this critical area. We have spent considerable time throughout this book focusing on managing our emotions and our thoughts. You could also move to Element 23, *Master Your Thoughts and Emotions*, in *Your Lifebook* as it is a treasure chest of ways to minimize our stress by improving our emotional management, as well as levels of awareness and focus. If you're experiencing health-robbing stress, it's worth your time to seek someone who can help you reduce and eliminate chronic stress from your life. Take a yoga class, re-read Part 2.16, *Creating Optimal Wellbeing: Aligning habits with what Matters Most,* on wellbeing, learn to say no, use your support network, get a pet, or find a soul mate and fall in love! And if you find you can't harness stress on your own, please seek professional help.

You can't live long and thrive if your mind isn't in its natural state—relaxed.

Connecting to Other Habits of Health

The Habits of Healthy Motion and the Habits of Healthy Eating and Hydration play crucial roles in your brain health, so as you incorporate the practices in this part into your daily routine, refer back to our discussions on nutrition and movement. Additionally, you can find a whole section on brain health in our supplementary guide in *Your LifeBook* within Element 26, *Ultrahealth™: Living Longer Full Out* and at HabitsofHealth.com!

A Habit of Health:
Practicing the relaxation response.

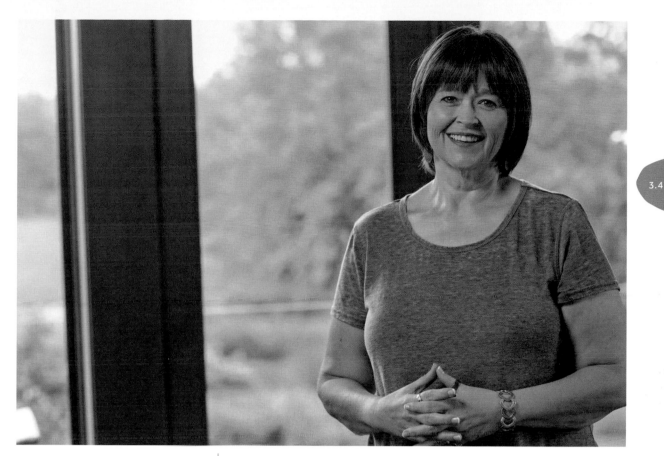

> "
> *The Habits of Health changed the way I look at everything, and it has allowed me to actually create the life that I truly believe I was created to live.*
> "

TRANSFORMATION: SHIRLEY MAST

I first started on this journey back in August of 2010 at my physician's recommendation and at that point I weighed close to 400 lbs*. My health was at a very desperate place. I am a registered nurse. I know what you need to do to get healthy. You eat less. You exercise more. But I could never put that together in a way that was effective or sustainable over time. And, honestly, I carried a lot of guilt and a lot of shame because of that. So, when my physician recommended the Habits of Health to me, I was skeptical at best, but I wasn't willing to tell him that I wouldn't try.

When I think about what my life was like back in August of 2010 and what it's like now, it's really hard to make a comparison between the two. The Habits of Health changed the way I looked at everything, and it has allowed me to actually create the life that I truly believe I was created to live. Because what I can do now—even on the most stressful days—is come back to the small healthy decisions that the Habits of Health taught me.

*Average weight loss on the Optimal Weight 5 & 1 Plan® is 12 lbs.

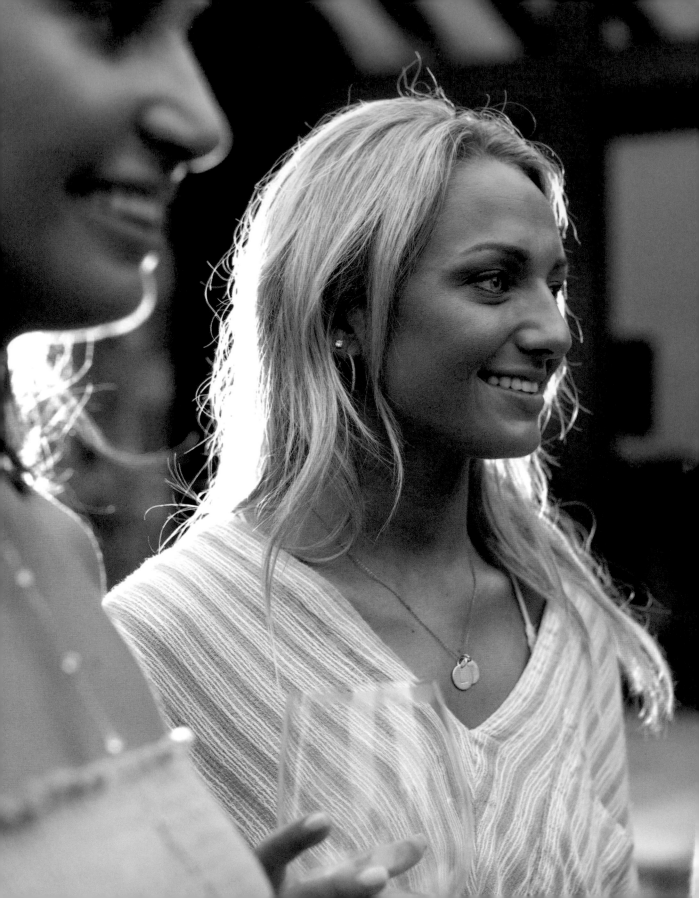

PART 3.5

REACHING A STATE OF ULTRAHEALTH™: LIVING THE FUTURE OF WELLBEING

Once you settle into your Ultrahealth™ program, you'll want to track your progress closely, especially for the first year. I suggest quarterly visits to your physician to make sure your body is responding properly. Your healthcare provider will be very interested in your progress, because you represent a new type of patient, with outstanding health parameters because of your optimal weight management and the installation of the MacroHabits of Health into your life.

Let's focus on three critical parameters that together really serve to define your Ultrahealth™ state:

- Your hs-CRP
- Your body mass index (BMI)
- Your percentage of body fat (body composition)

Major Ultrahealth™ Goals

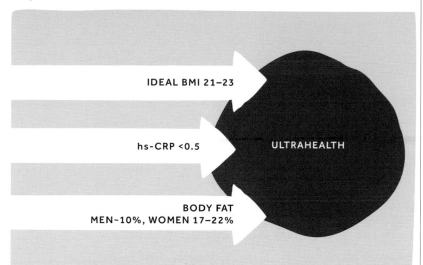

Achieving a state of Ultrahealth™ puts you in an elite group of individuals whose most critical parameters of health—hs-CRP, BMI, and body fat percentage—put them on target for the very best health and longevity.

Your hs-CRP
Initial goal: less than 1.0 mg/l
Ultrahealth™ goal: less than 0.5 mg/l

The hs-CRP test (high-sensitivity C-reactive protein) is probably the best single indicator of how well your body is performing in terms of cellular aging. A low level lets you know that your body is negotiating successfully through our complex world and that you're in the best possible condition for long-term health and longevity.

If your goal is to reach optimal health, an hs-CRP level of less than one is a great start. But, with Ultrahealth™ enhancements, you have a system that can help you reach an even healthier state. When your CRP reaches less than 0.5, you'll know that your body is positioned to thrive for a very long time indeed.

Your Body Mass Index
Initial goal: under 25
Ultrahealth™ goal: 21–23

The American Heart Association and Centers for Disease Control have defined the following categories for disease risk based on CRP level:

Low risk: less than 1.0 mg/l
Average risk: 1.0 to 3.0 mg/l
High risk: above 3.0 mg/l

3.5

" *Warning: This recommended* BMI *range (and indeed, the Ultrahealth™ program) is not intended for pregnant women and nursing mothers.* "

At the beginning of your journey, we checked your body mass index (BMI) to assess your risk for cardiovascular disease, diabetes, and a variety of cancers, and we worked to get your BMI into a healthy range of just under 25. But now we're returning to BMI from a completely different orientation—to move you into and keep you in the zone of Ultrahealth™.

So what does this mean? The World Health Organization and the National Institutes of Health have proposed a normal BMI range of between 20–24.9.[1] Values above or below this range increase the risk of premature death—above, because being overweight or obese leads to a whole host of serious diseases; and below, because a very low BMI probably reflects weight loss that's a result of diseases already present. I have evaluated many large studies completed in the last couple of years in terms of the ideal weight to live as long as possible. Based on this latest research I have constructed the following diagram which shows the ideal BMI for Ultrahealth™.

Many of the studies I've shared with you throughout the book support an association between high BMI and risk for diseases such as diabetes which can lead to an earlier demise. Conversely, there's a proven connection between the BMI at the low-normal end of the range and optimum metabolic and cardiovascular health. And, research studies aside, I can tell you personally that I've had the opportunity to evaluate Calorie Restriction Society members who enjoy incredible cardiovascular and metabolic parameters and are thriving, happy human beings.

BMI and Risk of Dying Early

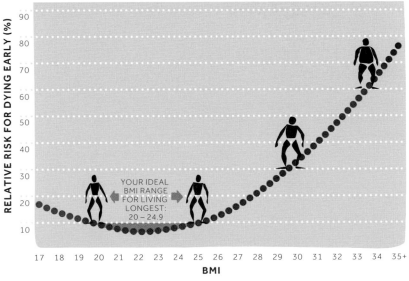

As you can see from the chart, as your BMI goes down, so does your risk of dying early. That's one of the reasons that a BMI of around 21–23 is ideal for ultimate health and disease resistance.[1]

While there may be some advantages to a BMI slightly lower than 20, I believe it's important to give the body a buffer and a bit of reserve. (In fact, I actually think you're better off focusing on CRP reduction as a goal.) That's why we've set your Ultrahealth™ BMI goal in the range of 20 to less than 24.9 with an ideal as a BMI of 21–23, a range that provides leeway for genetic and lifestyle differences and reinforces an important point—that weight reduction is not the focus, but rather the result of obtaining Ultrahealth™.

Just remember to get a check-up and have blood work done by your healthcare provider as you approach the lower end of this range (around 20). We're exploring new ground here, and you and your lab results will help us find out more as we move to the next level and redefine health for the 21st century.

Your Percentage of Body Fat

Initial goal: 15–18% for men and 22–25% for women
Ultrahealth™ goal: around 10% for men and 17–22% for women

The amount of body fat we have varies according to genetics, culture, and environment, but our general goal is around 10% for men and between 17–22% for women.

This significant difference between the sexes is because, in addition to storage fat (the fat we gain or lose as our weight changes, which normally makes up about 12–15% of a woman's total body weight), women carry gender-specific essential fat in their breasts, pelvis, hips, and thighs. This essential fat is biologically necessary for childbearing and other hormone-related functions, and should account for at least 10–12% of a woman's total weight. Together, these two types of fat make up the total percentage for women. But, as always, for the best analysis of your individual needs, see your healthcare provider.

Body Fat Percentage by Body Type, From the American Council on Exercise

BODY TYPE	FEMALE BODY FAT	MALE BODY FAT
ATHLETIC	17%	10%
LEAN	17–22%	10–15%
NORMAL	22–25%	15–18%
OVERWEIGHT	25–29%	18–20%
OVERFAT	29–35%	20–25%
OBESE	>35%	>25%

As we become lean and fit, our percentage of body fat decreases. For Ultrahealth™, you should aim for a percentage in the "lean" category.

WHAT ABOUT DIETARY (CALORIE) RESTRICTION?

Throughout this book, we've discussed the importance of gaining command over your calorie intake, and have used that control as an essential element to guide you on this journey.

First, we used it to help you reach a healthy weight. Then, as your body became able to move more freely, we found a balance between energy in and energy out. And then we set our sights on helping you reach optimal health. At each of these levels, we've also added many Habits of Health, thereby building a foundation of behaviors that will last you a lifetime.

Now, through the Habits of Longevity, we've taken your newfound mastery of energy intake, as well as those important supporting MacroHabits of Health, and given you access to a state of health that few adults have ever experienced, or ever will. The final verdict on dietary (calorie) restriction as a longevity enhancer isn't in, nor do we yet know the absolute optimal intake needed to slow the aging process. But what we do know is this: dietary restriction, when accompanied by a balanced, nutrient-dense diet, should provide the same benefits of disease reduction and metabolic adaptation in humans as it does in animal studies.[3]

Even if it turns out that dietary restriction doesn't extend mankind's maximum lifespan, its ability to help us spend more time in a healthier state is enough to be excited about. After all, who knows what possibilities are about to unfold? By living and thriving in Ultrahealth™, you'll be in a great position to take advantage of all the new advancements that science will gradually reveal.

A number of other opportunities for longevity show promise on the level of calorie restriction. For example, red wine might be part of the reason why we see consistently higher rates of longevity in the Mediterranean. I'm following this research closely, and you can go online to read the latest insights (my guide to wine and longevity included) by visiting HabitsofHealth.com.

A FINAL WORD

One of the leading cultural anthropologists of our time, a woman named Inga Treitler, evaluated a group of individuals who had mastered successful weight loss by losing at least 60 lbs and keeping it off for at least five years.

Although the subjects had lost weight in many different ways, these long-term success stories had one thing in common—every one of them had changed the way they lived their lives. They made a 180-degree change in orientation, in the way they experience the world. In fact Treitler describes this phenomenon as a "rite of passage." For some, this meant leaving their old jobs to become coaches, teachers, and mentors. They went from being passive to active participants in their own lives.[4]

As you know, this book is a compilation of the lessons I've learned over almost the last two decades, from people who've been successful at losing weight and reaching optimal health and creating wellbeing in their lives and the lives of others. By studying their successes—and the failures of others—the Habits of Health provides a path that many are following in order to reach and maintain optimal health.

Many of these very same people, who are living the Habits of Health, are now helping others which, as Treitler observed, is also helping them maintain optimal health and wellbeing. Working together, staying connected through an environment that inspires and creates long-term success, is a great way to give yourself the gift of comprehensive support and a lifetime of personal health and fulfillment.

Now that you recognize the importance of support as you install and master the MacroHabits you have learned to date, you're hopefully seeking more support and a community of kindred spirits.

Your Optimal Health and Longevity Bubble

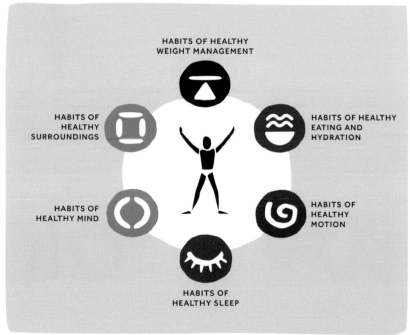

WHAT'S ON THE HORIZON?

As a young boy, I loved reading Jules Verne's books about submarines, airplanes, and space travel, as well as a host of science fiction stories that featured inventions that, at the time, seemed way outside the realms of possibility. Verne's books, including *Journey to the Center of* the Earth, *Around the World in Eighty Days* and, my favorite, *Twenty Thousand Leagues Under the Sea* have been translated more often than nearly any other author's work (only Disney productions and Agatha Christie's works can boast more). Clearly, we're all fascinated by the ability of science to create endless possibilities. Although, the fire hose of technological advances is also threatening our mental and emotional health, as we discussed in Part 1.1, *It's Not Your Fault That You're Struggling.*

Anyway, Futurist and author Ray Kurzweil reminds me a lot of Jules Verne. He believes that the cavalry who are going to help us live forever are just around the corner. He has vision, creativity and, most importantly, he's living a healthy lifestyle. Here's an extract from an interview he gave on CNN.[1]

Futurist and author Ray Kurzweil pops a couple hundred supplements a day, eats an extremely healthy diet, and exercises. Kurzweil says he plans to live long enough to live forever.

Kurzweil's strategy for immortality is based on the premise that science moves forward exponentially, with breakthroughs building on each other and coming at a faster and faster rate. As a result, he thinks life expectancy will start extending to the point where he can live indefinitely.

Kurzweil is dead serious about this. "It's going to be a very different situation 10 or 15 years from now," says Kurzweil, author of The Singularity Is Near: When Humans Transcend Biology. "We have very sharply designed interventions that can stop disease. So for baby boomers, we'd like to be in good shape 10 or 15 years from now when we have the full flowering of the biotechnological revolution."

Science is indeed making progress decoding the factors necessary to extend life. We're beginning to learn how telomeres unravel—a discovery that could teach us how to increase the production of telomerase and perhaps prevent this built-in aging process, as we mentioned when discussing a recent study.

We're learning more about several potent inducers of cell survival, such as the class of enzymes called sirtuins, which have the ability to specifically change NAD-dependent histone deacetylases, thereby protecting our DNA and helping our mitochondria become more resilient to aging.

Using complex computers, we're identifying genes that play a role in longevity. In just the past few years, Dr. Nir Barzilia of Albert Einstein College of Medicine has discovered, by studying the genes of centenarians, three longevity genes that shield against heart disease.

Eventually we'll unlock the secrets of aging, just as sure as we've created submarines that can visit shipwrecks 10,000 feet below sea level, learned to fly faster than the speed of sound, and put a man on the moon.

For certain, Ray Kurzweil's advice is accurate in at least one regard. In order for any of these wonderful scientific advancements to help us live longer, we must do our part to fulfill that destiny by maintaining a healthy lifestyle and optimal health, for today and for that boundless future.

Dr. A's Habits of Health provides that for you today, tomorrow, and I hope into a long and happy future. You now have a comprehensive system with this book, *Your LifeBook*, and your daily habit installer to start, continue, and thrive in every aspect of your health and wellbeing.

Use this system, along with our growing community, to place yourself and those you care about on a path to optimal health and wellbeing that will transform you from today onward, while others wait for the magic pill.

I wish you good luck and a bountiful lifetime of health and wellbeing.

DR. A, JANUARY 2019

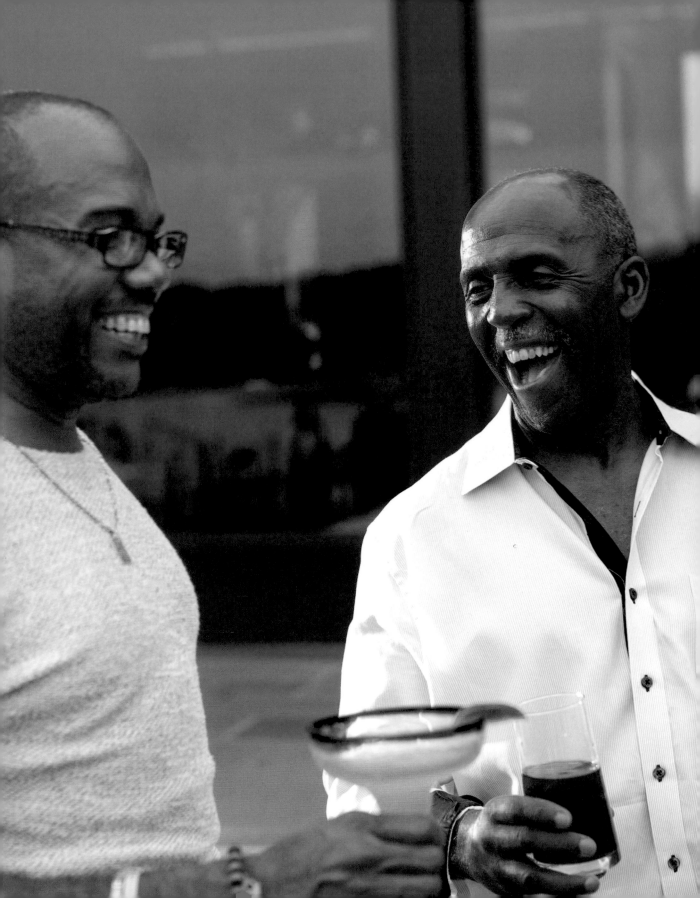

EPILOGUE

OUR FULL POTENTIAL

A better understanding of the key role that our emotional management plays in our health, wellbeing, and longevity has fueled the evolution of this transformational system. And the fabric of the new Habits of Health Transformational System has been fully immersed in helping you become the master of your thoughts and emotions.

Taking the opportunity to revise the original book, written over 10 years ago, has been deeply rewarding for me. When I left critical care to pursue what I saw as the new frontier for medicine, the future was uncertain, and many of my colleagues thought I was making the biggest mistake of my career. The first edition of *Dr. A's Habits of Health* showed the world that we were on to something. Today, there are tens of thousands of people who have transformed their lives and are helping create optimal wellbeing for themselves and their families. Each of them has helped us to uncover even more powerful insights into health.

The second edition of *Dr. A's Habits of Health* has given me the chance to incorporate new and exciting developments in the worlds of nutrition, psychology, human biology, and sustainable transformation. This opportunity has allowed me to think again, even more deeply, about my own experiences and how I can use these insights and evolved thinking in service of your journey to optimal health and wellbeing.

We've talked about the challenges presented to us in our daily lives by technology. We've taken a hard look at parts of the food industry who put profits over the health of their customers. And we've considered the dangers of a sedentary lifestyle.

Even though this epilogue marks the end of the book, it also signifies the start of an incredibly exciting journey, one that has the potential to transform your life. What is critical to me is that you understand that the transformation is—ultimately—up to you. You are the single most important force in achieving optimal health.

You can surround yourself with people who support you and who might even join you in the pursuit of Ultrahealth™. You can master the development of your brain and mind. You can move more, and eat tasty, nutritious food six times a day. You might even strike up a powerful relationship with a coach within the supportive community I've been part of building. But, in truth, even with all that's around you, only a fully motivated you can make it happen.

If you can align what matters most to you in life, with your health and wellbeing at the heart of it, you will not only become your best self but you'll also be more connected and more present for those around you.

I know, as do the hundreds of thousands of people whose lives have already been transformed by the original version of *Dr. A's Habits of Health*, that the systems and practices contained here can work.

The stories—of people who were in many ways just like you when they first began their journeys—are there for inspiration. Like you, these people decided there was a better, healthier future for themselves—and sometimes—for those around them. Hearing these stories will hopefully give you added incentive to stick to the path that has been laid out here, and I also hope that you now see that you are the author of your own story. Make sure you utilize *Your LifeBook* to break the habit of being yourself and write your new story that will fulfill all of your potential. Years from now, your success story could be the final push that someone else, who feels very much like you did before you began building the Habits of Health, needs to start their own journey.

You can be that example. You can be that leader, in your own way. I know you can. By picking up this book, you have already made the first of a series of decisions that will—if you persevere—change your life for the better.

So, I want to close by wishing you well on the journey you're embarking on, and to say it's truly a privilege to help you take control of your future health and wellbeing.

IN HEALTH,
DR WAYNE SCOTT ANDERSEN

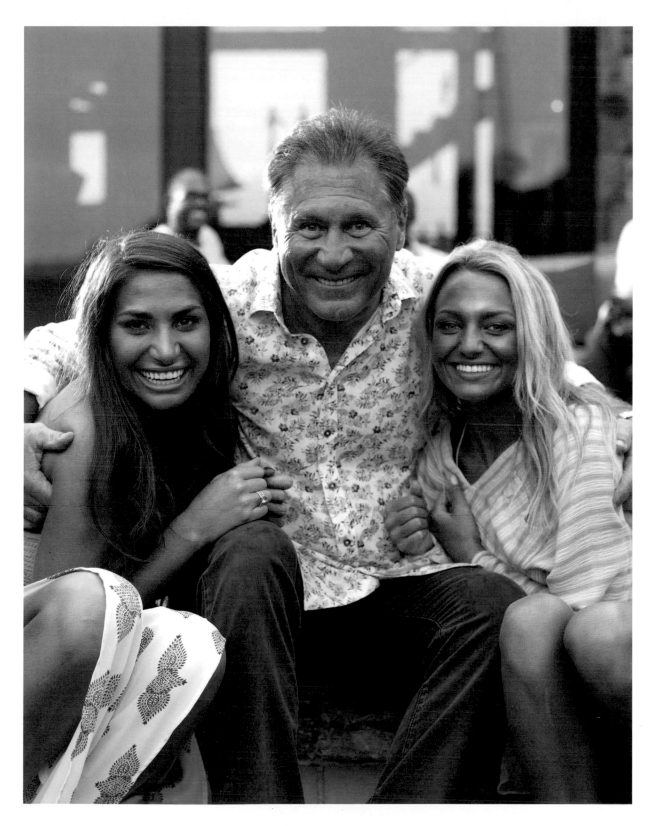

RESOURCES

Dr. A's Habits of Health Transformational System
www.HabitsofHealth.com
An in-depth resource on the Habits of Health Transformational System including support, tips, activities, exercises, links, and additional information on creating optimal health and wellbeing. Information on enhanced support, training, and coaching through the bionetwork for those who currently do not have a personal coach, as well as information on becoming a coach yourself. In addition, you can visit the website to order *Your LifeBook* and other tools to help you on your journey.

Dr. Wayne Andersen
www.drwayneandersen.com
Find out more about Dr. Andersen and his work as a visionary and global-thought leader, who helps individuals create transformational change in their lives. His goal is to foster optimal health and wellbeing and expand that mission around the world.

OPTAVIA®
www.optavia.com
Learn how to become part of the OPTAVIA® Community, a powerful support team made up of health-conscious, coach-supported people dedicated to optimizing their health through the Habits of Health Transformational system. The site also provides information on ordering OPTAVIA® portion-controlled fuelings, Purposeful Hydration™, eicosanoids (omega-3 dietary supplements), information about becoming a coach, and how to connect with your own free personal coach.

Alzheimer's Association
www.alz.org
Valuable information on ways to protect your brain.

American College of Sports Medicine
www.acsm.org
Information on movement and musculoskeletal health.

America on the Move
www.americaonthemove.org
Nonprofit initiative dedicated to helping people avoid weight gain by increasing their activity levels.

The American Institute of Stress
www.stress.org/americas
Information and problem-solving on stress-related health issues.

Johns Hopkins Health Site
www.hopkinsmedicine.org
An excellent resource for information on all aspects of health.

Mayo Clinic
www.mayoclinic.com
Information to help you live a healthier life.

National Heart, Lung, and Blood Institute
www.nhlbi.nih.gov
Information on lowering risk for disease.

The Obesity Society
www.obesity.org
A source of information for weight-challenged individuals.

National Sleep Foundation
www.sleepfoundation.org
Education on the importance of sleep and sleep issues.

World Health Organization
www.who.int
Information on the prevention and treatment of disease at a global level.

Choose My Plate
www.choosemyplate.gov
Information to help you understand MyPlate's simple-to-use tools and graphics on eating properly.

Nutrition.gov
www.nutrition.gov
U.S.-based nutrition resource.

EXPLANATION OF HABITS OF HEALTH PROGRAM FOR HEALTH CARE PROVIDERS

Your patient has made the fundamental choice to create health in his or her life by taking part in a comprehensive health improvement program.

This program is intended to help people reach a healthy weight and develop the habits that will create lifelong transformation in their health and wellbeing. As health care providers, we know that lifestyle change is the only thing that creates sustainable weight management and long-term health. Diets by themselves have no lasting value and the statistics on recidivism are very high. We provide the strategies, tactics, tools, and support to awaken; guidance by providing each patient a coach, a community of support, the Habits of Health Transformational System (educational and blueprint for long term health and wellbeing); and scientifically-proven products and programs.

I have asked your patient to share this program with you, the patient's personal health care provider, so that you are aware of the changes they will be making to their diet and lifestyle (as this can affect certain health conditions and medications), so you can properly advise and monitor as you deem appropriate. This may include potentially adjusting or eliminating medications which they may no longer need as they improve their health and their wellbeing.

The following is a brief description of the phases of the system and program and some suggested medical support you can provide that I hope is helpful.

Phase I: Reaching a Healthy Weight
Most of our patients and clients start in the weight loss and management phase:
- Nutritionally-balanced meal plans that incorporate six portion-controlled meals per day: one every two to three hours.
- These healthy fuelings are low glycemic and soy based, although non-soy options are available as well as non-GMO options, and they do not contain colors, flavors, or sweeteners from artificial sources.
- Eat one healthy lean and green meal per day, which teaches them how to pick healthy foods and create healthy meals. This leads to the ability to create long-term habits of shopping and eating for success.
- Plate and color-coded eating system for permanent healthy-eating habits.
- Progressive daily movement program.

Phase II: Lifestyle Change
Once we have the patient in a fat burning state and losing weight they will experience more energy and self-efficacy, we then use

this teachable moment to start introducing other healthy habits installation:

- Healthy eating for life using a plate and color coded eating system.
- Increased movement through a daily walking program with progressive resistance and cardio training at the patient's pace and perceived difficulty of exertion and target heart rate as a guideline.
- Improved sleeping rituals, routines, and environment modification.
- Support from their free personal coach, online webinars, and podcasts.
- Connections to our health community.
- Ongoing instruction through the Habits of Health System, the book, *Your Lifebook*, which is an interactive journal, and the daily habit installer feedback on the Habits of Health App.
- Focus on motivation and ability to provide microHabits to increase installation by creating consistency.

Phase III: Optimization
We will continue to work on healthy weight management, eating, and sleeping, but we will also help develop individual responsibility emotional agility, and stress management.

- Stop. Challenge. Choose.™ and relaxation exercises
- Meditation
- We know that by changing the underlying environment we can have a profound effect on behavior and health in this phase we will
  1. Remove inflammatory stimulants, water, air, home toxins
  2. Improve pantry/ bedroom environment
- Enhancement of healthy nutrients

Patient Progress
Your patient will be eating a reduced amount of balanced calories, protein, and fat during phase I. They will lose weight at a steady pace while conserving muscle.

As soon as a diabetic individual starts the program their blood sugar will probably start to drop because of the reduced calories and low glycemic fuelings. It is important for them to increase their blood sugar monitoring and also talk to their health care provider about lowering their medications such as oral agents and/or insulin.

This is imperative to prevent hypoglycemia.

Other Suggested Diagnostics
In addition to routine blood chemistry, suggested labs include lipid profile for baseline, hs-CRP, and an EKG. A cardiovascular assessment is suggested for high-risk individuals, especially if they have considerable weight to lose or if they have been inactive.

Significant Disease Precaution
Our program uses healthy food and common sense habit installation as its principle tools. There are no pharmaceuticals so it can be used on a wide range of patients, in terms of age and comorbidity.

That said, our program is not appropriate for women who are pregnant or anyone under the age of 13, and our program for teens is the only program appropriate for those aged 13 to 17 years.

Since your patient may lose weight, we also want to identify that some patients should be evaluated more thoroughly before beginning the program. If your patient has a serious acute or chronic illness (e.g., heart attack, diabetes, cancer, liver disease, kidney disease, anorexia, bulimia) they should not use our program until you feel they have recovered or stabilized. Examples would be within three months of an Myocardial Infarction (MI) or recent or reoccurring stroke or mini stroke, unstable angina, severe liver or kidney disease, clotting disorders, active cancers, eating disorders, severe psychiatric disturbances, current use of Lithium, or type 1 diabetes (Brittle). Patients taking prescription medications, especially Coumadin® (warfarin), lithium, diabetes medication, or medications for high blood pressure, may need to be monitored more closely. We offer specialized programs for nursing mothers, people with gout, some people with diabetes, and those who exercise more than 45 minutes per day.

Note: Rapid weight loss may cause gallstones or gallbladder disease for those at high risk. While adjusting to intake of a lower-calorie level and diet changes, some people may experience temporary lightheadedness, dizziness, or gastrointestinal disturbances.

We recommend drinking 64 ounces of water each day. Patients are to consult with you prior to changing the amount of water they drink as it can affect certain health conditions and medications.

For more information on our program, please go to www.habitsofhealth.com or contact one of our coaches. This document can also be downloaded on the website.

APPENDIX B:
CAFFEINE IN COMMONLY CONSUMED PRODUCTS

COFFEE	CAFFEINE (mg)
CARIBOU CAPPUCINO, 12 oz	160–200
DECAFFEINATED, INSTANT, 8 oz	2
DECAFFEINATED, BREWED, 8 oz	2
ESPRESSO, 1 fl oz	64
INSTANT, 8 oz	62
PLAIN, BREWED, 9 oz	95
STARBUCKS CAFFE LATTE, 16 oz	150

TEA	CAFFEINE (mg)
BLACK TEA, BREWED, 8 oz	47
DECAFFEINATED BLACK TEA, 8 oz	2
GREEN TEA, 8 oz	30–50
LIPTON BRISK ICED TEA, LEMON FLAVORED, 12 oz	10
NESTEA, SWEETENED OR UNSWEETENED, 12 oz	17
SNAPPLE ICED TEA, 16 oz	18
STARBUCKS TAZO CHAI TEA LATTE, 12 oz	75

FOODS	CAFFEINE (mg)
EXCEDRIN, EXTRA STRENGTH, 2 TABLETS	13
FOOSH ENERGY MINTS, 1 MINT	10
HAAGEN-DAZS COFFEE ICE CREAM, ½ CUP	30
HERSHEY'S CHOCOLATE BAR, 1.55 oz	9
HERSHEY'S SPECIAL DARK CHOCOLATE BAR	18
JOLT CAFFEINATED GUM, 1 STICK	33
NODOZ MAXIMUM STRENGTH, 1 TABLET	20

SOFT DRINKS	CAFFEINE (mg)
7Up	0
A&W CREME SODA	29
BARQ'S ROOT BEER	23
CHERRY COCA-COLA, DIET CHERRY COCA-COLA	35
COCA-COLA CLASSIC	35
CODE RED MOUNTAIN DEW	54
DIET BARQ'S ROOT BEER	0
DIET COKE	47
DR. PEPPER, DIET DR. PEPPER	41
DIET PEPSI	35
DIET WILD CHERRY PEPSI	38
FANTA	0
MELLO YELLO	53
RED BULL, 12 oz	111
MONSTER ENERGY, 24 oz	240
MOUNTAIN DEW, DIET MOUNTAIN DEW	54
PEPSI	38
SPRITE, SPRITE ZERO	0
SUNKIST ORANGE SODA	41
TAB	47
WILD CHERRY PEPSI	38

CITATIONS

Preface: Welcome to Habits of Health

1. CDC percent of adults aged 20 and over who are overweight, including obesity: 71.6% (2015–2016).
2. John Spengler, Harvard School of Public Health, (online).
3. Louise Jack, "'Children spend less time outdoors than prisoners, according to new Persil ad", Fast Company.
4. Murray CJL, Lopez AD. The Global Burden of Disease: A Comprehensive Assessment of Mortality and Disability from Diseases, Injuries and Risk Factors in 1990 and Projected to 2020. Geneva, Switzerland; World Health Organization, 1996.
5. The World Happiness Report is an annual publication of the United Nations Sustainable Development Solutions Network which contains rankings of national happiness and analysis of the data from various perspectives. NY Times Citation: "We're Making Life Too Hard for Millennials" By Steven Rattner.

Introduction: Beating the Odds

1. Up to 50% of women are on a diet at any given time, according to Judy Mahle Lutter in her book The Bodywise Woman.
2. CDC percent of adults aged 20 and over who are overweight, including obesity: 71.6% (2015–2016).
3. CDC The Health Effects of Overweight and Obesity. People who have obesity, compared to those with a normal or healthy weight, are at increased risk for many serious diseases and health conditions, including the following: 1, 2, 3
   - All-causes of death (mortality)
   - High blood pressure (Hypertension)
   - High LDL cholesterol, low HDL cholesterol, or high levels of triglycerides (Dyslipidemia)
   - Type 2 diabetes
   - Coronary heart disease
   - Stroke
   - Gallbladder disease
   - Osteoarthritis (a breakdown of cartilage and bone within a joint)
   - Sleep apnea and breathing problems
   - Some cancers (endometrial, breast, colon, kidney, gallbladder, and liver)
   - Low quality of life
   - Mental illness such as clinical depression, anxiety, and other mental disorders 4, 5
   - Body pain and difficulty with physical functioning 6
4. BMC Public Health. 2014; 14: 143. Published online 2014 Feb 10. doi: [10.1186/1471-2458-14-143] PMCID: PMC3929131, PMID: 24512151

Pharmacoeconomics. 2015 Jul; 33(7): 673–689. doi: [10.1007/s40273-014-0243-x] PMCID: PMC4859313 NIHMSID: NIHMS780628 PMID: 25471927. "The Epidemiology of Obesity: A Big Picture", Adela Hruby, PhD, MPH and Frank B. Hu, MD, PhD, MPH.

Part 1.1, It's Not Your Fault That You're Struggling

1. Johnson, R.K., Appel, L., Brands, M., Howard, B., Lefevre, M., Lustig, R., Sacks, F., Steffen, L., & Wyllie-Rosett, J. (2009, September 15). "Dietary sugars intake and cardiovascular health: a scientific statement from the American Heart Association." Circulation, 120(11), 1011-20. doi:10.1161/CIRCULATIONAHA.109.192627. Retrieved from http://circ.ahajournals.org/content/120/11/1011.full.pdf.
2. Johnson, R.K., Appel, L., Brands, M., Howard, B., Lefevre, M., Lustig, R., Sacks, F., Steffen, L., & Wyllie-Rosett, J. (2009, September 15). "Dietary sugars intake and cardiovascular health: a scientific statement from the American Heart Association." Circulation", 120(11), 1011-20. doi:10.1161/CIRCULATIONAHA.109.192627. Retrieved from http://circ.ahajournals.org/content/120/11/1011.full.pdf.
3. A paper presented at the 2013 Canadian Neuroscience Meeting, the annual meeting of the Canadian Association for Neuroscience - Association Canadienne des Neurosciences (CAN-ACN), says the problem is addiction rather than food wealth—the authors claim that high-fructose corn syrup can cause behavioral reactions in rats similar to those produced by drugs of abuse such as cocaine.
4. More than 100 million U.S. adults are now living with diabetes or prediabetes, according to a new report released today by the Centers for Disease Control and Prevention (CDC). The report finds that as of 2015, 30.3 million Americans—9.4% of the U.S. population—have diabetes. Another 84.1 million have prediabetes, a condition that if not treated often leads to type 2 diabetes within five years.
5. Live Strong: The Typical American Family Diet in 1908 by RAE CASTO Oct. 03, 2017.
6. Statista: This statistic illustrates the number of people who visited McDonald's for breakfast within the last 30 days in the U.S. from autumn 2009 to spring 2017. In spring 2017, the number of people who visited McDonald's for breakfast within a period of 30 days amounted to 44.51 million.
7. Nutr J. 2013; 12: 45. Published online 2013 Apr 11. doi: [10.1186/1475-2891-12-45] PMCID: PMC3639863 PMID: 23577692: "Trends in U.S. home food preparation and consumption: analysis of national

nutrition surveys and time use studies from 1965–1966 to 2007–2008" Lindsey P Smith, 1 Shu Wen Ng, 1 and Barry M Popkin 1, 2.
8. A survey by the National Center For Substance Abuse at Columbia University found 32% of families spending 20 minutes or less eating dinner, while another survey found that children in families where dinner lasted 16.4 minutes on average were at greater risk for being overweight, compared with families that sat. Sep 18, 2013.
9. Child Dev. Author manuscript; available in PMC 2013 Nov 1. Published in final edited form as: Child Dev. 2012 Nov; 83(6): 2104–2120. Published online 2012 Aug 7. doi: [10.1111/j.1467-8624.2012.01825.x] PMCID: PMC3498594 NIHMSID: NIHMS385646 PMID: 22880815 "Family Meals and Child Academic and Behavioral Outcomes" Daniel P. Miller, PhD, Jane Waldfogel, PhD, and Wen-Jui Han, PhD "The Conversation: Academic rigor, journalistic flair Science says: eat with your kids", January 9, 2015 6.08am ES.
10. PDF Commentaries "Hepatotoxicity of fast food?". Giulio Marchesini, Valentina Ridolfi, Valentina Nepoti Author affiliations, http://dx.doi.org/10.1136/gut.2007.143958.
11. The average Millennial eats out five times a week, and between Starbucks runs and bar tabs, it's making it harder for them to develop a savings habit, according to a new study by Bankratecom. Princeton Survey Research Associates International obtained telephone interviews with a nationally representative sample of 1,003 adults living in the continental United States.
12. Demographics Of Food Spending: Here Come The Millennials, from The Food Institute, 25–34 year-old Millennial households spent 45% of their food expenditures away-from-home in 2013 compared to just 37% for 55–64-year households—the tail end of the Baby Boomer generation. Looking at it dollar-wise, Millennials spent $50.75 weekly on food consumed away from home, while Baby Boomers spent $47.67–6.5% more despite Millennials having overall expenditures 14% below those of Baby Boomers, according to Food Institute analysis of data from the Bureau of Labor Statistics.
13. Public Health Nutrition, Volume 15, Issue 3, 26 January 2012, pp. 424–432 "Fast-food and commercial baked goods consumption and the risk of depression", Almudena Sánchez-Villegas (a1) (a2), Estefania Toledo (a2), Jokin de Irala (a2),

Miguel Ruiz-Canela (a2).

14. Mayo Clinic WebsiteDiet. Studies indicate that certain dietary factors, including skim milk and carbohydrate-rich foods—such as bread, bagels and chips—may worsen acne. Chocolate has long been suspected of making acne worse. A small study of 14 men with acne showed that eating chocolate was related to a worsening of symptoms. Further study is needed to examine why this happens and whether people with acne would benefit from following specific dietary restrictions.

15. Zachary Ward, M.P.H., Ph.D. candidate in health policy, Center for Health Decision Science, Harvard T.H. Chan School of Public Health, Boston; Lona Sandon, Ph.D., R.D.N., program director and assistant professor, clinical nutrition, School of Health Professions, University of Texas Southwestern Medical Center, Dallas; Nov. 30, 2017, *New England Journal of Medicine.*

16. Credit Donkey, Updated May 30, 2015, "Fast Food Statistics: 23 Shocking Facts and Habits" By Rebecca Lake. It's estimated that in the U.S., fast food residents rake in somewhere in the neighborhood of $208 billion a year. Revenues have increased by about 1.2% between 2010 and 2015.

17. "The effects of fast food on the body" Medically reviewed by Natalie Butler, RD, LD on July 25, 2018. Ann Pietrangelo, Elea Carey, and Kimberly Holland.

18. JAMA. 1993 Nov 10;270(18):2207-12. Actual causes of death in the United States. McGinnis JM1, Foege WH.

19. Child Dev. Author manuscript; available in PMC 2013 Nov 1.Published in final edited form as: Child Dev. 2012 Nov; 83(6): 2104–2120. Published online 2012 Aug 7. doi: [10.1111/J.1467-8624.2012.01825.x] PMCID: PMC3498594 NIHMSID: NIHMS385646 PMID: 22880815 "Family Meals and Child Academic and Behavioral Outcomes", Daniel P. Miller, PhD, Jane Waldfogel, PhD, and Wen-Jui Han, PhD.

20. AyeT, LevitskyLL "Type 2 Diabetes: An epidemic disease in childhood" Opin Pediatr 2003;15 411–415.

21. Moore, T. J., et al., "Serious adverse Drug events reported to the food and Drug administration, 1998–2005," Archives of Internal Medicine 167 (September 10,2007): 1752–1759.

22. Moore, T. J., et al., "Serious adverse Drug events reported to the food and Drug administration, 1998–2005," Archives of Internal Medicine 167 (September 10,2007): 1752–1759.

23. J Diabetes Metab Disord. 2015; 14: 31. Published online 2015 Apr 17. doi: [10.1186/s40200-015-0154-1] PMCID: PMC4429709, PMID: 2597340. "Diet, exercise or diet with

exercise: comparing the effectiveness of treatment options for weight-loss and changes in fitness for adults (18–65 years old) who are overfat, or obese; systematic review and meta-analysis" James E Clark.

Part 1.2, The Path: The Creation of Optimal Health and Wellbeing

1. Ford ES, Bergmann MM, Kroger J, Schienkiewitz A, Weikert C, Boeing H. "Healthy living is the best revenge: findings from the European Prospective Investigation Into Cancer and Nutrition Postda study." Arch Intern Med. 2009. Aug 10;169(15):1355-62.

2. May 22, 2015, "More than a third of Americans have metabolic syndrome" Research Letter, May 19, 2015, "Prevalence of the Metabolic Syndrome in the United States", 2003–2012 Maria Aguilar, MD1; Taft Bhuket, MD2; Sharon Torres, PA2; et al.

3. Ford ES, Bergmann MM, Kroger J, Schienkiewitz A, Weikert C, Boeing H. "Healthy living is the best revenge: findings from the European Prospective Investigation Into Cancer and Nutrition Postda study." Arch Intern Med. 2009. Aug 10; 169(15): 1355–62.

4. Kvaavik E, Batty Gd, Ursin G, Huxley R, Gale CR. "Influence of individual and combined health behaviors on total and cause-specific mortality in men and women: the United Kingdom health and lifestyle survey." Arch Intern Med. 2010; 170: 711–8.

5. McCullough ML, Patel AV, Kushi LH, Patel R, Willett WC, Doyle C, Thun MJ, Gapstur SM. "Following cancer prevention guidelines reduces risk of cancer, cardiovascular disease, and all-cause mortality." Cancer Epidemiol Biomarkers Prev. 2011; 20: 1089–97.

6. Akesson A, Larsson SC, Discacciati A, Wolk A. "Low-Risk Diet and Lifestyle Habits in the Primary Prevention of Myocardial Infarction in Men: A Population-Based Prospective Cohort Study." J Am Coll Cardiol. 2014 Sep 30; 64(13): 1299–306.

7. Aleksandrova K, et al. "Combined impact of healthy lifestyle factors on colorectal cancer: a large European cohort Study." BMC Med. 2014 Oct 10; 12(1): 168.

8. Chomistek AK, Chiuve SE, Eliassen AH, Mukamal KJ, Willett WC, Rimm EB. "Health lifestyle in the primordial prevention of cardiovascular disease among young women." J Am Coll Cardiol. 2015 Jan 6; 65(1): 43–51.

9. Ornish D, Magbanua MJ, Weidner G, Weinberg V, Kemp C, Green C, Mattie MD, Marlin R, Simko J, Shinohara K, Haqq CM, Carroll PR. "Changes in prostate gene expression in men undergoing

an intensive nutrition and lifestyle intervention." Proc Natl Acad Sci USA. 2008 Jun 17; 105(24): 8369–74.

10. According to data from the National Health and Nutrition Examination Survey (NHANES), 2013–2014 2,3,4,5
   • More than one in three adults were considered to be overweight.
   • More than two in three adults were considered to be overweight or have obesity.

11. Br J Gen Pract. 2012 Dec; 62(605): 664–666. doi: [10.3399/bjgp12X659466] PMCID: PMC3505409, PMID: 23211256 "Making health habitual: the psychology of 'habit-formation' and general practice", Benjamin Gardner, Lecturer in Health Psychology.

Part 1.3, Are You Really Ready to Change?

1. "Energy Expenditure and Weight Control", Free Access "Persistent metabolic adaptation six years after *The Biggest Loser* competition", Erin Fothergill, Nearly 65% of dieters return to their pre-dieting weight within three years, according to Gary Foster, Ph.D., clinical director of the Weight and Eating Disorders Program at the University of Pennsylvania. The statistics for dieters who lose weight rapidly, according to Wellsphere, a website sponsored by Stanford University, is worse. Only five percent of people who lose weight on a crash diet will keep the weight off. Crash diets include any unhealthy diet, from severe calorie-restriction diets to diets that consist of only a few types of food.

2. Niemeier, H. M., et al., "Internal Disinhibition Predicts Weight Regain Following Weight Loss and Weight Loss Maintenance," *Obesity Research* 15 (October, 2007): 2485–2494.

3. Maier, S.U., et al, "Acute Stress Impairs Self-Control in Goal-Directed Choice by Altering Multiple Functional Connections within the Brain's Decision Circuits," Neuron, 87.3 (August, 2015): 621–631.

Part 1.4, Health is All About Choice

1. Robert Fritz, The Path of Least Resistance, Ballantine Books, 1984.

2. Edward Deci Handbook of self-determination research New York: University of Rochester Press.

Part 1.5, The Bedrock of Transformation: Successful Habit Installation

1. *Behavioral and Brain Sciences,* "Homing in on consciousness in the nervous system: An action-based synthesis" Ezequiel Morsella (a1), Christine A. Godwin (a2), Tiffany K. Jantz (a3), Stephen C. Krieger (a4).

2. A new study from IDC Research released

this week found that 80% of smartphone users check their mobile devices within 15 minutes of waking up each morning.

3. *New York Post, Living.* Americans check their phones 80 times a day: study by SWNS, November 8, 2017.
A study by global tech protection and support company Asurion found that the average person struggles to go little more than 10 minutes without checking their phone. And of the 2,000 people surveyed, one in 10 check their phones on average once every four minutes. Americans check their phone on average once every 12 minutes, thereby burying their heads in their phones 80 times a day, according to new research.

4. "In Data We Trust" Content Bootcamp Data Studio Tracker Data Visualization, Which Generation is Most Distracted by Their Phones? If you watch the news or read articles on the Internet from time to time, you've probably heard that teenagers and Millennials are digital natives who constantly use Snapchat and Instagram and apps that only people who can't legally drink know about. Teenagers check their phones 150 times per day, marketers tell us. They need instant gratification.

5. "One-In-Three Americans Would Rather Give Up Sex Than Their Smartphones", Alyson Shontell, *Business Insider*, Aug. 7, 2011, Kevin McShane via flickr, According to A Telenav national survey, one in three Americans would rather give up sex than their smartphones. IDC-Facebook Always Connected.pdf https:fb-public.app.box.com/s/3iq5x6uwnqtq7ki4q8wk Survey Finds one-third of Americans more willing to give up sex than their mobile phone http://TeleNav.com/about/pr-summer-travel/report-20110803.html.

6. *Psycho-Cybernetics, A New Way to Get More Living Out of Life Mass Market*— August 15, 1989 by Maxwell Maltz.

7. *European Journal of Social Psychology,* Eur. J. Soc. Psychol. 40, 998–1009 (2010) Published online 16 July 2009 in Wiley Online Library (wileyonlinelibrary.com), DOI: 10.1002/ejsp.67. Research article "How are habits formed: Modelling habit formation in the real world" Phillippa Lally, Cornelia H. M. Van Jaarsveld, Henry W. W. Potts And Jane Wardle, University College London, London, UK.

8. Original Research, 3 October 2017, "Patterns of Sedentary Behavior and Mortality in U.S. Middle-Aged and Older Adults: A National Cohort Study", Keith M. Diaz, PhD; Virginia J. Howard, PhD; Brent Hutto, MSPH; Natalie Colabianchi, PhD; John E. Vena, PhD; Monika M. Safford, MD; Steven N. Blair, PED; Steven P. Hooker, PhD.

Part 1.6, You in Charge of Yourself: Setting Up for Success

1. The Stanford marshmallow experiment was a series of studies on delayed gratification in the late 1960s and early 1970s led by psychologist Walter Mischel, then a professor at Stanford University.

Part 1.7, Optimizing Your Surroundings: Creating Your Microenvironment of Health

1. "Saving for the future self: Neural measures of future self-continuity predict temporal discounting", Hal Ersner-Hershfield G. Elliott Wimmer Brian Knutson, *Social Cognitive and Affective Neuroscience,* Volume 4, Issue 1, 1 March 2009, Pages 85–92, https://doi.org/10.1093/scan/nsn042 Published: 30 November 2008.

2. The Collective Dynamics of Obesity NEJM 357(4) 370–379.

3. J Health Soc Behav. Author manuscript; available in PMC 2011 Aug 4. Published in final edited form as: J Health Soc Behav. 2010; 51(Suppl): S54–S66. doi: [10.1177/0022146510383501] PMCID: PMC3150158, NIHMSID: NIHMS300162, PMID: 20943583 "Social Relationships and Health: A Flashpoint for Health Policy", Debra Umberson1 and Jennifer Karas Montez1.

4. J Health Soc Behav. Author manuscript; available in PMC 2011 Aug 4. Published in final edited form as: J Health Soc Behav. 2010; 51(Suppl): S54–S66. doi: [10.1177/0022146510383501] PMCID: PMC3150158, NIHMSID: NIHMS300162, PMID: 20943583, "Social Relationships and Health: A Flashpoint for Health Policy" Debra Umberson1 and Jennifer Karas Montez1.

5. Am J Public Health. 2012 Mar;102(3):527-33. doi: 10.2105/AJPH.2011.300391. Epub 2012 Jan 19. A 2-phase labeling and choice architecture intervention to improve healthy food and beverage choices.

6. Journal of Consumer Research, Healthy Side Salad Wilcox 36(3) 380–393.

7. www.NRPA.org, Children today spend less time outdoors than any other generation, devoting only four to seven minutes to unstructured outdoor play per day while spending an average of seven and a half hours in front of electronic media.

8. A 2014 study published in the *Journal Environment and Behavior,* "The iPhone Effect: The Quality of In-Person Social Interactions in the Presence of Mobile Devices".

Part 2, Your Journey to Optimal Health and Wellbeing

1. Dominican University of California, Study demonstrates that writing goals enhances goal achievement, January 5, 2017.

Part 2.1, The Habits of Healthy Weight Management

1. "CDC. Healthy Weight—it's not a diet, it's a lifestyle!" Centers for Disease Control and Prevention. N. Lasikiewicz, K. Myrissa, A. Hoyland, C.L. Lawton. " Psychological benefits of weight loss following behavioral and/or dietary weight loss interventions. A systematic research review." Appetite January 2014.
   • Nadia B. Pietrzykowska, MD, FACP. Benefits of 5–10% Weight-loss. Obesity Action Coalition.
   • NHS Choices. What are the benefits of losing weight? NHS England.
   • PubMed Health. Exercise, weight loss, and osteoarthritis. U.S. National Library of Medicine.

Harvard T.H. Chan School of Public Health, Your weight, your waist size, and the amount of weight gained since your mid-20s can have serious health implications. These factors can strongly influence your chances of developing the following diseases and conditions:
   • Cardiovascular disease, heart attack, stroke
   • Diabetes
   • Cancer
   • Arthritis
   • Gallstones
   • Asthma
   • Cataracts
   • Infertility
   • Snoring
   • Sleep apnea

If your weight is in the healthy range and isn't more than 10 lbs over what you weighed when you turned 21, focus on maintaining that weight by watching what you eat and exercising. Because most adults between the ages of 18 and 49 gain one to two pounds each year (1), stopping and preventing weight gain should be a priority. Gaining weight as you age increases the chances of developing one or more chronic diseases.
   • In the Nurses' Health Study and the Health Professionals Follow-up Study, middle-aged women and men who gained 11–22 lbs after age 20 were up to three times more likely to develop heart disease, high blood pressure, type 2 diabetes, and gallstones than those who gained five pounds or fewer.
   • Those who gained more than 22 lbs had an even larger risk of developing these diseases. (2–6)
   • Another analysis of Nurses' Health Study data found that adult weight gain—even after menopause—can increase the risk of postmenopausal breast cancer. (7)
   • Encouragingly, for women who had never used hormone replacement

therapy, losing weight after menopause—and keeping it off—cut their risk of post-menopausal breast cancer in half.

2. Reference for 5%: Blackburn G. (1995). "Effect of degree of weight loss on health benefits." Obesity Research 3: 211S–216S. Reference for 10%: NIH, NHLBI Obesity Education Initiative. Clinical Guidelines on the Identification, Evaluation, and Treatment of Overweight and Obesity in Adults. Available online: http://www.nhlbi.nih.gov/guidelines/obesity/ob_gdlns.pdf. In one national study, for example, patients who lost a mere seven percent of their total body weight reduced their risk for diabetes by 58%. A study in Finland found the same benefit with only a five percent weight loss. Similar improvements have been documented for hypertension and even sleep apnea.

3. Reference for 5%: Blackburn G. (1995). Effect of degree of weight loss on health benefits. Obesity Research 3: 211S-216S. Reference for 10%: NIH, NHLBI "Obesity Education Initiative. Clinical Guidelines on the Identification, Evaluation, and Treatment of Overweight and Obesity in Adults." Available online: http://www.nhlbi.nih.gov/guidelines/obesity/ob_gdlns.pdf.

4. Table 53. "Selected health conditions and risk factors, by age: United States, selected years 1988–1994 through 2015–2016" https://www.cdc.gov/nchs/hus/contents2017.htm#053.

5. *The Lancet: Diabetes & Endocrinology*, "Association of BMI with overall and cause-specific mortality: a population-based cohort study of 3·6 million adults in the UK", Krishnan Bhaskaran, PhD; Prof Isabel dos-Santos-Silva, PhD; Prof David A Leon, PhD; Ian J Douglas, PhD; Prof Liam Smeeth, PhD. Open Access, Published: October 30, 2018 DOI:https://doi.org/10.1016/S2213-8587(18)30288-2.

Part 2.2, *Your Blueprint: Safe Weight Loss and Health Gain*

1. "Nibbling versus Gorging: Metabolic Advantages of Increased Meal Frequency", David J.A. Jenkins, M.D., Ph.D., Thomas M.S. Wolever, M.D.., Ph.D., Vladimir Vuksan, Ph.D., Furio Brighenti, Ph.D., Stephen C. Cunnane, Ph.D., A. Venketeshwer Rao, Ph.D., Alexandra L. Jenkins, R.P.DT., Gloria Buckley, M.SC, Robert Patten, M.D., William Singer, M.B., B.S., Paul Corey, Ph.D., and Robert G. Josse, M.B., B.S. N Engl J Med 1989; 321:929-934.

2. "The Effects of 6 Isocaloric Meals Pattern on Blood Lipid Profile, Glucose, Hemoglobin A1c, Insulin and Malondialdehyde in Type 2 Diabetic Patients: A Randomized Clinical Trial" Article (PDF Available) in *Iranian Journal of Medical Sciences* 39(5): 433-9 September 2014, Source: PubMed.

3. The Effects of 6 Isocaloric Meals Pattern on Blood Lipid Profile, Glucose, Hemoglobin A1c, Insulin and Malondialdehyde in Type 2 Diabetic Patients: A Randomized Clinical Trial Article (PDF Available) in Iranian Journal of Medical Sciences 39(5):433-9 September 2014, Source: PubMed.

4. Anderson, J. W., Konz, E. C., Frederich, R. C., & Wood, C. L. (2001). "Long-term weight-loss maintenance: A meta-analysis of U.S. studies", *American Journal of Clinical Nutrition*, 74, 579 – 584. Anderson, J. W., Vichitbandra, S., Qian, W., & Kryscio, R. J. (1999). "Long-term weight maintenance after an intensive weight-loss program'" *Journal of the American College of Nutrition*, 18, 620 – 627. Andres, R., Muller, D. C., & Sorkin, J. D. (1993). Long-term effects of change in body weight on all-cause mortality. *Annals of Internal Medicine*, 119, 737–743. Astrup, A., & Rossner, S. (2000). "Lessons from obesity management programmes: Greater initial weight loss improves long-term maintenance", *Obesity Reviews*, 1, 17 – 19. Avenell, A., Brown, T. J., McGee, M. A., Campbell, M. K., Grant, A. M., Broom, J., et al. (2004). "What interventions should we add to weight reducing diets in adults with obesity? A systematic review of randomized controlled trials of adding drug therapy, exercise, behaviour therapy or combinations of these interventions", *Journal of Human Nutrition and Dietetics*, 17, 293 – 316.

5. "Medicare's Search for Effective Obesity Treatments Diets Are Not the Answer" Traci Mann, A. Janet Tomiyama, Erika Westling, Ann-Marie Lew, Barbra Samuels, and Jason Chatman, University of California, Los Angeles.

6. Klem ML, Wing RR, McGuire MT, Seagle HM & Hill JO (1997). "A descriptive study of individuals successful at long-term maintenance of substantial weight loss", *American Journal of Clinical Nutrition*, 66, 239–246. Shick SM, Wing RR, Klem ML, McGuire MT, Hill JO & Seagle HM (1998). "Persons successful at long-term weight loss and maintenance continue to consume a low calorie, low fat diet", *Journal of the American Dietetic Association*, 98, 408–413.

7. McGuire MT, Wing RR, Klem ML, Seagle HM & Hill JO (1998). "Long-term maintenance of weight loss: Do people who lose weight through various weight loss methods use different behaviors to maintain their weight?" *International Journal of Obesity*, 22, 572-577 Ann Epidemiol. 2016 Aug;26(8): 527–533.

doi: 10.1016/j.annepidem.2016.06.006. Epub 2016 Jun 15. "Relationship between frequency of eating and cardiovascular disease mortality in U.S. adults: the NHANES III follow-up study." Chen HJ1, Wang Y2, Cheskin LJ3.

8. "The Effects of 6 Isocaloric Meals Pattern on Blood Lipid Profile, Glucose, Hemoglobin A1c, Insulin and Malondialdehyde in Type 2 Diabetic Patients: A Randomized Clinical Trial" Article (PDF Available) in *Iranian Journal of Medical Sciences* 39(5): 433–9, September 2014, Source: PubMed.

9. Schoenfeld BJ, Aragon AA, Krieger JW. Nutr Rev. 2015 Feb;73(2):69-82. doi: 10.1093/nutrit/nuu017. Review. PMID: 26024494. "Highlighting the positive impact of increasing feeding frequency on metabolism and weight management", Louis-Sylvestre J1, Lluch A, Neant F, Blundell JE.

10. Proc Nutr Soc. 2000 Aug;59(3):349-58. "Role of dietary carbohydrate and frequent eating in body-weight control", Kirk TR1.

Part 2.3, *The Catalyst to Reaching a Healthy Weight*

1. This statistic shows the revenue of quick service restaurants in the United States from 2002 to 2014, with a forecast to 2020. In 2014, the revenue of the QSR restaurant industry in the United States was 198.9 billion U.S. dollars. www.statista.com/statistics/196614/revenue.

2. According to a report in the September 2014 *American Journal of Medicine* that pooled results from 19 different studies, fish eaters were less likely to have a heart attack or unstable angina (unexpected chest pain that usually happens at rest) than non–fish eaters.

3. Bucher H, Hengstler P, Schindler C, Meier G. "N-3 polyunsaturated fatty acids in coronary heart disease: a meta-analysis of randomized controlled trials", Am J Med. 2002;112(4): 298 – 304. [PubMed].

4. Carroll D, Roth MT. "Evidence for the cardioprotective effects of omega-3 Fatty acids", Ann Pharmacother. 2002; 36(12): 1950 – 6. [PubMed].

5. Chen Q, Cheng LQ, Xiao TH, Zhang YX, Zhu M, Zhang R, Li K, Wang Y, Li Y. "Effects of omega-3 fatty acid for sudden cardiac death prevention in patients with cardiovascular disease: a contemporary meta-analysis of randomized, controlled trials: Cardiovasc Drugs Ther." 2011; 25(3): 259 – 65. [PubMed].

6. Di Minno M, Tremoli E, Tufano A, Russolillo A, Lupoli R, Di Minno G. "Exploring newer cardioprotective strategies: Omega-3 fatty acids in perspective", Thromb Haemost. 2010; 104(4): 664 – 80. [PubMed].

7. Filion K, El Khoury F, Bielinski M, Schiller I, Dendukuri N, Brophy JM. "Omega-3 fatty acids in high-risk cardiovascular patients: a meta-analysis of randomized controlled trials. BMC Cardiovasc Disord", 2010; 10(24) [PMC free article] [PubMed].

8. Hooper L, Thompson RL, Harrison RA, Summerbell CD, Ness AR, Moore HJ, Worthington HV, Durrington PN, Higgins JP, Capps NE, Riemersma RA, Ebrahim SB, Davey Smith G. "Risks and benefits of omega-3 fats for mortality, cardiovascular disease, and cancer: systematic review", BMJ. 2006; 332(7544): 752–60. [PMC free article] [PubMed].

9. Oomen C, Feskens EJ, Räsänen L, Fidanza F, Nissinen AM, Menotti A, Kok FJ, Kromhout D. "Fish consumption and coronary heart disease mortality in Finland, Italy, and The Netherlands", Am J Epidemiol. 2000; 151(10): 999–1006. [PubMed].

10. von Schacky C, Harris WS. "Cardiovascular benefits of omega-3 fatty acids", Cardiovasc Res. 2007; 73(2): 310–5. [PubMed].

11. Whelton S, He J, Whelton PK, Muntner P. Meta-analysis of observational studies on fish intake and coronary heart disease. Am J Cardiol. 2004; 93(9): 1119–23. [PubMed].

12. Yzebe D, Lievre M. "Fish oils in the care of coronary heart disease patients: a meta-analysis of randomized controlled trials", Fundam Clin Pharmacol. 2004;18(5):581–92. [PubMed].

13. Physiol Behav. Author manuscript; available in PMC 2011 Apr 26. Published in final edited form as: Physiol Behav. 2010 Apr 26; 100(1): 22–32. Published online 2010 Jan 11. doi: [10.1016/j.physbeh.2009.12.026] PMCID: PMC2849909, NIHMSID: NIHMS175763, PMID: 20060847, "Hunger and Thirst: Issues in measurement and prediction of eating and drinking", Richard D. Mattes, MPH, PhD, RD.

14. J Clin Endocrinol Metab. 2003 Dec;88(12):6015-9. "Water-induced thermogenesis", Boschmann M1, Steiniger J, Hille U, Tank J, Adams F, Sharma AM, Klaus S, Luft FC, Jordan J.

Part 2.5, Choosing Wisely: Dr. A's Color-Coded Shopping System

1. "Gliadin protein-derived opiates that increase appetite by binding to the opiate receptors of the human brain", J Health Popul Nutr. 2015; 33: 24. Published online 2015 Nov 24. doi: [10.1186/s41043-015-0032-y] PMCID: PMC5025969, PMID: 26825414 "The opioid effects of gluten exorphins: asymptomatic celiac disease", Leo Pruimboom1,2 and Karin de Punder 1, 3. Gliadin is a hard-to-digest protein found in wheat that can negatively impact your appetite; it can stimulate your appetite and cause you to eat more carb-rich foods. Cardiologist and author William Davis, MD.

2. Vena, N., Rada, P., & Hoebel, B. (2008). "Evidence for sugar addiction: behavioral and neurochemical effects of intermittent, excessive sugar intake", Neuroscience Behavior Review, 52(1), 20-39. Retrieved from http://www.ncbi.nlm.nih.gov/pubmed/17617461.

3. Ervin, R.B., & Ogden, C.L. U.S. Department of Health and Human Services, Centers for Disease Control and Prevention. (2013). "NCHS Data Brief, No. 122: Consumption of Added Among U.S. Adults, 2005–2010" Retrieved from http://www.cdc.gov/nchs/data/databriefs/db122.pdf.

4. A Murakami, K Ohnishi. "Target molecules of food phytochemicals: Food science bound for the next dimension", Food Funct. 2012 May; 3(5): 462–76.

5. J Putnam, J Allshouse, L S Kantor. "U.S. Per Capita Food Supply Trends: More Calories, Refined Carbohydrates, and Fats". Food Review, Vol 25, Issue 3.

6. Br J Health Psychol. 2015 May;20(2):413-27. doi: 10.1111/bjhp.12113. Epub 2014 Jul 30. "On carrots and curiosity: eating fruit and vegetables is associated with greater flourishing in daily life", Conner TS1, Brookie KL, Richardson AC, Polak MA.

7. A study by Vanderbilt-Ingram Cancer Center and Shanghai Center for Disease Control and Prevention investigators reveals that breast cancer survivors who eat more cruciferous vegetables may have improved survival. The study of women in China was presented by postdoctoral fellow Sarah J. Nechuta, Ph.D., M.P.H., at the American Association for Cancer Research Annual Meeting in Chicago, Ill. Women who were in the highest quartiles of intake of vegetables per day had a 62% reduced risk of total mortality, 62% reduced risk of breast cancer mortality, and 35% reduced risk of breast cancer recurrence, compared to women with the lowest quartile of intake.

8. "Disparities in State-Specific Adult Fruit and Vegetable Consumption", United States, 2015, Weekly / November 17, 2017 / 66(45);1241–1247.

9. New York Times: "Told to Eat Its Vegetables, America Orders Fries" ,Kim Severson, Sept. 24, 2010.

10. Bucher H, Hengstler P, Schindler C, Meier G. "N-3 polyunsaturated fatty acids in coronary heart disease: a meta-analysis of randomized controlled trials", Am J Med. 2002; 112(4): 298–304. [PubMed].

11. Carroll D, Roth MT. "Evidence for the cardioprotective effects of omega-3 Fatty acids", Ann Pharmacother. 2002; 36(12): 1950–6. [PubMed].

12. Chen Q, Cheng LQ, Xiao TH, Zhang YX, Zhu M, Zhang R, Li K, Wang Y, Li Y. Effects of omega-3 fatty acid for sudden cardiac death prevention in patients with cardiovascular disease: a contemporary meta-analysis of randomized, controlled trials. Cardiovasc Drugs Ther. 2011;25(3): 259–65. [PubMed].

13. Di Minno M, Tremoli E, Tufano A, Russolillo A, Lupoli R, Di Minno G. "Exploring newer cardioprotective strategies: omega-3 fatty acids in perspective". Thromb Haemost. 2010; 104(4): 664–80. [PubMed].

14. Filion K, El Khoury F, Bielinski M, Schiller I, Dendukuri N, Brophy JM. Omega-3 fatty acids in high-risk cardiovascular patients: a meta-analysis of randomized controlled trials. BMC Cardiovasc Disord. 2010;10(24) [PMC free article] [PubMed].

15. Hooper L, Thompson RL, Harrison RA, Summerbell CD, Ness AR, Moore HJ, Worthington HV, Durrington PN, Higgins JP, Capps NE, Riemersma RA, Ebrahim SB, Davey Smith G. "Risks and benefits of omega-3 fats for mortality, cardiovascular disease, and cancer: systematic review", BMJ. 2006; 332(7544): 752–60. [PMC free article] [PubMed].

16. Oomen C, Feskens EJ, Räsänen L, Fidanza F, Nissinen AM, Menotti A, Kok FJ, Kromhout D. "Fish consumption and coronary heart disease mortality in Finland, Italy, and The Netherlands", Am J Epidemiol. 2000; 151(10): 999–1006. [PubMed].

17. von Schacky C, Harris WS. "Cardiovascular benefits of omega-3 fatty acids", Cardiovasc Res. 2007;73(2):310–5. [PubMed].

18. Whelton S, He J, Whelton PK, Muntner P. Meta-analysis of observational studies on fish intake and coronary heart disease. Am J Cardiol. 2004; 93(9): 1119–23. [PubMed].

19. Yzebe D, Lievre M. "Fish oils in the care of coronary heart disease patients: a meta-analysis of randomized controlled trials", Fundam Clin Pharmacol. 2004; 18(5): 581–92. [PubMed].

20. "Red Meat consumption and Mortality", Archives of Internal Medicine, 172(7)555-563 2011.

21. Researchers at the Mount Sinai School of Medicine in New York found that frying, roasting, searing or grilling certain foods at high temperatures produces compounds called advanced glycation end products (AGES). Your body produces AGES, also known as glycotoxins, as part of the metabolic process. AGES are also present in raw animal products, including meat. Cooking, especially at high temperatures, forms new AGES in foods. Although some AGES are not bad, high levels of the compounds in the tissues

and blood can trigger an inflammatory response and have been linked to the recent epidemics of diseases like diabetes and cardiovascular disease.

22. "Unlocking the heart-protective benefits of soy", February 21, 2017 Source: University of Pittsburgh Schools of the Health Sciences Summary: A product of digesting a micronutrient found in soy may old the key to why some people seem to derive a heart-protective benefit from eating soy foods, while others do not.

23. J Nutr. 1999 Mar;129(3):758S-767S. "Dietary isoflavones: biological effects and relevance to human health", Setchell KD1, Cassidy A.

24. Penn State. "Whole Grain Diets Lower Risk Of Chronic Disease, Study Shows." *ScienceDaily*, 11 February 2008. www.sciencedaily.com/ releases/2008/02/080205161231.htm.

25. J Nutr. 2010 Mar; 140(3): 587–594. doi: [10.3945/jn.109.116640] PMCID: PMC2821887, PMID: 20089789, Whole and Refined Grain Intakes Are Related to Inflammatory Protein Concentrations in Human Plasma 1, 2.

26. "HHS and USDA Release New Dietary Guidelines to Encourage Healthy Eating Patterns to Prevent Chronic Diseases".

27. Hooper L, Abdelhamid A, Bunn D, Brown T, Summerbell CD, Skeaff CM. "Effects of total fat intake on body weight", Cochrane Database Syst Rev. 2015; (8):CD011834. (2) "Diet, nutrition and the prevention of chronic diseases: report of a Joint WHO/FAO Expert Consultation", WHO Technical Report Series, No. 916. Geneva: World Health Organization; 2003. (3) "Fats and fatty acids in human nutrition: report of an expert consultation", FAO Food and Nutrition Paper 91. Rome: Food and Agriculture Organization of the United Nations; 2010.

28. Brain Behav Immun. Author manuscript; available in PMC 2012 Nov 1. Published in final edited form as: Brain Behav Immun. 2011 Nov; 25(8): 1725–1734. Published online 2011 Jul 19. doi: [10.1016/j.bbi.2011.07.229] PMCID: PMC3191260, NIHMSID: NIHMS312102, PMID: 21784145, "Omega-3 Supplementation Lowers Inflammation and Anxiety in Medical Students: A Randomized Controlled Trial".

29. Physiol Behav. Author manuscript; available in PMC 2011 Apr 26. Published in final edited form as: Physiol Behav. 2010 Apr 26; 100(1): 22–32. Published online 2010 Jan 11. doi: [10.1016/j.physbeh.2009.12.026] PMCID: PMC2849909, NIHMSID: NIHMS175763, PMID: 20060847 "Hunger and Thirst: Issues in measurement and prediction of eating and drinking", Richard D. Mattes, MPH, PhD, RD.

30. J Clin Endocrinol Metab. 2003 Dec; 88(12): 6015–9. "Water-induced thermogenesis", Boschmann M1, Steiniger J, Hille U, Tank J, Adams F, Sharma AM, Klaus S, Luft FC, Jordan.

31. Chin Med. 2010; 5: 13. Published online 2010 Apr 6. doi: [10.1186/1749-8546-5-13] PMCID: PMC2855614, PMID: 20370896, "Beneficial effects of green tea: A literature review", Sabu M Chacko,1 Priya T Thambi,1 Ramadasan Kuttan,2 and Ikuo Nishigaki J Ethnopharmacol. 2018 Jan 10;210:296-310. doi: 10.1016/j.jep.2017.08.035. Epub 2017 Aug 31. "Molecular understanding of Epigallocatechin gallate (EGCG) in cardiovascular and metabolic diseases." Free Radic Biol Med. Author manuscript; available in PMC 2011 Dec 1. Published in final edited form as: Free Radic Biol Med. 2010 Dec 1; 49(11): 1603–1616. Published online 2010 Sep 16. doi: [10.1016/j.freeradbiomed.2010.09.006] MCID: PMC2990475, NIHMSID: NIHMS236168, PMID: 20840865 "Oxidative stress, inflammation, and cancer: How are they linked?" Simone Reuter, Subash C. Gupta, Madan M. Chaturvedi, and Bharat B. Aggarwal.

32. J Nutr. 2008 Aug;138(8):1572S-1577S. "L-theanine and caffeine in combination affect human cognition as evidenced by oscillatory alpha-band activity and attention task performance." Kelly SP1, Gomez-Ramirez M, Montesi JL, Foxe JJ.

33. Arch Intern Med. 2011 Sep 26;171(17):1571-8. doi: 10.1001/archinternmed.2011.393. "Coffee, caffeine, and risk of depression among women", Lucas M1, Mirzaei F, Pan A, Okereke OI, Willett WC, O'Reilly ÉJ, Koenen K, Ascherio A. "The impact of caffeine on mood, cognitive function, performance and hydration: a review of benefits and risks", C. H. S. Ruxton, First published: 13 February 2008 https://doi.org/10.1111/j.1467-3010.2007.00665. *Diabetologia*, December 2009, Volume 52, Issue 12, pp 2561–2569 "Coffee and tea consumption and risk of type 2 diabetes" S. van Dieren, C. S. P. M. Uiterwaal, Y. T. van der Schouw, D. L. van der A, J. M. A. Boer, A. Spijkerman, D. E. Grobbee, m J Clin Nutr. 2012 Aug;96(2):374-81. doi: 10.3945/ajcn.111.031328. Epub 2012 Jun 13. "Caffeinated and decaffeinated coffee and tea intakes and risk of colorectal cancer in a large prospective study".

34. .35. Park S, McGuire LC, Galuska DA. "Regional differences in sugar-sweetened beverage intake among U.S. adults", J Acad Nutr Diet. 2015;115(12): 1996–2002.

36. "New evidence: Sugary soft drinks could increase cancer risk, no matter your weight", Thursday 22 February, 2018 The findings are based on a research study of more than 35,000 Australians who developed 3283 cases of obesity-related cancers."We were surprised to find this increased cancer risk was not driven completely by obesity. Our study found that the more sugary soft drinks participants drank, the higher their risk of cancer. This was not the case with those who drank diet soft drinks, suggesting sugar is a key contributor," said A/Prof Hodge.

37. Live Science, Health, "Daily Soda Consumption Increases Stroke Risk", By Live Science Staff | April 20, 2012 01:55pm ET. The study was published online April 4 in the *American Journal of Clinical Nutrition*.

38. PLOS, Peer-reviewed Research Article, "No Evidence of Dehydration with Moderate Daily Coffee Intake: A Counterbalanced Cross-Over Study in a Free-Living Population", Sophie C. Killer, Andrew K. Blannin.

Part 2.6, Choosing Wisely: Building Healthy Meal Plans for Optimal Health

1. Another study published in the *Journal of Agricultural and Food Chemistry* in 2002 showed that cooking carrots increases their level of beta-carotene. One 2002 study he did (published in the *Journal of Agriculture and Food Chemistry*) found that cooking actually boosts the amount of lycopene in tomatoes, cooked carrots, spinach, mushrooms, asparagus, cabbage, peppers and many other vegetables also supply more antioxidants, such as carotenoids and ferulic acid, to the body than they do when raw, Liu says. At least, that is, if they're boiled or steamed. A January 2008 report in the *Journal of Agriculture and Food Chemistry* said that boiling and steaming better preserves antioxidants, particularly carotenoid, in carrots, zucchini and broccoli, than frying, though boiling was deemed the best.

2. J Zhejiang Univ Sci B.2009 Aug;10(8):580-8. doi: 10.1631/jzus.B0920051.Effects of different cooking methods on health-promoting compounds of broccoli Pharmacol Res. Author manuscript; available in PMC 2009 Sep 4. Published in final edited form as: Pharmacol Res. 2007 Mar; 55(3): 224–236. Published online 2007 Jan 25. doi: [10.1016/j.phrs.2007.01.009] PMCID: PMC2737735, NIHMSID: NIHMS22145, PMID: 17317210, "Cruciferous Vegetables and Human Cancer Risk: Epidemiologic Evidence and Mechanistic Basis".

3. De Graff, Mia. (2016, August 17). From cataracts to cancer: The REAL dangers of microwave ovens and how to test if yours is leaking. Retrieved from http://www.dailymail.co.uk/health/article-3745308/

From-cataracts-cancer-REAL-dangers-microwave-ovens-test-leaking.html#ixzz5B0My1kRe, Lens Eye Toxic Res. 1989;6(1-2):379 - 86. Effects of microwave radiation on the eye: the occupational health perspective. Cutz A1.

Part 2.7, The Science of Healthy Eating and Weight Loss

1. http://www.diabetes.org/diabetes-basics/statistics/
   Last Edited: March 22, 2018 Undiagnosed: Of the 30.3 million adults with diabetes, 23.1 million were diagnosed, and 7.2 million were undiagnosed.

2. http://www.diabetes.org/diabetes-basics/statistics/
   Last Edited: March 22, 2018Undiagnosed: Of the 30.3 million adults with diabetes, 23.1 million were diagnosed, and 7.2 million were undiagnosed.

3. New CDC report: More than 100 million Americans have diabetes or prediabetes For Immediate Release: Weekday, July 18, 2017.

4. "Insulin Resistance" Andrew M. Freeman; Nicholas Pennings. June 26, 2018. Criteria proposed by the National Cholesterol Education Program Adult Treatment Panel III national survey data suggests insulin resistance syndrome is very common, affecting about 24% of United States (US) adults older than 20 years.

5. Heart. 2004 Jan; 90(1): 107–111. PMCID: PMC1768013, PMID: 14676260, The French paradox: lessons for other countries, Jean Ferrières.

6. Adv Nutr. 2015 Nov; 6(6): 712–728. Published online 2015 Nov 10. doi: [10.3945/an.115.009654] PMCID: PMC4642426, PMID: 26567196 "Plant Protein and Animal Proteins: Do They Differentially Affect Cardiovascular Disease Risk?" 1, 2.

7. David Katz, M.D., M.P.H., director, Yale-Griffin Prevention Research Center, Derby, Conn., and president, American College of Lifestyle Medicine; Samantha Heller, M.S., R.D., senior clinical nutritionist, New York University Medical Center, New York City; BMJ Open, Feb. 12, 2018, online They often contain hidden additives, like salt in breakfast cereal or sugar in some tomato sauces and salad dressings, says David Katz, MD, founding director of the Yale University Prevention Research Center. Barbara Rolls, PhD, professor of nutritional sciences at Pennsylvania State University and author of The Ultimate Volumetrics Diet. "It's called sensory-specific satiety," she explains, "and it happens when you eat one type of food to the point where you don't want any more, yet you can still be hungry for foods with other flavors, textures and smells."

8. "A high-protein diet induces sustained reductions in appetite, ad libitum caloric intake, and body weight despite compensatory changes in diurnal plasma leptin and ghrelin concentrations" David S, Weigle, Patricia A Breen, Colleen C Matthys, Holly S Callahan, Kaatje E Meeuws, Verna R Burden, Jonathan Q Purnell, The American Journal of Clinical Nutrition, Volume 82, Issue 1, 1 July 2005, Pages 41 – 48, https://doi.org/10.1093/ajcn/82.1.41, Published: 01 July 2005.

9. Rolls, B. J., et al., "Reductions in Portion Size and Energy Density of Foods," American Journal of Clinical Nutrition, 83 (January 2006): 11 – 17.

Part 2.8, Healthy Eating for Life: Your Transition to Permanent Health

1. Cell Metab. Author manuscript; available in PMC 2016 Oct 31. Published in final edited form as: Cell Metab. 2014 Mar 4; 19(3): 418 – 430. doi: [10.1016/j.cmet.2014.02.009] PMCID: PMC5087279, NIHMSID: NIHMS824753, PMID: 24606899, "The Ratio of Macronutrients, Not Caloric Intake, Dictates Cardiometabolic Health, Aging, and Longevity in Ad Libitum-Fed Mice". Samantha M. Solon-Biet,1,2,3,4,13 Aisling C. McMahon,1,2,3,13 J. William O. Ballard,5 Kari Ruohonen,6 Lindsay E. Wu,7 Victoria C. Cogger,1,2,3 Alessandra Warren,1,2,3 Xin Huang,1,2,3 Nicolas Pichaud,5 Richard G. Melvin,8 Rahul Gokarn,2,3 Mamdouh Khalil,3 Nigel Turner,9 Gregory J. Cooney,9 David A. Sinclair,7,10 David Raubenheimer,1,4,11,12 David G. Le Couteur, 1,2,3,* and Stephen J. Simpson.

2. "Eating attentively: a systematic review and meta-analysis of the effect of food intake memory and awareness on eating", Eric Robinson Paul Aveyard Amanda Daley Kate Jolly Amanda Lewis Deborah Lycett Suzanne Higgs, The American Journal of Clinical Nutrition, Volume 97, Issue 4, 1 April 2013, Pages 728 – 742, https://doi.org/10.3945/ajcn.112.045245, Bellisle Dalix, "Cognitive restraint can be offset by distraction, leading to increased meal intake in women", Am J Clin Nutr 2001 74 197 200.

3. "Fruit, vegetable, and legume intake, and cardiovascular disease and deaths in 18 countries (PURE): a prospective cohort study", Miller V1, Mente A2, Dehghan M2, Rangarajan S2, Zhang X2, Swaminathan S3, Dagenais G4, Gupta R5, Mohan V6, Lear S7, Bangdiwala SI2, Schutte AE8, Wentzel-Viljoen E8, Avezum A9, Altuntas Y10, Yusoff K11, Ismail N12, Peer N13, Chifamba J14, Diaz R15, Rahman O16, Mohammadifard N17, Lana F18, Zatonska K19, Wielgosz A20, Yusufali A21, Iqbal R22, Lopez-Jaramillo P23, Khatib R24, Rosengren A25, Kutty VR26, Li W27, Liu J28, Liu X27, Yin L27, Teo K2, Anand S2, Yusuf S2; Prospective Urban Rural Epidemiology (PURE) study investigators.

4. Arch Intern Med. 2012 Apr 9;172(7):555-63. doi: 10.1001/archinternmed.2011.2287. Epub 2012 Mar 12. "Red meat consumption and mortality: results from 2 prospective cohort studies." Pan A1, Sun Q, Bernstein AM, Schulze MB, Manson JE, Stampfer MJ, Willett WC, Hu FB. Circulation. 2010 Jun 1;121(21):2271-83. doi: 10.1161/CIRCULATIONAHA.109.924977. Epub 2010 May 17. "Red and processed meat consumption and risk of incident coronary heart disease, stroke, and diabetes mellitus: a systematic review and meta-analysis", Micha R1, Wallace SK, Mozaffarian D. "Intestinal microbiota metabolism of l-carnitine, a nutrient in red meat, promotes atherosclerosis", Robert A Koeth, Zeneng Wang, Bruce S Levison, Jennifer A Buffa, Elin Org, Brendan T Sheehy, Earl B Britt, Xiaoming Fu, Yuping Wu, Lin Li, Jonathan D Smith, Joseph A DiDonato, Jun Chen, Hongzhe Li, Gary D Wu, James D Lewis, Manya Warrier, J Mark Brown, Ronald M Krauss, W H Wilson Tang, Frederic D Bushman, Aldons J Lusis, & Stanley L Hazen, Nature Medicine volume 19, pages 576 – 585 (2013).

5. The United States topped the list as the biggest eaters, according to calorie intake data released by The Food and Agriculture Organization in 2018. Americans eat an average of over 3,000 calories a day, according to the report. This is well above the U.S. Department of Agriculture recommendations.

6. Wellbeing by Rath Reference 85: Journal of Consumer Research, 36 (3),380 – 393 Vicarious goal fulfilment.

7. The United States topped the list as the biggest eaters, according to calorie intake data released by The Food and Agriculture Organization in 2018. Americans eat an average of over 3,000 calories a day, according to the report. This is well above the U.S. Department of Agriculture recommendations.

8. health.gov Dietary Guidelines, 2015 – 2020 Dietary Guidelines for Americans.

9. Wellbeing by Rath Reference 85: Journal of Consumer Research, 36 (3),380-393 "Vicarious goal fulfilment", Mac Evilly C & Kelly C. (2001). Conference report on 'Mood and Food'. Nutrition Bulletin 26 (no 4). Margetts BM, et al. (1998). Factors which influence 'healthy' eating patterns: results from the 1993 Health Education Authority health and lifestyle survey in England. Public Health Nutrition 1(3):193-198. Nestle M, et al. (1998). "Behavioural and social influences on food choice", Nutrition Reviews 56(5):S50 – S64.

10. Rolls, B. J., et al., "Reductions in Portion Size and Energy Density of Foods," American Journal of Clinical Nutrition 83 (January 2006): 11–17.

Part 2.9, Active Living: Inside and Out

1. "Don't Just Sit There", December 1, 2015 by Katy Bowman.

2. "Astronaut muscles waste in space", August 17, 2010, Wiley, Astronaut muscles waste away on long space flights reducing their capacity for physical work by more than 40%, according to research published online in the Journal of Physiology. Read more at: https://phys.org/news/2010-08-astronaut-muscles-space.html#jCp.

3. Boscia, Ted. (2014, January 10). Study: Prolonged sitting jeopardizes older women's health. Retrieved from http://news.cornell.edu/stories/2014/01/study-prolonged-sitting-jeopardizes-older-women-s-health. Am J Epidemiol. 2010 Aug 15;172(4):419-29. doi: 10.1093/aje/kwq155. Epub 2010 Jul 22.

4. J Clin Endocrinol Metab. 2003 Dec;88(12):6015–9. "Water-induced thermogenesis", Boschmann M1, Steiniger J, Hille U, Tank J, Adams F, Sharma AM, Klaus S, Luft FC, Jordan J. The Journal of Clinical Endocrinology & Metabolism, Volume 88, Issue 12, 1 December 2003, Pages 6015–6019, https://doi.org/10.1210/jc.2003-030780.

5. "Sedentary Time and Its Association With Risk for Disease Incidence, Mortality, and Hospitalization in Adults: A Systematic Review and Meta-analysis", Mayo Clinic: An analysis of 13 studies of sitting time and activity levels found that those who sat for more than eight hours a day with no physical activity had a risk of dying similar to the risks of dying posed by obesity and smoking.

6. Am J Epidemiol. Author manuscript; available in PMC 2012 Dec 21, Published in final edited form as: Am J Epidemiol. 2008 Apr 1; 167(7): 875–881. Published online 2008 Feb 25. doi: [10.1093/aje/kwm390] PMCID: PMC3527832, NIHMSID: NIHMS209987, PMID: 18303006, Amount of Time Spent in Sedentary Behaviors in the United States, 2003–2004, Charles E. Matthews,1 Kong Y. Chen,2 Patty S. Freedson,3 Maciej S. Buchowski,4 Bettina M. Beech,1 Russell R. Pate,5 and Richard P. Troiano6.

7. Am J Epidemiol. 2010 Aug 15;172(4):419-29. doi: 10.1093/aje/kwq155. Epub 2010 Jul 22.

8. "Prolonged Sitting and the Risk of Cardiovascular Disease and Mortality" Article (PDF Available)in Current Cardiovascular Risk Reports 5(4):350-357 · August 2011, DOI: 10.1007/s12170-011-0174-4.

9. U.S. Department Of Health And Human Services Centers for Disease Control and Prevention, National Center for Health Statistics, National Health Statistics Reports, Number 112, June 28, 2018, "State Variation in Meeting the 2008 Federal Guidelines, for Both Aerobic and Muscle-strengthening Activities, Through Leisure-time Physical Activity Among, Adults Aged 18–64: United States, 2010–2015", Debra L. Blackwell, Ph.D., and Tainya C. Clarke, Ph.D., M.P.H. CDC, CDC.

Part 2.10, First Steps: Introduction to Dr. A's Habits of Motion System

1. U.S. Department Of Health And Human Services Centers for Disease Control and Prevention, National Center for Health Statistics, National Health Statistics Reports, Number 112, June 28, 2018, "State Variation in Meeting the 2008 Federal Guidelines, for Both Aerobic and Muscle-strengthening Activities, Through Leisure-time Physical Activity Among, Adults Aged 18–64: United States, 2010–2015", Debra L. Blackwell, Ph.D., and Tainya C. Clarke.

2. Sobering Statistics on Physical Inactivity in the U.S.Approximately 36% of adults in the U.S. do not engage in any leisure-time physical activity. Lack of physical activity accounts for 22% of coronary heart disease, 22% of colon cancer, 18% of osteoporotic fractures, 12% of diabetes and hypertension, and 5% of breast cancer. Sources: Debra Blackwell, Ph.D., statistician/demographer, U.S. National Center for Health Statistics.

3. Steven Lewis, Charles H. Hennekens, Regular Physical Activity: Forgotten Benefits. The American Journal of Medicine, 2015; DOI: 10.1016/j.amjmed.2015.07.016.

4. Lifehack, "90% of People Quit After 3 Months of Hitting the Gym, Here's How to Be the Exception".

5. Dansinger, M. L., and Schaefer, e. J., Journal of the American Medical Association 295: pp. 94–95.

6. Wellbeing,Rath, Reference 78, "Immediate increase in Mood, Attention, Performance, Creativity", Mayo Clinic (2008) Moderate exercise. Mayo Clinic Health Letter, 26 (1) 13.

7. Citations: Int J MS Care. 2016 Jan-Feb;18(1):1-8. doi: 10.7224/1537-2073.2014-104. Effects of Single Bouts of Walking Exercise and Yoga on Acute Mood Symptoms in People with Multiple Sclerosis.Ensari I1, Sandroff BM1, Motl RW1. Front Psychiatry. 2013 Apr 23;4:27. doi: 10.3389/fpsyt.2013.00027. eCollection 2013. Effects of exercise and physical activity on anxiety. Anderson E1, Shivakumar G Iran J Public Health. 2016 Dec;45(12):1545-1557. "Influence of Adolescents' Physical Activity on Bone Mineral Acquisition: A Systematic Review Article", Zulfarina MS1, Sharkawi AM1, Aqilah-S N ZS2, Mokhtar SA2, Nazrun SA1, Naina-Mohamed I1. Curr Protein Pept Sci. 2018;19(7):649-667. doi: 10.2174/1389203717666161227144349 "Nutrition and Exercise in Sarcopenia", Anton SD1,2, Hida A1,3, Mankowski R1, Layne A1, Solberg LM1, Mainous AG4,5, Buford T1, Sports Med. 2006;36(9):767–80. "Physical activity and feelings of energy and fatigue: epidemiological evidence", Puetz TW1. Ann Intern Med. 2000 Jul 18;133(2):92-103, "Reduction in obesity and related comorbid conditions after diet-induced weight loss or exercise-induced weight loss in men. A randomized, controlled trial".

8. Levine, J.A., "Nonexercise Activity Thermogenesis (NEAT): Environment and Biology," American Journal of Physiology, Endocrinology and Metabolism 286: E675-E685.

9. Hill, J. O., et al., "Obesity and the environment," Science 299: 853–855.

10. According to the Bureau of Labor Statistics, the average American works 44 hours per week, or 8.8 hours per day. A 2014 national Gallup poll put the average number at 47 hours per week, or 9.4 hours per day, with many saying they work 50 hours per week. May 3, 2017.

11. "Cardiovascular Risk of High- Versus Moderate-Intensity Aerobic Exercise in Coronary Heart Disease Patients" Article in Circulation 126(12):1436-40 · August 2012, DOI: 10.1161/CIRCULATIONAHA.112.123117 · Source: PubMed, Marijon E, Uy-Evanado A, Reinier K, et al, Sudden cardiac arrest during sports activity in middle age. Circulation. 2015;131(16):1384-1391.

2. Centers for Disease Control and Prevention. Physical Activity. Physical activity and health. Benefits of physical activity. https://www.cdc.gov/physicalactivity/basics/pa-health/index.htm. Accessed January 20, 2018.

3. Lavie CJ, Milani RV, Marks P, de Gruiter H. "Exercise and the heart: risks, benefits, and recommendations for providing exercise prescriptions". Ochsner J. 200;3(4): 207–213.

Part 2.11, Dr. A's Habits of Healthy Motion Part 1: NEAT System

1. Through three decades of research funded by the NIH, Dr. Levine's team has pioneered the science of nonexercise activity thermogenesis (NEAT) and harm associated with sedentariness. Low NEAT and sedentariness are major causes of obesity, diabetes, breast cancer, and two dozen other chronic disease and conditions. This work, published in journals such as Science and Nature, has

resulted in broad societal impact and policy change. "Get Up!: Why Your Chair is Killing You and What You Can Do About It", James A. Levine.

Part 2.12, Dr. A's Habits of Healthy Motion Part 2: EAT System

1. Int J Behav Nutr Phys Act. 2011; 8: 80. Published online 2011 Jul 28. doi: [10.1186/1479-5868-8-80] PMCID: PMC3169444, PMID: 21798044, "How many steps/day are enough? For older adults and special populations" Catrine Tudor-Locke, 1, 2 Cora L Craig, 2, 3 Yukitoshi Aoyagi, 4 Rhonda C Bell, 5 Karen A Croteau, 6 Ilse De Bourdeaudhuij, 7 Ben Ewald, 8 Andrew W Gardner, 9 Yoshiro Hatano, 10 Lesley D Lutes, 11 Sandra M Matsudo, 12, 13 Farah A Ramirez-Marrero, 14 Laura Q Rogers, 15 David A Rowe, 16 Michael D Schmidt, 17, 18 Mark A Tully, 19 and Steven N Blair20.

2. BMC Musculoskelet Disord. 2011; 12: 105. Published online 2011 May 20. doi: [10.1186/1471-2474-12-105] PMCID: PMC3118151, PMID: 21599967 "Mortality and cause of death in hip fracture patients aged 65 or older—a population-based study" Jorma Panula, 1 Harri Pihlajamäki, 2 Ville M Mattila, 3 Pekka Jaatinen, 4 Tero Vahlberg, 5 Pertti Aarnio, 6, 7 and Sirkka-Liisa Kivelä 8, 9, 10.

3. J Sports Sci. 2006 Dec;24(12):1247-64. "Effects of exercise intensity and duration on the excess post-exercise oxygen consumption", LaForgia J1, Withers RT, Gore CJ.

4. "Going for a walk at an average to brisk pace can provide people with a tremendous health benefit. It's free, easy, and can be done anywhere," says Alpa Patel, PhD, Strategic Director, CPS-3, American Cancer Society, and lead investigator of the study. The study was published online on October 19 in the *American Journal of Preventive Medicine*, "The Benefits of Walking for 30 Minutes a Day", July 2, 2015
Taking a 30-minute walk a day is kind of like that proverbial apple: There's a good chance it'll keep the doctor away. From helping you lose weight and de-stress to lowering your blood pressure and reducing your risk of many chronic diseases, going for regular walks is one of the best and easiest things you can do for your health, says Melina B. Jampolis, MD, author of The Doctor on Demand Diet.

5. Based on guidelines from the American College of Sports Medicine, Centers for Disease Control and Prevention, American Heart Association, U.S. Surgeon General, and U.S. Dietary Guidelines 2005.

6. Int J Environ Res Public Health. 2017 Aug; 14(8): 851. Published online 2017 Jul

28. doi: [10.3390/ijerph14080851], PMCID: PMC5580555, PMID: 28788101, Shinrin-Yoku (Forest Bathing) and Nature Therapy: A State-of-the-Art Review, Margaret M. Hansen,* Reo Jones, and Kirsten Tocchini.

7. Maslar, P.M., "The Effect of Music on the Reduction of Pain: A Review of the Literature," The Arts in Psychotherapy 13:215-219.

8. *Metabolism*. 1994 Jul;43(7):814–8. "Impact of exercise intensity on body fatness and skeletal muscle metabolism." Tremblay A1, Simoneau JA, Bouchard C.

9. J Obes. 2011;2011:868305. doi: 10.1155/2011/868305. Epub 2010 Nov 24. "High-intensity intermittent exercise and fat loss", Boutcher SH1.

Part 2.13, Healthy Sleep and Unlimited Energy

1. "Lack of Sleep is Affecting Americans, Finds the National Sleep Foundation", Washington, D.C. (December 2014), 45% of Americans say that poor or insufficient sleep affected their daily activities at least once in the past seven days, according to the National Sleep Foundation's inaugural Sleep Health Index™ CDC Update: 1 in 3 adults don't get enough sleep, A good night's sleep is critical for good health.

2. Sleep Med Clin. Author manuscript; available in PMC 2016 Dec 1. Published in final edited form as: Sleep Med Clin. 2015 Dec; 10(4): 413–421. doi: [10.1016/j.jsmc.2015.08.007] PMCID: PMC4758938, NIHMSID: NIHMS726533, PMID: 26568119 "Genetics of Circadian Rhythms", Tomas S. Andreani, BA,1 Taichi Q. Itoh, PhD,2 Evrim Yildirim, PhD,3 Dae-Sung Hwangbo, PhD,4 and Ravi Allada, MD5 2017-10-02. The Nobel Assembly at Karolinska Institutet has today decided to award the 2017 Nobel Prize in Physiology or Medicine jointly to Jeffrey C. Hall, Michael Rosbash and Michael W. Young for their discoveries of molecular mechanisms controlling the circadian rhythm.

3. Dialogues Clin Neurosci. 2008 Sep; 10(3): 329–336. PMCID: PMC3181883 PMID: 18979946, Language: English | Spanish | French, Sleep disorders as core symptoms of depression, David Nutt, DM, FRCP, FRCPsych, FMedSci,* Sue Wilson, PhD, and Louise Paterson, PhD.

4. Neuropsychiatr Dis Treat. 2007 Oct; 3(5): 553–567. PMCID: PMC2656292 PMID: 19300585 "Sleep deprivation: Impact on cognitive performance".

5. Occup Environ Med. 2000 Oct; 57(10): 649–655. doi: 10.1136/oem.57.10.649] PMCID: PMC1739867 PMID: 10984335 "Moderate sleep deprivation produces

impairments in cognitive and motor performance equivalent to legally prescribed levels of alcohol intoxication", A Williamson and A. Feyer, National Sleep Foundation. "Drowsy Driving vs. Drunk Driving: How Similar Are They?".

6. Knutson KL, Ryden AM, Mander VA, Van Cauter E. "Role of sleep duration and quality in the risk and severity of type 2 diabetes mellitus", Arch Intern Med 2006;166:176–1764.

7. Kasasbeh E, Chi DS, Krishnaswamy G. Inflammatory aspects of sleep apnea and their cardiovascular consequences. South Med J 2006;99:58–67.

8. Taheri S. The link between short sleep duration and obesity: We should recommend more sleep to prevent obesity. Arch Dis Child 2006;91:881–884.

9. Zimmerman M, McGlinchey JB, Young D, Chelminski I. Diagnosing major depressive disorder I: A psychometric evaluation of the DSM-IV symptom criteria. J Nerv Ment Dis 2006;194:158–163.

10. Schwartz DJ, Kohler WC, Karatinos G. Symptoms of depression in individuals with obstructive sleep apnea may be amenable to treatment with continuous positive airway pressure. Chest 2005;128:1304–1306.

11. Wheaton AG, Chapman DP, Presley-Cantrell LR, Croft JB, Roehler DR. "Drowsy driving—19 states and the District of Columbia, 2009-2010",[630 KB] MMWR Morb Mortal Wkly Rep. 2013; 61:1033. Wheaton AG, Shults RA, Chapman DP, Ford ES, Croft JB. "Drowsy driving and risk behaviors—10 states and Puerto Rico, 2011-2012", [817 KB] MMWR Morb Mortal Wkly Rep. 2014; 63:557–562. National Highway Traffic Safety Administration. Research on Drowsy Driving. Accessed October 20, 2015. Klauer SG, Dingus TA, Neale VL, Sudweeks JD, Ramsey DJ. "The Impact of Driver Inattention on Near-Crash/Crash Risk: An Analysis Using the 100-Car Naturalistic Study Data, 2006", Springfield, VA: DOT; year. DOT HS 810 594. Tefft BC, AAA Foundation for Traffic Safety. "Prevalence of Motor Vehicle Crashes Involving Drowsy Drivers, United States, 2009—2013" [457 KB].Washington, DC: AAA Foundation for Traffic Safety; 2014. October 19, 2015. Institute of Medicine. "Sleep Disorders and Sleep Deprivation: An Unmet Public Health Problem", Washington, DC: The National Academies Press; 2006 PLoS One. 2017; 12(8): e0184002. Published online 2017 Aug 31. doi: [10.1371/journal.pone.0184002], PMCID: PMC5578645 PMID: 28859144 "The effects of sleep loss on young drivers' performance: A systematic review", Shamsi Shekari Soleimanloo,

Conceptualization, Formal analysis, Investigation, Methodology, Project administration, Writing—original draft, Writing—review & editing, 1, 2, 3, Melanie J. White, Investigation, Methodology, Project administration, Supervision, Writing—review & editing, #2, 3 Veronica Garcia-Hansen, Investigation, Methodology, Project administration, Supervision, Writing—review & editing, #4 and Simon S. Smith, Conceptualization, Investigation, Methodology, Project administration, Supervision, Writing—review & editing 5.

12. Arch Intern Med. Author manuscript; available in PMC 2010 Jan 12. Published in final edited form as: Arch Intern Med. 2009 Jan 12; 169(1): 62–67. doi: [10.1001/archinternmed.2008.505] PMCID: PMC2629403 NIHMSID: NIHMS82203, PMID: 19139325, "Sleep Habits and Susceptibility to the Common Cold", Sheldon Cohen, PhD, William J. Doyle, PhD, Cuneyt M. Alper, MD, Denise Janicki-Deverts, PhD, and Ronald B. Turner, MD *NewsWeek*, "Lack of Sleep Makes You More Prone to Colds by Weakening Your Immune System", Jessica Firger On 8/31/15 at 5:16 PM.

13. Sleep. 2012 Aug 1; 35(8): 1173–1181. Published online 2012 Aug 1. doi: [10.5665/sleep.2012] PMCID: PMC3397790, PMID: 22851813, "Sleep Problems: An Emerging Global Epidemic? Findings From the INDEPTH WHO-SAGE Study Among More Than 40,000 Older Adults From Eight Countries Across Africa and Asia", Saverio Stranges, MD, PhD,1 William Tigbe, MD, PhD,1 Francesc Xavier Gómez-Olivé, MD,2,3 Margaret Thorogood, PhD,1,2,3 and Ngianga-Bakwin Kandala, PhD1 April 25, 2017, "Sleep Deprivation—A Global Epidemic", In just the past 50 years, the average sleep duration has decreased by almost two hours per day. Over the course of a lifespan, that's A LOT of sleep. During the same time period, the medical community has seen a leap in the prevalence of chronic diseases and conditions including obesity and diabetes. Could it be that sleep deprivation is a fueling factor of these epidemics?

14. Gilberg M, Akerstedt T. "Sleep restriction and SWS-suppression: effects on daytime alertness and night-time recovery", *Journal of Sleep Research* 1994;3: 144–151.

15. "Poor Sleep More Dangerous For Women", March 11, 2008, Duke University Medical Center, Researchers say they may have figured out why poor sleep does more harm to cardiovascular health in women than in men. Their study, in the journal, Brain, Behavior and Immunity, found that poor sleep is associated with greater psychological distress and higher levels of biomarkers associated with elevated risk of heart disease and type 2 diabetes. They also found that these associations are significantly stronger in women than in men. Duke University Medical Center. "Poor Sleep More Dangerous For Women", *ScienceDaily*, 11 March 2008. www.sciencedaily.com/releases/2008/03/080310131529.html.

16. 1545. Published online 2016 September. doi: [10.2105/AJPH.2016.303343] PMCID: PMC4981811, PMID: 27459441, "The Impact of the Nurses' Health Study on Population Health: Prevention, Translation, and Control" Graham A. Colditz, MD, DrPH, Sydney E. Philpott, BS, and Susan E. Hankinson, ScD.

17. CDC Prevalence of Healthy Sleep Duration among Adults—United States, 2014, February 19, 2016 / 65(6);137–141, Yong Liu, MD1; Anne G. Wheaton, PhD1; Daniel P. Chapman, PhD1; Timothy J. Cunningham, ScD1; Hua Lu, MS1; Janet B. Croft, PhD1 (View author affiliations).

18. Gilberg M, Akerstedt T. Sleep restriction and SWS-suppression: effects on daytime alertness and night-time recovery. *Journal of Sleep Research* 1994;3:144–151.

19. According to a research study earlier this year which got little attention on this side of the Atlantic, mobile phones send out radiation that hampers people's ability to sink into the deep stages of sleep. Scientists from Karolinska Institute and Uppsala University in Sweden, and from Wayne State University in Michigan, gathered 35 men and 36 women between the ages of 18 and 45 and exposed about half of them to 884-megaherz wireless signals identical to those emitted by cell phones. The other half got no radiation. The result: The people who had been subjected to the radiation took longer to enter the deep stage of sleep that refreshes and restores, and spent less time there, than the other group.

20. Subst Abus. Author manuscript; available in PMC 2009 Nov 10. Published in final edited form as: Subst Abus. 2005 Mar; 26(1):1–13. PMCID: PMC2775419, NIHSID: NIHMS150204, PMID: 16492658, "Disturbed Sleep and Its Relationship to Alcohol Use" Michael D. Stein, MD and Peter D. Friedmann, MD, MPH.

21. According to The Cleveland Clinic, two-thirds of patients referred to sleep disorders centers have a psychiatric disorder. "Anxiety is an emotion that actually wakes us up," Dr. Steve Orma, author of "Stop Worrying and Go to Sleep: How to Put Insomnia to Bed for Good", told *The Huffington Post*.

22. *Well-Being*, December 19, 2013 "In U.S., 40% Get Less Than Recommended Amount of Sleep Hours of sleep similar to recent decades, but much lower than in 1942" by Jeffrey M. Jones PRINCETON, NJ -- 59% of Americans get seven or more hours of sleep at night, while 40% get less than seven hours. Those figures are largely unchanged from Gallup polls in the 1990s and 2000s, but Americans, on average, slept much more in the 1940s. Americans currently average 6.8 hours of sleep at night, down more than an hour from 1942.

23. Epstein, L. J. & Mardon, S. (2007). The Harvard Medical School Guide to A Good Night's Sleep. New York: McGraw Hill "The 20-Minute Break" by Ernest Lawrence Rossi, Ph.D "Chronobiology by Bruno Dubuc" at TheBrain.McGill. ca Basic Rest-Activity Cycle at *Wikipedia*, Kleitman, Father of Sleep Research at The University of Chicago Chronicle The Pomodoro Technique by Cirillo Company at CirilloCompany. de.

24. Lumley M, Roehrs T, Zorick F, Lamphere J, Roth T. The alerting effects of naps in sleep-deprived subjects. Psychophysiology 1986;23(4):403–408.

Part 2.14, *Inflammation: Dousing the Flame*

1. Pai, J. K., et al., "Inflammatory Markers and the Risk of Coronary Heart Disease in Men and Women," New England Journal of Medicine 351 (December 16, 2004): 2599–2610.

2. Effect of physical inactivity on major non-communicable diseases worldwide The Lancet 380 219–229.

3. Fishing" for the origins of the "Eskimos and heart disease" story. Facts or wishful thinking? A review" George J. Fodor, MD, PhD, FRCPC, FAHA Eftyhia Helis, MSc Narges Yazdekhasti, MSc Branislav Vohnout, MD 10.1016/j.cjca.2014.04.007, Reference; CJCA 1183 *Canadian Journal of Cardiology*.

4. Sabatine MS, Morrow DA, Jablonski KA, et al. "Prognostic significance of the Centers for Disease Control/American Heart Association high-sensitivity C-reactive protein cut points for cardiovascular and other outcomes in patients with stable coronary artery disease", Circulation 2007; 115:1528. Zouridakis E, Avanzas P, Arroyo-Espliguero R, et al. "Markers of inflammation and rapid coronary artery disease progression in patients with stable angina pectoris", Circulation 2004; 110:1747. Liuzzo G, Buffon A, Biasucci LM, et al. "Enhanced inflammatory response to coronary angioplasty in patients with severe unstable angina", Circulation 1998; 98:2370. Berk BC, Weintraub WS, Alexander RW. Elevation of C-reactive protein in "active" coronary artery disease. Am J Cardiol 1990; 65:168. http://mayoclinic.org/tests-procedures/c-

reactive-protein/basics/definition/prc-20014480, nlm.nih.gov/medlineplus/ency/article/003356.htm, webmd.com/a-to-z-guides/c-reactive-protein-crp Ridker PM, Rifai N, Rose L, et al. "Comparison of C-reactive protein and low-density lipoprotein cholesterol levels in the prediction of first cardiovascular events", N Engl J Med 2002; 347:1557. Cushman M, Arnold AM, Psaty BM, et al. "C-reactive protein and the 10-year incidence of coronary heart disease in older men and women: the cardiovascular health study", Circulation 2005; 112:25. Rifai N, Buring JE, Lee IM, et al. Is C-reactive protein specific for vascular disease in women? Ann Intern Med 2002; 136:529.

5. *The Big Book,* "Processed foods make up 70% of the U.S. diet", BMJ Open. 2018; 8(3): e020574. Published online 2018 Mar 9. doi: [10.1136/bmjopen-2017-020574] PMCID: PMC5855172 PMID: 29525772 "Consumption of ultra-processed foods and associated sociodemographic factors in the USA between 2007 and 2012: evidence from a nationally representative cross-sectional study", Larissa Galastri Baraldi,1,2 Euridice Martinez Steele,1,2 Daniela Silva Canella, 2 ,3 and Carlos Augusto Monteiro 1, 2.

6. Int J Immunopathol Pharmacol.2009 Oct-Dec;22(4):951-9."Effect of phytoncide from trees on human natural killer cell function", Li Q1, Kobayashi M, Wakayama Y, Inagaki H, Katsumata M, Hirata Y, Hirata K, Shimizu T, Kawada T, Park BJ, Ohira T, Kagawa T, Miyazaki Y.

Part 2.15, *The Best You Can Be: Optimizing Your Life at Any Age*

1. *The Big Book,* "Processed foods make up 70% of the U.S. diet", BMJ Open. 2018; 8(3): e020574. Published online 2018 Mar 9. doi: [10.1136/bmjopen-2017-020574] PMCID: PMC5855172 PMID: 29525772 "Consumption of ultra-processed foods and associated sociodemographic factors in the USA between 2007 and 2012: evidence from a nationally representative cross-sectional study", Larissa Galastri Baraldi,1,2 Euridice Martinez Steele,1,2 Daniela Silva Canella,2,3 and Carlos Augusto Monteiro 1, 2.

2. PLoS One. 2014 Feb 5;9(2):e88103. doi: 10.1371/journal.pone.0088103. eCollection 2014. "Effect of marine-derived n-3 polyunsaturated fatty acids on C-reactive protein, interleukin 6 and tumor necrosis factor: a meta-analysis", Li K1, Huang T1, Zheng J1, Wu K1, Li D1. J Am Coll Nutr. 2009 Oct;28(5):525-42. EPA but not DHA appears to be responsible for the efficacy of omega-3 long chain polyunsaturated fatty acid supplementation in depression:

evidence from a meta-analysis of randomized controlled trials. Martins JG1.

3. Am J Clin Nutr. 2007 May;85(5): 1267 – 74. "Combining fish-oil supplements with regular aerobic exercise improves body composition and cardiovascular disease risk factors", *Nutrients,* 2010 Dec; 2(12): 1212–1230. Published online 2010 Dec 9. doi: [10.3390/nu2121212] PMCID: PMC3257626 PMID: 22254005
"Long-Chain Omega-3 Polyunsaturated Fatty Acids May Be Beneficial for Reducing Obesity—A Review", Jonathan D. Buckley1,2,* and Peter R. C. Howe1,2 Appl Physiol Nutr Metab. 2014 Sep;39(9):1083-91. doi: 10.1139/apnm-2014-0049. Epub 2014 Apr 23. "Variable effects of 12 weeks of omega-3 supplementation on resting skeletal muscle metabolism", Gerling CJ1, Whitfield J, Mukai K, Spriet LL.

4. Atherosclerosis.2007 Jul;193(1):159-67. Epub 2006 Aug 1."Age/ dose-dependent effects of an eicosapentaenoic acid-rich oil on cardiovascular risk factors in healthy male subjects", Cazzola R1, Russo-Volpe S, Miles EA, Rees D, Banerjee T, Roynette CE, Wells SJ, Goua M, Wahle KW, Calder PC, Cestaro B.

5. *Nutrition,* 2010 Feb;26(2):168-74. doi: 10.1016/j.nut.2009.04.002. Epub 2009 May 31. "Moderate consumption of fatty fish reduces diastolic blood pressure in overweight and obese European young adults during energy restriction", Ramel A1, Martinez JA, Kiely M, Bandarra NM, Thorsdottir I.

6. Int J Cardiol.2009 Jul 24;136(1):4-16. doi: 10.1016/j.ijcard.2008.03.092. Epub 2008 Sep 6. "Benefits of fish oil supplementation in hyperlipidemia: a systematic review and meta-analysis",
Eslick GD1, Howe PR, Smith C, Priest R, Bensoussan A.

7. Circulation.2002 Apr 23;105(16):1897 – 903. "Early protection against sudden death by n-3 polyunsaturated fatty acids after myocardial infarction: time-course analysis of the results of the Gruppo Italiano per lo Studio della".

8. Atherosclerosis.2012 Apr;221(2):536-43. doi: 10.1016/j.atherosclerosis.2012.01.006. Epub 2012 Jan 20. "Effect of omega-3 fatty acids supplementation on endothelial function: a meta-analysis of randomized controlled trials", Wang Q1, Liang X, Wang L, Lu X, Huang J, Cao J, Li H, Gu D.

9. J Nutr Biochem.2003 Sep;14(9):513-21. Dietary fish oil decreases C-reactive protein, interleukin-6, and triacylglycerol to HDL-cholesterol ratio in postmenopausal women on HRT.

10. Arch Intern Med.2012 May 14;172(9):686-94. doi: 10.1001/archinternmed.2012.262."Efficacy of omega-3 fatty acid supplements

(eicosapentaenoic acid and docosahexaenoic acid) in the secondary prevention of cardiovascular disease: a meta-analysis of randomized, double-blind, placebo-controlled trials", Kwak SM1, Myung SK, Lee YJ, Seo HG; Korean Meta-analysis Study Group.

11. Am J Clin Nutr.2006 Jun;83(6 Suppl):1505S-1519S.n-3 polyunsaturated fatty acids, inflammation, and inflammatory diseases. Calder PC1.

12. Brain Behav Immun.2011 Nov, 25(8):1725-34. doi: 10.1016/j.bbi.2011.07.229. Epub 2011 Jul 19. "Omega-3 supplementation lowers inflammation and anxiety in medical students: a randomized controlled trial", Kiecolt-Glaser JK1, Belury MA.

13. J Sleep Res.2014 Aug;23(4):364-88. doi: 10.1111/jsr.12135. Epub 2014 Mar 8. "Fatty acids and sleep in UK children: subjective and pilot objective sleep results from the DOLAB study—a randomized controlled trial",Montgomery P1, Burton JR, Sewell RP, Spreckelsen TF, Richardson AJ.

14. Food Nutr Res. 2012; 56: 10.3402/fnr. v56i0.17252. Published online 2012 Jul 20. doi: 10.3402/fnr.v56i0.17252, "Dietary factors and fluctuating levels of melatonin", Katri Peuhkuri,*Nora Sihvola, and Riitta Korpela.

15. J Sleep Res.2014 Aug;23(4):364-88. doi: 10.1111/jsr.12135. Epub 2014 Mar 8. "Fatty acids and sleep in UK children: subjective and pilot objective sleep results from the DOLAB study--a randomized controlled trial", Montgomery P1, Burton JR.

16. Oxid Med Cell Longev. 2014; 2014: 313570. Published online 2014 Mar 18. doi: 10.1155/2014/313570Omega-3, "Fatty Acids and Depression: Scientific Evidence and Biological Mechanisms", Giuseppe Grosso,1 ,*Fabio Galvano,1 Stefano Marventano,2 Michele Malaguarnera,1 Claudio Bucolo,1 Filippo Drago,1 and Filippo Caraci3, 4.

17. Psychiatry ResearchVolume 229, Issues 1–2, 30 September 2015, Pages 485–489 "Short-term supplementation of acute long-chain omega-3 polyunsaturated fatty acids may alter depression status and decrease symptomology among young adults with depression: A preliminary randomized and placebo controlled trial".

18. Eur Neuropsychopharmacol.2013 Jul;23(7):636-44. doi: 10.1016/j. euroneuro.2012.08.003. Epub 2012 Aug 19. "Eicosapentaenoic acid versus docosahexaenoic acid in mild-to-moderate depression: a randomized, double-blind, placebo-controlled trial".

19. *Australian and New Zealand Journal of Psychiatry* Volume 42, 2008 – Issue 3, "Comparison of therapeutic effects of omega-3 fatty acid eicosapentaenoic acid and fluoxetine, separately and in combination, in major depressive

disorder".

20. Mark Hyman MD is the Director of Cleveland Clinic's Center for Functional Medicine, the Founder of The UltraWellness Center, and a ten-time #1 New York Times Bestselling author.

21. Am J Epidemiol.2007 Jul 15;166(2):181-95. Epub 2007 May 9. "Dietary fatty acids and colorectal cancer: a case-control study", Theodoratou E1, McNeill G, Cetnarskyj R, Farrington SM, Tenesa A, Barnetson R, Porteous M, Dunlop M, Campbell H.

22. J Nutr.2004 Dec;134(12 Suppl):3412S-3420S. "Long-chain (n-3) fatty acid intake and risk of cancers of the breast and the prostate: recent epidemiological studies, biological mechanisms, and directions for future research", Epidemiology Branch, National Institute of Environmental Health Sciences, Research Triangle Park, NC 27709, USA. terry2@niehs.nih.gov.

23. Pediatrics.2003 Jan;111(1):e39-44. "Maternal supplementation with very-long-chain n-3 fatty acids during pregnancy and lactation augments children's IQ at four years of age", Helland IB1, Smith L, Saarem K, Saugstad OD, Drevon CA.

24. Ophthalmol Vis Sci.2014 Mar 28;55(3):2010-9. doi: 10.1167/iovs.14-13916. "Circulating omega-3 Fatty acids and neovascular age-related macular degeneration", Merle BM1, Benlian P, Puche N, Bassols A, Delcourt C, Souied EH; Nutritional AMD Treatment 2 Study Group.

25. J Am Acad Child Adolesc Psychiatry.2011 Oct;50(10):991-1000. doi: 10.1016/j.jaac.2011.06.008. Epub 2011 Aug 12. "Omega-3 fatty acid supplementation for the treatment of children with attention-deficit/hyperactivity disorder symptomatology: systematic review and meta-analysis". Bloch MH1, Qawasmi A.

26. PLoS One. 2013; 8(11); e80048. Published online 2013 Nov 12. doi: 10.1371/journal.pone.0080048 "Fish and Fish Oil Intake in Relation to Risk of Asthma: A Systematic Review and Meta-Analysis", Huan Yang,1 , 2, 3, 4 Pengcheng Xun,2 , 3 , 4 and Ka He 2, 3, 4 , Lynette Kay Rogers, Editor.

27. Acta Cardiol.2009 Jun;64(3):321–7. "Omega-3 fatty acid supplements improve the cardiovascular risk profile of subjects with metabolic syndrome, including markers of inflammation and auto-immunity".Ebrahimi M1, Ghayour-Mobarhan M, Rezaiean S, Hoseini M, Parizade SM, Farhoudi F, Hosseininezhad SJ, Tavallaei S, Vejdani A, Azimi-Nezhad M, Shakeri MT, Rad MA, Mobarra N, Kazemi-Bajestani SM, Ferns GA.

28. Oxid Med Cell Longev. 2014; 2014: 313570. Published online 2014 Mar 18. doi: 10.1155/2014/313570. "Omega-3 Fatty Acids and Depression: Scientific Evidence and Biological Mechanisms". Giuseppe

Grosso,1 ,*Fabio Galvano,1 Stefano Marventano,2 Michele Malaguarnera,1 Claudio Bucolo,1 Filippo Drago,1 and Filippo Caraci 3, 4. Am J Prev Med.2014 Oct;47(4):444-51. doi: 10.1016/j.amepre.2014.05.037. Epub 2014 Jul 29. "Regular fish consumption and age-related brain gray matter loss". Raji CA1, Erickson KI2, Lopez OL3, Kuller LH4, Gach HM2, Thompson PM5, Riverol M6, Becker JT7.

29. Prog Lipid Res.1997 Sep;36(2-3):131-51.

30. Prog Lipid Res.1997 Sep;36(2-3):131-51. "Calcium metabolism, osteoporosis and essential fatty acids: a review". Kruger MC1, Horrobin DF. J Natl Med Assoc.J Natl Med Assoc.1959 Jul;51(4):266–70 passim. J Natl Med Assoc.1959 Jul;51(4):266-70 passim. "A new dietary regimen for arthritis: value of cod liver oil on a fasting stomach". Brusch CA, Johnson ET. 1959 Jul;51(4):266–70 passim.

31. Caspian J Intern Med. 2011 Summer; 2(3): 279–282. Comparison of the effect of fish oil and ibuprofen on treatment of severe pain in primary dysmenorrhea" Mandana Zafari, MSc,1Fereshteh Behmanesh, MSc,*,2and Azar Agha Mohammadi, MSc1.

32. Int J Dermatol.2009 Apr;48(4):339-47. doi: 10.1111/j.1365-4632.2009.04002.x. "Diet and acne: a review of the evidence". Spencer EH1, Ferdowsian HR, Barnard ND.

33. Anderson JW, et al. "Health benefits of dietary fiber". *Nutrition Reviews.* 2009;67:188.

34. "Dietary, functional and total fiber". Institute of Medicine. http://www.nap.edu/openbook.php?record_id=10490&page=339. Accessed Aug. 30, 2015.

35. Colditz GA. Healthy diet in adults. http://www.uptodate.com/home. Accessed Aug. 30, 2015.

36. "Position of the American Dietetic Association: Health implications of dietary fiber". *Journal of the American Dietetic Association.* 2008;108:1716.

37. "Whole grains and fiber". American Heart Association. http://www.heart.org/HEARTORG/GettingHealthy/NutritionCenter/HealthyDietGoals/Whole-Grains-and-Fiber_UCM_303249_Article.jsp. Accessed Aug. 30. 2015.

38. Duyff RL. Carbs: Sugar, starches, fiber. In: American Dietetic Association Complete Food and Nutrition Guide. 4th ed. Hoboken, N.J.: John Wiley & Sons; 2012.

39. Zeratsky KA (expert opinion). Mayo Clinic, Rochester, Minn. Sept. 10, 2015.

40. Arch Latinoam Nutr. 2007 Mar;57(1):94–8. "Characterization of the acai or manaca (Euterpe oleracea Mart.): a fruit of the Amazon". Neida S1, Elba S.

41. "USDA Database for the Oxygen Radical, Absorbance Capacity (ORAC) of Selected

Foods, Release 2", David B. Haytowitz and Seema Bhagwat, Nutrient Data Laboratory Beltsville Human Nutrition Research Center (BHNRC), Agricultural Research Service (ARS), U.S. Department of Agriculture (USDA), May 2010 "Potent Antioxidant and Anti-Inflammatory Flavonoids in the Nutrient-Rich Amazonian Palm Fruit, Açaí (Euterpe spp.)". Int J Food Sci Nutr. 2005 Feb;56(1):53–64. Total oxidant scavenging capacities of Euterpe oleracea Mart. (Açaí) fruits. Lichtenthäler R1, Rodrigues RB, Maia JG, Papagiannopoulos M, Fabricius H, Marx F. J Agric Food Chem. 2008 Sep 10;56(17):7796-802. doi: 10.1021/jf8007037. Epub 2008 Aug 12.

42. J Agric Food Chem. 2008 Sep 10;56(17):7796-802. doi: 10.1021/jf8007037. Epub 2008 Aug 12. "Pharmacokinetics of anthocyanins and antioxidant effects after the consumption of anthocyanin-rich acai juice and pulp (Euterpe oleracea Mart.) in human healthy volunteers." Mertens-Talcott SU1, Rios J, Jilma-Stohlawetz P, Pacheco-Palencia LA, Meibohm B, Talcott ST, Derendorf H. Nutritio,. 2010 Jul-Aug;26(7-8):804-10. doi: 10.1016/j.nut.2009.09.007. Epub 2009 Dec 22. "Diet supplementation with acai (Euterpe oleracea Mart.) pulp improves biomarkers of oxidative stress and the serum lipid profile in rats". de Souza MO1, Silva M, Silva ME, Oliveira Rde P, Pedrosa ML.

43. "Ultra-processed foods and cancer" BMJ 2018; 360 doi: https://doi.org/10.1136/bmj.k599 (Published 14 February 2018) Cite this as: BMJ 2018;360:k599. "Prevention of Chronic Disease by Means of Diet and Lifestyle Changes". Walter C. Willett, Jeffrey P. Koplan, Rachel Nugent, Courtenay Dusenbury, Pekka Puska, and Thomas A. Gaziano,

44. Acta Cir Bras. 2015 May;30(5):366–70. doi: 10.1590/S0102-865020150050000009. "Fructo-oligosaccharide effects on serum cholesterol levels. An overview". Costa GT1, Abreu GC2, Guimarães AB2, Vasconcelos PR3, Guimarães SB4.

45. Gut. 2006 Oct; 55(10): 1512–1520. doi: [10.1136/gut.2005.085373] PMCID: PMC1856434, PMID: 16966705, "Alterations in intestinal permeability" J Exp Med. 2006 Mar 20;203(3):541-52. Epub 2006 Feb 27. "The primary defect in experimental ileitis originates from a nonhematopoietic source". Olson TS1, Reuter BK, Scott KG, Morris MA, Wang XM, Hancock LN, Burcin TL, Cohn SM, Ernst PB, Cominelli F, Meddings JB, Ley K, Pizarro TT.

46. Exp Gerontol. 2013 Oct;48(10):1018-24. doi: 10.1016/j.exger.2013.04.005. Epub 2013 Apr 25. "Resveratrol vs. calorie restriction: data from rodents to humans". Lam YY1,

Peterson CM, Ravussin E. *Nature*. 2003 Sep 11;425(6954):191-6. Epub 2003 Aug 24. "Small molecule activators of sirtuins extend Saccharomyces cerevisiae lifespan". Howitz KT1, Bitterman KJ, Cohen HY, Lamming DW, Lavu S, Wood JG, Zipkin RE, Chung P, Kisielewski A, Zhang LL, Scherer B, Sinclair DA. *Science*. Author manuscript; available in PMC 2013 Oct 19. Published in final edited form as: Science. 2013 Mar 8; 339(6124): 1216–1219. doi: [10.1126/science.1231097] PMCID: PMC3799917, NIHMSID: NIHMS504463, PMID: 23471411, "Evidence for a Common Mechanism of SIRT1 Regulation by Allosteric Activators". Basil P. Hubbard,1 Ana P. Gomes,1,2 Han Dai,3 Jun Li,1 April W. Case,3 Thomas Considine,3 Thomas V. Riera,3 Jessica E. Lee,4 E Sook Yen,4 Dudley W. Lamming,1,* Bradley L. Pentelute,5 Eli R. Schuman,3 Linda A. Stevens,6 Alvin J. Y. Ling,1 Sean M. Armour,1 Shaday Michan,1,† Huizhen Zhao,7 Yong Jiang,7 Sharon M. Sweitzer,7 Charles A. Blum,3 Jeremy S. Disch,3 Pui Yee Ng,3 Konrad T. Howitz,8,‡ Anabela P. Rolo,2,9 Yoshitomo Hamuro,4 Joel Moss,6 Robert B. Perni,3 James L. Ellis,3 George P. Vlasuk,3 and David A. Sinclair,10,§ *Nature*. 2004 Aug 5;430(7000):686-9. Epub 2004 Jul 14. "Sirtuin activators mimic caloric restriction and delay ageing in metazoans." Wood JG1, Rogina B, Lavu S, Howitz K, Helfand SL, Tatar M, Sinclair D.

47. Articles| Volume 392, ISSUE 10145, P387-399, August 04, 2018. "Effects of aspirin on risks of vascular events and cancer according to bodyweight and dose: analysis of individual patient data from randomised trials". Prof Peter M Rothwell, FMedSci, Prof Nancy R Cook, ScD, Prof J Michael Gaziano, MD, Prof Jacqueline F Price, PhD. Prof Jill F F Belch, MD, Maria Carla Roncaglioni, PhD, et al. "Effect of Aspirin on Disability-free Survival in the Healthy Elderly" Richard Grimm, M.D., Ph.D., M.P.H. and Anne M. Murray, M.D. NEJM September 23, 2018.

Part 3.1, The Principles of Longevity: The Secret of Life Extension

1. Appl Transl Genom. 2015 Mar; 4: 23–32. Published online 2015 Feb 4. doi: [10.1016/j.atg.2015.01.001] PMCID: PMC4745363 PMID: 26937346. "Genetics, lifestyle and longevity: Lessons from centenarians" Diddahally Govindaraju,a,b, Gil Atzmon,b,c and Nir Barzilaib.

2. "A healthy lifestyle increases life expectancy by up to seven years". July 20, 2017, Max-Planck-Gesellschaft. Summary: Maintaining a normal weight, not smoking, and drinking alcohol at moderate levels are factors that add

healthy years to life.

3. https://www.ssa.gov/cgi-bin/longevity.cgi.

4. "Hidden secret of immortality enzyme telomerase. Can we stay young forever, or even recapture lost youth?". February 27, 2018, Source: Arizona State University.

5. Lane M, Black A and Ingram D. Calorie restriction in nonhuman primates: implications for age-related disease risk. *Journal of Anti-Aging*, 1998.

6. Morley JE, Chahla E and Alkaade S. "Antiaging, longevity and calorie restriction. Current Opinion in Clinical Nutrition and Metabolic Care". 2010;13(1): 40–45.

7. McCay CM, Crowell MF and Maynard LA. "The effect of retarded growth upon the length of life span and upon the ultimate body size." *Nutrition*. 1935;10(1): 63–79.

8. Lane MA, Ingram DK. and Roth, GS. "2-Deoxy-D-glucose feeding in rats mimics physiologic effects of calorie restriction". *Journal of Anti-Aging Medicine*, 1998;1(4): 327–337.

9. Spindler SR. "Caloric restriction: from soup to nuts". Ageing Res Rev. 2010;9(3): 324–353.

10. Masoro EJ. Dietary restriction-induced life extension: a broadly based biological phenomenon. Biogerontology. 2006;7(3):153-155.

11. Bodkin NL, Alexander TM, Ortmeyer HK, Johnson E and Hansen BC. Mortality and morbidity in laboratory-maintained Rhesus monkeys and effects of long-term dietary restriction. J Gerontol A Biol Sci Med Sci. 2003;58(3):212-219.

12. Yankner BA, Lu T and Loerch P. The aging brain. Annu Rev Pathol. 2008;3: 41–66.

13. Colman RJ, Anderson RM, Johnson SC, et al. "Caloric Restriction Delays Disease Onset and Mortality in Rhesus Monkeys". *Science*. 2009;325(5937): 201–204.

14. Colman RJ, Anderson RM, Johnson SC, et al. "Caloric Restriction Delays Disease Onset and Mortality in Rhesus Monkeys". *Science*. 2009;325(5937): 201–204.

15. Rodriguez NA, Garcia KD, Fortman JD, Hewett TA, Bunte RM and Bennett BT. "Clinical and histopathological evaluation of 13. cases of adenocarcinoma in aged rhesus macaques (Macaca mulatta)". J Med Primatol. 2002;31(2):7 4–83.

16. Bodkin NL, Alexander TM, Ortmeyer HK, Johnson E and Hansen BC. "Mortality and morbidity in laboratory-maintained Rhesus monkeys and effects of long-term dietary restriction". J Gerontol A Biol Sci Med Sci. 2003;58(3):212–219.

17. Bodkin NL, Ortmeyer HK and Hansen BC. A comment on the comment: relevance of nonhuman primate dietary restriction to aging in humans. J Gerontol A Biol Sci Med Sci. 2005;60(8): 951–952.

18. Oeppen, Vaupel. "Demography.

Broken limits to life expectancy." Science.2002;296(5570):1029-1031.

19. Lane M, Black A and Ingram D. Calorie restriction in nonhuman primates: implications for age-related disease risk. *Journal of Anti-Aging*, 1998.

20. Kalimi M, Regelson W, eds. "Dehydroepiandrosterone (DHEA): Biochemical, Physiological and Clinical Aspects". New York , NY : Walter de Gruyter; 1999.

21. Lane MA, Ingram DK, Ball SS and Roth GS. "Dehydroepiandrosterone sulfate: a biomarker of primate aging slowed by calorie restriction". J Clin Endocrinol Metab. 1997;82(7): 2093–2096.

22. N. W. Shock et al., Eds., "Normal Human Aging: The Baltimore Longitudinal Study on Aging" (U.S. Government Printing Office, Washington, DC, 1984).

23. Roth GS, Lane MA, Ingram DK, et al. Biomarkers of caloric restriction may predict longevity in humans. *Science*. 2002;297(5582):811.

24. Kagawa Y. Impact of Westernization on the nutrition of Japanese: changes in physique, cancer, longevity and centenarians. Prev Med. 1978;7(2): 205–217.

25. Vallejo EA. Hunger diet on alternate days in the nutrition of the aged. Prensa Med Argent. 1957; 44(2): 119–120.

26. Walford RL, Mock D, Verdery R and MacCallum T. "Calorie restriction in biosphere two alterations in physiologic, hematologic, hormonal, and biochemical parameters in humans restricted for a two-year period". J Gerontol A Biol Sci Med Sci. 2002;57(6):B211–224.

27. Fontana L, Meyer TE, Klein S and Holloszy JO. Long-term calorie restriction is highly effective in reducing the risk for atherosclerosis in humans. Proc Natl Acad Sci USA. 2004;101(17): 6659–6663.

28. Fontana L, Klein S, Holloszy JO and Premachandra BN. "Effect of long-term calorie restriction with adequate protein and micronutrients on thyroid hormones". J Clin Endocrinol Metab. 2006;91(8):3232-3235.

29. Meyer TE, Kovács SJ, Ehsani AA, Klein S, Holloszy JO and Fontana L. "Long-term caloric restriction ameliorates the decline in diastolic function in humans". J Am Coll Cardiol. 2006;47(2):398-402.

30. Sci Transl Med. 2017 Feb 15;9(377). pii: eaai8700. doi: 10.1126/scitranslmed.aai8700. "Fasting-mimicking diet and markers/risk factors for aging, diabetes, cancer, and cardiovascular disease." Wei M1, Brandhorst S1, Shelehchi M1, Mirzaei H1, Cheng CW1, Budniak J1, Groshen S2, Mack WJ2, Guen E1, Di Biase S1, Cohen P1, Morgan TE1, Dorff T3, Hong K4, Michalsen A5, Laviano A6, Longo VD7,8.

31. Nat Commun. 2017 Jan 17;8:14063. doi:

10.1038/ncomms14063. Healthcare provider. "Caloric restriction improves health and survival of rhesus monkeys". Mattison JA1, Colman RJ2, Beasley TM3,4, Allison DB3, Kemnitz JW2,5, Roth GS6, Ingram DK7, Weindruch R8,9, de Cabo R1, Anderson RM8,9.

32. Sci Transl Med. 2017 Feb 15;9(377). pii: eaai8700. doi: 10.1126/scitranslmed.aai8700. Fasting-mimicking diet and markers/risk factors for aging, diabetes, cancer, and cardiovascular disease.
Wei M1, Brandhorst S1, Shelehchi M1, Mirzaei H1, Cheng CW1, Budniak J1, Groshen S2, Mack WJ2, Guen E1, Di Biase S1, Cohen P1, Morgan TE1, Dorff T3, Hong K4, Michalsen A5, Laviano A6, Longo VD 7, 8.

33. Evert, J., et al., "Morbidity Profiles of Centenarians: Survivors, Delayers, and escapers," *The Journals of Gerontology Series A: Biological Sciences and Medical Sciences* 58 (2003): M232–M237.

34. *Time Magazine,* By Jamie Ducharme, February 15, 2018, Loma Linda, Calif., U.S.A. The U.S.'s only Blue Zone is a haven for the Seventh-day Adventist Church, a Protestant denomination. A shared set of principles, emphasis on community and adherence to the Sabbath—a day of rest, reflection, and recharging— help Loma Linda Adventists live 10 years longer than their fellow Americans. Many avoid meat and eat plenty of plants, whole grains, and nuts.

Part 3.2, The Habits of Longevity: Living Longer in Ultrahealth

1. Nat Commun. 2017 Jan 17;8:14063. doi: 10.1038/ncomms14063. "Caloric restriction improves health and survival of rhesus monkeys". Mattison JA1, Colman RJ2, Beasley TM3,4, Allison DB3, Kemnitz JW2,5, Roth GS6, Ingram DK7, Weindruch R8,9, de Cabo R1, Anderson RM8,9.

2. Centers for Disease Control and Prevention. Overweight and obesity. https://www.cdc.gov/obesity/index.html . Accessed July 25, 2017.

3. CNN: U.S. life expectancy drops for second year in a row, By Ben Tinker, CNN, NCHS Data Brief No. 293, December 2017, U.S. Department Of Health and Human Services, Centers for Disease Control and Prevention, National Center for Health Statistics, Mortality in the United States, 2016, Kenneth D. Kochanek, M.A., Sherry L. Murphy, B.S., Jiaquan Xu, M.D., and Elizabeth Arias, Ph.D. Key findings: Data from the National Vital Statistics System, Life expectancy for the U.S. population in 2016 was 78.6 years, a decrease of 0.1 year from 2015.

4. CNN: U.S. life expectancy drops for second year in a row, By Ben Tinker, CNN, NCHS Data Brief No. 293, December 2017, U.S. Department Of Health and Human Services, Centers for Disease Control and Prevention, National Center for Health Statistics, Mortality in the United States, 2016, Kenneth D. Kochanek, M.A., Sherry L. Murphy, B.S., Jiaquan Xu, M.D., and Elizabeth Arias, Ph.D. Key findings: Data from the National Vital Statistics System, Life expectancy for the U.S. population in 2016 was 78.6 years, a decrease of 0.1 year from 2015.

5. Am J Public Health. 2012 March; 102(3): 411–418. Published online 2012 March. doi: [10.2105/AJPH.2011.300362] PMCID: PMC3487659 PMID: 22390504."Burden of Oral Disease Among Older Adults and Implications for Public Health Priorities". Susan O. Griffin, PhD, Judith A. Jones, DDS, MPH, DScD, Diane Brunson, RDH, MPH, Paul M. Griffin, PhD, and William D. Bailey, DDS, MPH.

6. https://www.hsph.harvard.edu/healthy weight, Front Endocrinol (Lausanne). 2014; 5: 121. Published online 2014 Jul 30. Prepublished online 2014 Jun 3. doi: [10.3389/fendo.2014.00121] PMCID: PMC 4115619. PMID: 25126085. "How Much Should We Weigh for a Long and Healthy Life Span? The Need to Reconcile Caloric Restriction versus Longevity with Body Mass Index versus Mortality Data".

7. "A healthy lifestyle increases life expectancy by up to seven years".July 20, 2017, Source: Max-Planck-Gesellschaft. Summary: Maintaining a normal weight, not smoking, and drinking alcohol at moderate levels are factors that add healthy years to life.

8. Nat Commun. 2017 Jan 17;8:14063. doi: 10.1038/ncomms14063. "Caloric restriction improves health and survival of rhesus monkeys." Mattison JA1, Colman RJ2, Beasley TM3,4, Allison DB3, Kemnitz JW2,5, Roth GS6, Ingram DK7, Weindruch R8,9, de Cabo R1, Anderson RM8,9.

Part 3.4, Brain and Mind Longevity: Protecting and Enhancing Your Future

1. ISRN Neurol. 2011; 2011: 953818. Published online 2011 Oct 1. doi: [10.5402/2011/953818] PMCID: PMC3263535 PMID: 22389836 "Physical Activity in the Prevention and Treatment of Stroke". Siobhan Gallanagh, 1 Terry J. Quinn, 2 Jen Alexander, 3 and Matthew R. Walters 2.

2. Wilson, R.S., et al., "Participation in Cognitively Stimulating Activities and Risk of Incident Alzheimer's Disease," *Journal of the American Medical Association* 287 (2002): 742–748.

3. March 14, 2018, Article Open Access, "Midlife cardiovascular fitness and dementia, A 44-year longitudinal population study in women".Helena Hörder, Lena Johansson, XinXin Guo, Gunnar Grimby, Silke Kern, Svante Östling, Ingmar Skoog. *Neurology.* 2012 Apr 24;78(17):1323-9. doi: 10.1212/ NL.0b013e3182535d35. Epub 2012 Apr 18.

5 "Total daily physical activity and the risk of AD and cognitive decline in older adults." Buchman AS1, Boyle PA, Yu L, Shah RC, Wilson RS, Bennett DA.

4. Sci Rep. 2016; 6: 33212. Published online 2016 Sep 15. doi: [10.1038/srep33212] PMCID: PMC5024122 PMID: 27628682. "The Impact of Cognitive Training on Cerebral White Matter in Community-Dwelling Elderly: One-Year Prospective Longitudinal Diffusion Tensor Imaging Study" Transl Neurosci. 2015; 6(1): 13 –19. Published online 2014 Nov 14. doi: [10.1515/ tnsci-2015-0003] PMCID: PMC4936611 PMID: 28123787, "Online cognitive training in healthy older adults: a preliminary study on the effects of single versus multi-domain training", Courtney C Walton,1,2 Alexandra Kavanagh,1,3 Luke A. Downey,1,4 Justine Lomas,1 David A Camfield,1,5 and Con Stough1, "Review: Healthy minds 0–100 years: Optimising the use of European brain imaging cohorts ("Lifebrain")". Kristine B. Walhovd, Anders M. Fjell, René Westerhausen, Lars Nyberg, Klaus P. Ebmeier, Ulman Lindenberger, David Bartrés-Faz, William F.C. Baaré, Hartwig R. Siebner, Richard Henson, Christian A. Drevon, Gun Peggy Strømstad Knudsen, Isabelle Budin Ljøsne, Brenda W.J.H. Penninx, Paolo Ghisletta, Ole Rogeberg, Lorraine Tyler, Lars Bertram, Lifebrain Consortium.

5. Int J MS Care. 2016 Jan-Feb;18(1):1-8. doi: 10.7224/1537-2073.2014-104. "Effects of Single Bouts of Walking Exercise and Yoga on Acute Mood Symptoms in People with Multiple Sclerosis." Ensari I1, Sandroff BM1, Motl RW1.

6. "Alzheimer's disease: Can exercise prevent memory loss and improve cognitive function?" Jonathan Graff-Radford, M.D.

7. J Physiol. 2016 Aug 15;594(16):4485-98. doi: 10.1113/JP271270. Epub 2016 Jan 6. "Promoting brain health through exercise and diet in older adults: a physiological perspective". Jackson PA1, Pialoux V2, Corbett D3,4, Drogos L5,6, Erickson KI7, Eskes GA5,8, Poulin MJ5,6,9,10,11.

8. Clin Interv Aging. 2014;9:51-62. doi: 10.2147/ CIA.S39506. Epub 2013 Dec 18. "Physical exercise and cognitive performance in the elderly: current perspectives". Kirk-Sanchez NJ1, McGough EL2.

9. Ann N Y Acad Sci. 2015 Mar;1337:1-6. doi: 10.1111/nyas.12682. "Cognitive plasticity in

older adults: effects of cognitive training and physical exercise". Bherer L1.

10. Ann N Y Acad Sci. 2015 Mar;1337:1-6. doi: 10.1111/nyas.12682. "Cognitive plasticity in older adults: effects of cognitive training and physical exercise". Bherer L1.

11. "Brain MRI fiber-tracking reveals white matter alterations in hypertensive patients without damage at conventional neuroimaging". Lorenzo Carnevale Valentina D'Angelosante Alessandro Landolfi Giovanni Grillea Giulio Selvetella Marianna Storto Giuseppe Lembo Daniela Carnevale Cardiovascular Research, Volume 114, Issue 11, 1 September 2018, Pages 1536–1546, https://doi.org/10.1093/cvr/cvy104.

12. J Epidemiol Community Health. 2010 Dec;64(12):1029-35. doi: 10.1136/jech.2008.081034. Epub 2009 Oct 23. "The importance of community education for individual mortality: a fixed-effects analysis of longitudinal multilevel data on 1.7 million Norwegian women and men." PLoS One. 2018; 13(1): e0190033. Published online 2018 Jan 4. doi: [10.1371/journal.pone.0190033] PMCID: PMC5754055 PMID: "Association of loneliness with all-cause mortality: A meta-analysis Laura Alejandra Rico-Uribe, Conceptualization, Data curation, Formal analysis, Investigation, Methodology, Writing—original draft". Writing—review & editing, 1,2,3 Francisco Félix Caballero, Data curation, Formal analysis, Methodology, Validation, Writing—review & editing, 1, 2, 3 Natalia Martín-María, Data curation, Investigation, Methodology, Writing—review & editing, 1, 2, 3 María Cabello, Data curation, Investigation, Writing—review & editing, 1, 2, 3 José Luis Ayuso-Mateos, Conceptualization, Funding acquisition, Project administration, Supervision, Writing—review & editing, 1, 2, 3 and Marta Miret, Conceptualization, Project administration, Supervision, Validation, Writing—review & editing 1, 2, 3,*

Part 3.5, Reaching a State of Ultrahealth™: Living the Future of Wellbeing

1. N Engl J Med. 2010 Dec 2; 363(23): 2211–2219. doi: [10.1056/NEJMoa1000367] PMCID: PMC3066051 NIHMSID: NIHMS278498 PMID: 21121834, Lancet. 2016 Aug 20; 388(10046): 776– 786. doi: [10.1016/S0140-6736(16)30175-1] PMCID: PMC4995441 PMID: 27423262 "BMI and Mortality: Results From a National Longitudinal Study of Canadian Adults". Heather M. Orpana, Jean Marie Berthelot, Mark S. Kaplan, David H. Feeny, Bentson McFarland, Nancy A. Ross.

2. "BMI and all cause mortality: systematic review and non-linear dose-response meta-analysis of 230 cohort studies with 3.74 million deaths among 30.3 million participants", BMJ 2016; 353 doi: https://

doi.org/10.1136/bmj.i2156 (Published 04 May 2016) Cite this as: BMJ 2016;353:i2156 N Engl J Med. Author manuscript; available in PMC 2011 Jun 2. Published in final edited form as: N Engl J Med. 2010 Dec 2; 363(23): 2211–2219. doi: [10.1056/NEJMoa1000367] PMCID: PMC3066051 NIHMSID: NIHMS278498 PMID: 21121834 Lancet. 2016 Aug 20; 388(10046): 776–786. doi: [10.1016/S0140-6736(16)30175-1] PMCID: PMC4995441 PMID: 27423262 "Body-mass index and all-cause mortality: individual-participant-data meta-analysis of 239 prospective studies in four continents". The Global BMI Mortality Collaboration. "Body-Mass Index and Mortality among 1.46 Million White Adults". Amy Berrington de Gonzalez, D.Phil., Patricia Hartge, Sc.D., James R. Cerhan, Ph.D., Alan J. Flint, Dr.P.H., Lindsay Hannan, M.S.P.H., Robert J. MacInnis, Ph.D., Steven C. Moore, Ph.D., Geoffrey S. Tobias, B.S., Hoda Anton-Culver, Ph.D., Laura Beane Freeman, Ph.D., W. Lawrence Beeson, Dr.P.H., Sandra L. Clipp, M.P.H., Dallas R. English, Ph.D., Aaron R. Folsom, M.D., D. Michal Freedman, Ph.D., Graham Giles, Ph.D., Niclas Hakansson, Ph.D., Katherine D. Henderson, Ph.D., Judith Hoffman-Bolton, Jane A. Hoppin, Sc.D., Karen L. Koenig, Ph.D., I-Min Lee, Sc.D., Martha S. Linet, M.D., Yikyung Park, Sc.D., Gaia Pocobelli, M.S., Arthur Schatzkin, M.D., Howard D. Sesso, Sc.D., Elisabete Weiderpass, Ph.D., Bradley J. Willcox, M.D., Alicja Wolk, Dr.Med.Sci., Anne Zeleniuch-Jacquotte, M.D., Walter C. Willett, M.D., Dr.P.H., and Michael J. Thun, M.D.

3. "BMI and Mortality: Results From a National Longitudinal Study of Canadian Adults". Heather M. Orpana, Jean Marie Berthelot, Mark S. Kaplan, David H. Feeny, Bentson McFarland, Nancy A. Ross.

4. http://edition.cnn.com/2007/LIVING/personal/06/29/in.your.head/When Treitler listened to subjects' stories, something stood out. They'd all gone through an inner transformation, almost like those celebrated in traditional rites of passage. Each had found a coach, mentor or guide for the journey; had pulled back and separated somewhat from his or her old environment and was then "reborn" into a different way of life. The newly thin person became a leader rather than a follower, which was a change that opened the door to further goals and achievements, often in fields completely unrelated to weight loss.

5. David S. Martin, "The Future of Longevity," interview with Ray Kurzweil, CNN, May 9, 2007, http://www.cnn.com/2007/HEALTH/03/23/chasinglife.fountainyouth/index.html.

INDEX

ACKNOWLEDGEMENTS

This book and the evolution of the Habits of Health over the last decade into a transformational system would not have been possible without many individual contributions.

First, I want to thank all of you who have taken this journey of transformation yourselves and have served as my teachers.

Your stories, your experiences, your passion, and your ideas have helped blaze this path to optimal health and wellbeing. Those stories are woven in throughout this new edition as validation that reaching and sustaining optimal health and wellbeing is not only possible but probable if you follow the principles outlined in these pages. We have spent almost two decades understanding and developing this system, and many of those featured in the first edition over 10 years ago are once again featured here. These individuals validate everything that the Habits of Health stands for by living life-long transformations. I would be remiss if I did not call them out by name as they have not only been great disciples but have gone beyond and developed into powerful leaders in advancing this mission forward. In order of their appearance in this version: Rita Tarinelli, Dr. Mark Nelson, Dominic Tarinelli, Greg Rex, and Lisa Castro.

Beyond those featured in the first version, we have many other amazing stories of transformations from many of our top leaders, who are also dedicated to this mission of changing the world. They are featured either relating their stories or by providing the action photos featured throughout the book and website. They are Dan and Mary Bell, Terri and David Miller, Bekah and Kevin Tinter (and family), Doug and Thea Wood, Brad and Ashley Miller (and family), Whitney Kell, Amber and Jared Smithson, Dr. JC Doornick, Jaime Castro, Patti and Mike Glick, Gina and Adam Echols, Michelle and Brad Heyman, Shirley and Cliff Mast, Suzy Heyman, Megan and Dan Valentine, Nancy Strauss, Sam and Harold Prestenbach, and Marcus Caillet. And we have some of those that are just in the beginning of their journey: Jean and John Jeffreys, Savannah Andersen, and Molly Kim.

All of these individuals—each on their own transformational journeys—have added to the uniqueness of this book which features only authentic users of the Habits of Health system. No stock photos. No dramatizations. No paid actors. These are real people with real stories.

I also want to thank everyone that has given feedback during the making of this book, *Your LifeBook*, and the Habits of Health App over the last four years of development. And thanks to all of our coaches who believe that we can make a difference in the world. I am in awe of you for getting up every day with the desire help to others improve their lives. Thank you!

One of the reasons this system has evolved to be the world class system that it is today is the influence of several people I would like to personally mention.

First, the continual impact that my close friend, colleague, and mentor Robert Fritz has had by teaching me the craft of creating at a progressively higher level has been critical.

Second, the addition of Helen Urwin into my life has been invaluable. As a fellow traveler on the path to conscious leadership, our connection from our parallel worlds has been instrumental in accelerating my development. As a creator, she has helped connect me to co-creators from other disciplines. Helen, thank you for turning me on to some of the most amazing talented graphic designers in the world.

That team is Gardiner Richardson, led by my English mate Darren Richardson. His team's design of the Habits of Health Transformational System is truly brilliant. My thanks start with the project managers Jen Mason, Emma Douglas, and their Director, Peter Kane. Thank you for putting up with my nuances and for assembling and delivering this complex project. And to my Italian Da Vinci, Gino Di Meo, Head of Design, who has brought the habits alive and created a body of art work that I am so proud to share with the world: Thank you for your work. And Chris Stephenson, Designer, also extremely talented, you rocked the *LifeBook*. And of course, thank you Angela Trainor who built an amazing web portal to support the Habits of Health Transformational System. And also, I want to give a shout out to Andrea Murphy, the Studio Manager, and Dom Aldred, Darren's partner. Thank you for everything.

I want to give special thanks to Patrick Baglee, an amazing colleague, sounding board, and insightful critic, who has helped the content of the book really take on a special flair. Patrick has been crucial in every aspect of the project, and I have relied on his judgement and editing to create the end product that you are holding in your hands.

And then there is Marshal Carper who has handled my communications to the world for almost a decade. From the inception of the Habits of Health 2.0, he has been there to provide the logistical backbone, keeping me on track, and always saying "yes" to some of my outrageous demands on his time and talents. He has always been there to help me provide these ideas and skills of health that I so much want to share with the world. Thank you for your tireless effort and many sleepless nights to help this project become a reality. And special thanks to your team to their daily effort to spread the idea of health: Nina Musser for her help on the website and Averi Clements for her editing contributions.

Also, I want a shout out to the hedgehog lab team who developed our new Habits of Health App, adding a valuable tool to our transformational system. Designed to facilitate and create daily consistent habit installation, the speed and predictability of transformation will increase because of their work. Thanks to Patrick Richardson for taking the lead on this incredible new App and quarterbacking it through to reality. I want to especially thank "Hutch" (Michael Hutchinson) for his innovation, and Lizzie Hodgkiss for her adaptability to take over mid-project and deliver with precision what

ACKNOWLEDGEMENTS

I felt was necessary for our users. I also want to thank Bryce DelGrande for his design insights.

The incredible photography that brings this book to life was created by Michael Heffernan, whose talent needs no explanation. I desired to create complete authenticity by using only our community of coaches whose lives have been forever changed by the Habits of Health. His mastery depicts a vibrant representation of what is possible with this system. Thank you to you and your team for bringing it to life.

Also to equally talented, David Burroughs of Dirt Media for your contributions with your beautiful photography and videography in producing the transformational stories. Your work in bringing the Habits of Health to life has helped to make this system what it is today.

And my long-term friends and business partners over at Springfield Printing, led by their CEO Mark Sandersen, MaryAnne Culver, and Ruth Sargent: Your support has been incredible. You have been amazing partners over the last 10 years bringing the Habits of Health alive with consistent quality.

As the Co-Founder of OPTAVIA®, our health network, I want to thank those that have helped since its inception and have all played a vital role in building it into the formidable force for change that it is today. It all started with the MacDonald family and Brad and Shirley, Mike and Jean, and Meg and Guy. I first met Brad nearly two decades ago and, as a fellow entrepreneur, we shook hands and ventured out with lots of ambition (and not much else) to fight an obesity epidemic. Brad, you and your family's almost two decades of contributions has provided the financial strength and value-based leadership that will set the standard for years to come. The contributions along the way from General Leo Williams, Rick Logsdail, Mike McDevitt, and Mona Ameli have been immeasurable as well.

In bridging the contributions of the past and the exciting anticipation of the future are those that are currently working hard in the present. Dan Bell has been with me for 17 years and has helped so much in building us to this point. His contributions have been instrumental, and I want to thank him for the thousands of hours of sacrifice and expertise that he has poured into this idea that we can change the world. Thank you, Dan, from the bottom of my heart.

I am excited about the future of our mission, especially with our growing corporate partnership, which is now led by Dan Chard, our CEO, who deeply understands the magnitude of our mission. He has already shown the capability of elevating the support of our mission to the level that will be required in order to help us help the human species to move from surviving to thriving. In his capable hands and supported by the strong executive team of our CFO Tim Robinson, our Chief Legal Counsel Jason Groves, our EVP of Technology Bill Baker, and our VP of Marketing Lisa Goldberg, we are preparing for global expansion and taking this idea of optimal health and wellbeing to the international stage.

A special thanks is also owed to our market U.S. President Nick

Johnson whose maturity and open-minded approach is facilitating our coaches guiding people to the Habits of Health in a more powerful and effective way. And to Clovis Lau, Vice President of Business Development, Asia Pacific and his team who will help us repair the damage done by U.S. exportation of globesity: Thank you for helping us to expand our global reach.

And the tireless effort of the staff have been so critical. Allison Quillen, Consultant; Terri Roberts, Creative Manager; Lisa Sery, Marketing Operations Manager; Kelly Rose McCann, Director; Field Marketing and Communications, have all been incredibly focused on the success of the new system and how we can be of service to all those that desire better health. And to our corporate legal staff that has reviewed all compliance and citation needs, led by Courtney Mattson, senior legal counsel, Pooja Kothari, Staff Council, and Jean Kelter, Paralegal and Compliance: Thank you for painstakingly reviewing the 1200 plus pages in this transformational system. And thank you for the contributions from Jen Christman, RDN, LDN, CPT, Clinical Director, Alexandra Miller, MS, RDN, LDN who reviewed and the provided nutritional oversight of our programs.

And a special call out goes out to Angilee Myers, Consultant, who is helping, with the educational curriculum and coaching guide, to train our coaches to assist those that desire to transform their health and wellbeing. And I want to thank Kelli Caudill, Lori's and now my assistant, who has provided amazing support to me throughout this project which has given me the ability to focus on this important body of work.

And last, but far from least, I thank my family who has sacrificed the most throughout this adventure. First, I want to thank my mom, and Lori's mom, Marilyn (who is my second mom), for supporting me through thick and thin. They have always been there to encourage and support me in every way possible.

And to my daughters who have been so supportive and understanding of the long hours away each day that were required to make this herculean undertaking a reality. They have grown into amazing young ladies and have made me so proud of them, especially in the last six months of the project despite the loss of their mom. They have taken on Lori's role and understood how to support and encourage me despite their devastating loss.

The final thank you goes to my wife, Lori, who contributed professionally from her vast nursing and coaching experience. She is alive in this system, and I feel her presence in every bit of advice and wisdom in these pages. She sacrificed so much to help so many, and I dedicate the Habits of Health Transformational System to the first health coach who has inspired a movement which we know will create a healthier world. We will miss you, and I know you are smiling as this beautiful change in the world becomes a reality.

IN HEALTH,
DR WAYNE SCOTT ANDERSEN

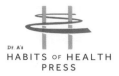

Dr. A's
HABITS OF HEALTH
PRESS

P.O. Box 3301
Annapolis, Maryland 21403
www.drwayneandersen.com
Copyright © 2019
by Dr. Wayne Scott Andersen